OXFORD MEDICAL PUBLICATIONS

Oxford Handbook of
ENT and
Head and Neck
Surgery

Published and forthcoming Oxford Handbooks

Oxford Handbook of Clinical Medicine 6/e (also available for PDAs and in a Mini Edition)
Oxford Handbook of Clinical Specialties 7/e
Oxford Handbook of Accident and Emergency Medicine 2/e
Oxford Handbook of Acute Medicine 2/e
Oxford Handbook of Anaesthesia 2/e
Oxford Handbook of Applied Dental Sciences
Oxford Handbook of Cardiology
Oxford Handbook of Clinical and Laboratory Investigation 2/e
Oxford Handbook of Clinical Diagnosis
Oxford Handbook of Clinical Haematology 2/e
Oxford Handbook of Clinical Immunology and Allergy 2/e
Oxford Handbook of Clinical Surgery 2/e
Oxford Handbook of Critical Care 2/e
Oxford Handbook of Dental Patient Care 2/e
Oxford Handbook of Dialysis 2/e
Oxford Handbook of Endocrinology and Diabetes
Oxford Handbook of ENT and Head and Neck Surgery
Oxford Handbook for the Foundation Programme
Oxford Handbook of Gastroenterology and Hepatology
Oxford Handbook of General Practice 2/e
Oxford Handbook of Genitourinary Medicine, HIV and AIDS
Oxford Handbook of Geriatric Medicine
Oxford Handbook of Medical Sciences
Oxford Handbook of Obstetrics and Gynaecology
Oxford Handbook of Oncology
Oxford Handbook of Ophthalmology
Oxford Handbook of Palliative Care
Oxford Handbook of Practical Drug Therapy
Oxford Handbook of Psychiatry
Oxford Handbook of Public Health Practice 2/e
Oxford Handbook of Rehabilitation Medicine
Oxford Handbook of Respiratory Medicine
Oxford Handbook of Rheumatology
Oxford Handbook of Tropical Medicine 2/e
Oxford Handbook of Urology

Oxford Handbook of
ENT and
Head and Neck
Surgery

Rogan Corbridge

and

Nicholas Steventon

OXFORD
UNIVERSITY PRESS

OXFORD
UNIVERSITY PRESS

Great Clarendon Street, Oxford OX2 6DP

Oxford University Press is a department of the University of Oxford.
It furthers the University's objective of excellence in research, scholarship,
and education by publishing worldwide in

Oxford New York

Auckland Cape Town Dar es Salaam Hong Kong Karachi
Kuala Lumpur Madrid Melbourne Mexico City Nairobi
New Delhi Shanghai Taipei Toronto

With offices in

Argentina Austria Brazil Chile Czech Republic France Greece
Guatemala Hungary Italy Japan Poland Portugal Singapore
South Korea Switzerland Thailand Turkey Ukraine Vietnam

Oxford is a registered trade mark of Oxford University Press
in the UK and in certain other countries

Published in the United States
by Oxford University Press Inc., New York

© Oxford University Press 2006

The moral rights of the authors have been asserted
Database right Oxford University Press (maker)

First published 2006
Reprinted 2008 (with corrections)

A Catalogue record for this title is available from the British Library

Library of Congress Cataloging in Publication Data
Corbridge, Rogan J.
Oxford handbook of ENT and head and neck surgery/Rogan Corbridge and
Nicholas Steventon.
(Oxford handbook series)
Includes bibliographical references and index.
1. Otolaryngology–Handbooks, manuals, etc. 2. Head–Surgery–Handbooks,
manuals, etc. 3. Neck–Surgery–Handbooks, manuals, etc. I. Steventon, Nicholas. II. Title.
III. Title: Handbook of ENT and head and neck surgery. IV. Series: Oxford handbooks.
[DNLM: 1. Otorhinolaryngologic Diseases–Handbooks. 2. Head–surgery–Handbooks.
3. Neck–surgery–Handbooks. 4. Otorhinolaryngologic Surgical Procedures–Handbooks.
WV 39 C792o 2006]
RF56.C67 2006   617.5'1–dc22   2005033087

Typeset by Newgen Imaging Systems (P) Ltd., Chennai, India
Printed in China
on acid-free paper through Asia Pacific Offset

ISBN 978–0–19–856492–8 (flexicover: alk.paper)

10 9 8 7 6 5 4 3 2

Oxford University Press makes no representation, express or implied, that the drug dosages in this book are correct. Readers must therefore always check the product information and clinical procedures with the most up to date published product information and data sheets provided by the manufacturers and the most recent codes of conduct and safety regulations. The authors and the publishers do not accept responsibility or legal liability for any errors in the text or for the misuse or misapplication of material in this work.

Contents

Detailed contents

Advisors

Sean Burrell, PRHO in ENT, University Hospital Aintree, UK
Nicholas Clifton, ENT Specialist Registrar, Nottingham, UK
Paul Hughes, Final Year Medical Sudent, Warwick, UK
Kay Seong Ngoo, SHO in ENT/Surgery, Aberdeen, UK
Carys Williams, Final Year Medical Student, Barts and the Royal London
Medical School, UK

Chapter 1 1

Overview

Using this book

The aim of this book, like all the other Oxford Handbooks, is to provide a compact but comprehensive guide to medical practice. It has been designed to slip inside the pocket of a white coat and to be rapidly retrieved for reference. There are many blank facing pages for notes, and for amending or annotating the text to fit in with local practice.

The core text is based on an anatomical list of ear nose and throat (ENT) diseases. There are separate sections on ENT examinations, investigations, common operations, ward care, and emergencies. There is also a separate section on the work of other ENT health professionals.

Chapter 3, 'Common methods of presentation'. is unique for this type of book. This chapter is a guide for dealing with patients as they present in clinical practice. It also provides a convenient way of accessing the relevant chapter in the anatomical list.

We hope that the book will be well used and will help guide you through the sometimes complex world of ENT.

ENT as a subject and career

ENT is a fantastic specialty that is every bit as exciting in practice as it is in theory. It is difficult to conceive of any specialty which can provide such diversity in medical practice.

- ENT conditions make up 25–50% of all general practice consultations.
- ENT conditions affect people of all ages from neonates to the elderly.
- Outpatient work is about 50% of the ENT workload. This gives a good balance between surgical and medical practice.
- Surgical skills are broad, from microsurgery on the smallest bones in the body, to major head and neck reconstructive surgery.
- ENT is an expanding surgical specialty that is taking over traditional general surgical areas such as salivary gland surgery and thyroid surgery.
- Cosmetic surgery is undertaken by ENT, in the form of facial plastics.
- Surgery is also performed on the skull base and pituitary gland.
- ENT offers enormous research potential from nasal polyps to congenital hearing loss.
- There are cutting edge developments occurring in ENT, such as cochlear implantation.

We hope that your experiences in ENT will fill you with enthusiasm for this specialty.

Further sources of information

British Association of Otolaryngologists
website: www.entuk.org
Royal College of Surgeons website: www.rcseng.ac.uk

Students and ENT

The subject of ENT can seem quite daunting to students. Particularly as this vast subject occupies such a small part of the curriculum, and has been dropped entirely from some medical schools.

In strong contrast to the time given to it in training, ENT conditions make up between 25–50% of all general practice consultations. As a student, it is important to have a firm idea in your mind of important topics you want to cover in ENT. These will form your learning aims and objectives—see the next section (p.8). There may be local variations.

You will find that ENT departments throughout the world are welcoming to students, but do not abuse their hospitality by being late or discourteous. Professional conduct is important whatever specialty you are studying.

There are particularly sensitive areas within ENT practice which require special tact as a student. Two of these are:

Head and neck cancer

These cancers form an important part of the ENT workload. You will need to be sensitive in dealing with these patients. They often have unique problems associated with their disease and treatment. These may include:

- Poor communication
- Disfiguring surgery
- Depression
- Alcohol withdrawal.

Hearing problems

The diagnosis of hearing loss in a child can be a devastating blow to parents. You will need to be sensitive to this. Another cause of great concern to parents is when a poorly performing child has a normal hearing test, as this may confirm the diagnosis of global developmental delay.

ENT learning aims and objectives for clinical medical students

Aims

- To acquire sufficient knowledge of ENT conditions to be able to recognize common problems and when and what to refer.
- To understand that ENT conditions are extremely common and form a large part of the workload of a general practitioner.
- To learn the skills required to examine patients with ear, nose, and throat diseases and to make a presumptive diagnosis.
- To learn how to prioritize and manage different ENT conditions.
- To become stimulated and interested in the specialty of ENT.

Objectives

- To learn the signs and symptoms of common ENT conditions.
- To learn the techniques of ear, nasal, and neck examination.
- To demonstrate an understanding of the basic anatomy and physiology of the ear and upper aero-digestive tract, and relate this knowledge to the signs and symptoms of ENT disease.
- To understand the medical and surgical treatment of common ENT conditions.
- To be familiar with the commonly used medications for treating ENT problems, and their side effects.
- To understand the risks and complications of surgery.
- To recognise the different ways in which head and neck malignancy can present, and to understand that early diagnosis of head and neck cancer leads to improved survival.
- To learn the ways in which ENT related communication difficulties can arise and be overcome.
- To appreciate and be sensitive to the impact of ENT conditions on patients and their families.

Student ENT curriculum

Practical skills

- Use of the auriscope to examine the external auditory meatus and tympanic membrane.
- Basic examination of the nose.
- Examination of the oral cavity and oropharynx.
- Examination of the neck.
- How to manage a nosebleed.
- How to deal with a tracheostomy.

Ear

- Basic anatomy and physiology of the ear.
- Presentation and management of common ear disease e.g. otitis externa, otitis media, glue ear, chronic suppurative otitis media with or without cholesteatoma, vertigo, and facial palsy.
- Examination of the ear including the pinna, ear canal, and otoscopy.
- Testing hearing with tuning fork tests.
- The advantages of the microscope and the fibreoptic otoscope.
- Basic interpretation of play audiometry, pure tone audiograms, and tympanograms.
- The principles of grommet insertion, mastoid surgery and the treatment of Menieres disease.
- Identifying postoperative problems following ear surgery i.e. sensorineural hearing loss, facial nerve palsy, and vestibular dysfunction.
- Understanding the differential diagnosis of facial nerve palsy and its treatment.

Nose

- Anatomy and physiology of the nose.
- Symptoms and signs of common sinonasal disease e.g. rhinitis, sinusitis, nasal polyps.
- Examination of the nose including an assessment of the appearance, the septum, the turbinates, and the mucosa.
- The endoscopic evaluation of the nose.
- Management of a fractured nose and the timing of intervention.
- Management of epistaxis from minor nosebleeds to torrential haemorrhage.
- The principles of common nasal operations including septal surgery, functional endoscopic sinus surgery, and rhinoplasty.

Head and neck—benign and malignant disease

- The basic anatomy and physiology of the oral cavity, salivary glands, pharynx, larynx, oesophagus, and lymph node drainage.
- The presentation of head and neck cancer.
- The presentation and management of salivary gland disease.
- Examining the oral cavity, larynx and pharynx including the use of the nasendoscope.
- Examining the neck with reference to the lymph nodes.
- The role of fine needle aspiration cytology (FNAC).
- The principles and limitations of radiological investigation of the head and neck region.
- Management of neck lumps, in particular the malignant lymph node with an unknown primary.
- The management of the airway in patients with a tracheostomy or end tracheostomy after laryngectomy.
- A basic knowledge of the principles of operative surgery, in particular the principles of reconstructive surgery and the surgery for salivary gland disease e.g. parotidectomy.
- The postoperative management of a patient who has undergone major head and neck surgery.
- The role of the multidisciplinary team in head and neck cancer and voice disorders.

Supplementary knowledge

- The role of otoacoustic emissions and evoked auditory potentials in managing hearing loss.
- The use of speech audiometry.
- The surgery for otosclerosis.
- Bone-anchored hearing aids for conductive hearing loss.
- Cochlear implantation and the reactions of the deaf community to this intervention.
- The use of sign language.
- Neuro-otology, in particular the presentation and management of acoustic neuromas.
- Craniofacial surgery and the interplay between ENT, plastic surgery and neurosurgery.
- The management of cleft palate and the increased risk of glue ear.
- Advanced endoscopic sinus surgery for the mangement of sinonasal malignancy, pituitary tumours and skull base tumours.
- Microlaryngeal surgery and surgical voice restoration.
- The use of chemotherapy and radiotherapy in head and neck malignancy.

Working in ENT

Working in ENT should be a very enjoyable experience, whether it is a temporary attachment or a long-term career plan. It is helpful if you have an understanding of what others expect of you. It is also important for you to think about your own career development.

Your duties

- Patient care and continuity.
- Professional development.
- Research.

Other staff

- Show courtesy and consideration to all staff on the ward.
- Always consider yourself to be part of a multidisciplinary team.

Communication

- It is essential to develop good communication skills, both written and verbal.
- You will need to liaise closely with junior and senior staff when on call.
- Always keep people informed if you have swapped your on call duties.

Timetable

- Be aware of your own and others' timetables.
- Never miss a clinic or theatre session.
- Always arrive in clinic or theatre with time to spare, and don't leave until the job is finished.

Rotas

- You will be expected to organize your own rota. Any disputes should be settled amicably without the involvement of senior staff if at all possible.
- Try to plan your annual and study leave in advance and arrange this at the beginning of the job, in consultation with your colleagues.
- If you are going to be away, make sure the administrative staff have cancelled your clinics and theatre lists.

▶ Always try to establish the best way of communicating with the team you are on call with. Obtain contact numbers directly rather than relying on switchboard to connect you each time. Always contact the other members of your team with your numbers when you are on call so they can contact you in an emergency. Write down all the numbers you are likely to need.

Research

▶ Make research a priority in your mind. It is important to keep your CV moving and improving. Aim to produce at least one publication every six months. Don't be distracted by trying to be involved in too many projects at once.

Work in a team if you can, to maximize your publications. Don't take on too many projects in a team—each team member should take on one research project at a time. Ask senior colleagues about possible projects, and affiliated University departments may be helpful. Involve a statistician before undertaking research. This will often help turn an idea into a first rate publication and avoid unnecessary work. Always check local ethics committee guidelines before you start. Research is expected but not everyone needs to produce a D. Phil.

Minimum requirements for entry into specialist training:

- One publication in a peer reviewed journal.
- Three presentations at national meetings.
- Full understanding of research methods, including statistical interpretation.
- Critical appraisal skills to evaluate published material.

Audit

Audit is often regarded as a poor relative of research. At its best, audit can be very informative and can lead to changes in practice. Involvement in audit is an expected part of professional practice. There are many opportunities available and help is often on hand from audit departments within the hospital.

Like research, make sure that you plan an audit that will achieve something with a tangible result. The best audits provide a completion of the audit cycle (see Fig. 1.1).

Types of audit

- Structure—how the system is set up.
- Process—how the system works.
- Outcome—the product of the system.
- Departmental—audits which are carried out in your department.
- Regional—audits carried out in your region.
- National—audits carried out by national organizations, such as the National Tonsillectomy Audit, NCEPOD.

Fig. 1.1. The audit cycle diagram

Chapter 2

The ENT examination

Equipment

A fully equipped ENT department will have all the necessary instruments for performing a full ENT examination. However, if you are a GP, or if you are working in another specialty, you will need to obtain a basic equipment kit. ENT SHOs or SpRs will also need to have such a kit when visiting patients at home or visiting peripheral hospitals.

Basic equipment

- A light source—a portable headlight that runs off batteries is ideal.
- Wooden tongue depressors.
- Thudicum nasal speculum.
- An otoscope with several speculae.
- Pneumatic attachment for the otoscope.
- Tuning fork 512Hz.
- Pen and paper.
- Gloves.

Advanced equipment

- Co-phenylcaine spray.
- A flexible nasendoscope with light source.
- Alcohol wipe to act as demist for the scope.
- Aqueous lubricating gel for the scope.

Emergency equipment

- Large nasal tampons (you can always cut 10cm ones to size).
- Silver nitrate sticks.
- Foley catheters.

▶ On call tip

Many SpRs are not resident on call. Therefore always pack an emergency kit box to leave in your car. This can be passed from SpR to SpR nightly. Even some of the most basic pieces of equipment are sometimes impossible to find in the middle of the night.

Basic requirements

How to master the use of a head mirror

The principle of the head mirror is that a light source is reflected from mirror onto the patient. The mirror is concave and the light is focused to a point. Also, it has a hole through which the examiner can look also allowing binocular vision. Correct positioning the examiner and the light source is important. Ensure that the light source is placed approximately level with the patients left ear. You must sit opposite the patient with the light shining directly at your mirror. Place the mirror over the right eye, close the left eye, adjust the mirror so that you can look through the hole directly at the patient's nose. Now adjust the light and mirror until the maximum amount of light is reflected onto the patient. When the left eye is opened, you should have binocular vision and reflected light shining to the patient's nose. The focal length of the mirror is approximately two feet. This means that the reflected light will be brightest and sharpest when the examiner and patient are this distance apart.

Examination of the ear

The examination should be practised and repeated regularly so that it becomes routine. It is equally important to document the findings of any examination accurately.

▶ Know your otoscope

Each type of otoscope is turned on in a slightly different way, usually by twisting it at the top of the body. Nothing inspires less confidence when you are examining a patient, than being unable to turn on the otoscope. It should be held like a pen with the little finger extended—like an affected tea drinker—to touch the patient's cheek. This enables an early warning of head turning, particularly in children. The right hand holds the otoscope for the right ear examination and vice versa. See Fig. 2.1.

Routine examination

- Ask the patient which is their better hearing ear and start by examining this ear.
- Check with the patient that their ear is not sore to touch.
- Examine the pinna and look for preauricular abnormalities.
- Examine for postauricular and endaural scars (see Fig. 2.2.).
- Straighten the EAC by pulling the pinna up and backwards (if you are examining a baby pull backwards only).
- Examine the EAC skin and document any changes using an otoscope.
- Systematically examine the tympanic membrane.
- Visualize the handle of the malleus and follow it up to the lateral process. Then you will not miss the superior part of the drum. You may need to kneel down to get the correct angle.
- Perform a pneumatic otoscopy. It will be more accurate if you have a soft tipped speculum which can occlude the EAC (see Fig. 2.3.).
- Repeat with the pathological ear.
- Perform tuning fork tests (see Chapter 2, p.23).
- Perform a free field test of hearing (see Chapter 2, p.26).
- Check facial nerve function—ask the patient to smile and close their eyes, while looking for facial weakness.
- Visualize the postnasal space with an endoscope.

Fig. 2.1. How to hold the otoscope

Post auricular approach

Ear turned forward

(a)

Hair line incision
Occasionally used to
harvest temporalis fascia

End aural
approach

Lobule incision
Used to harvest fat
in stapedectomy

(b)

Fig. 2.2. Common ear incisions

Fig. 2.3. The performance of pneumatic otoscopy

Using an otoendoscope

The use of this instrument is becoming more widespread in ENT. It is often attached to a camera and TV monitor. The patient may enjoy seeing their ear on screen, and it can help when explaining ear pathology or surgery. No anaesthetic is used. The end can fog-up, so use an alcohol wipe to demist (see Fig. 2.4.).

Tuning fork tests

These are simple tests of hearing which are most often used to differentiate between a conductive or a sensorineural hearing loss. They should be performed with a tuning fork of 512Hz. If the frequency is lower, then vibrations are produced which can mislead patients who think this is an auditory stimulus.

The ends of a tuning fork are known as tynes not prongs. The loudest sound from the tuning fork is produced at the end of the tyne.

Start the tuning fork by hitting your elbow or knee. Plucking the tynes produces less efficient sound and hitting a table or desk edge produces overtones. Weber's and Rinne's test's are performed together as a 'package' to help identify the type of hearing loss.

Weber's test

In this test (Fig. 2.5.), the tuning fork is placed at the top of the patient's head. The patient then says which ear hears the sound loudest, or if it is in the middle.

In normal hearing, sound is not localized to either ear. In sensorineural hearing loss the non-affected ear hears the sound loudest. In conductive loss the sound is heard loudest in the affected ear.

Fig. 2.4. Inserting the otoendoscope

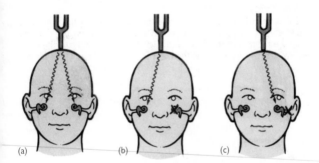

Fig. 2.5. Diagram of Weber's tests

Rinne's test

This test (Fig. 2.6.) compares air conduction with bone conduction. The activated tuning fork is placed behind the patient's ear, against the mastoid process. The patient is asked to say when they stop hearing the stimulus. The tuning fork is then moved to a position 2cm away from the EAM and held with the tips of the tynes level and in line with the ear canal. The patient is then asked if they can hear the sound.

This test can be modified by moving the tuning fork from the mastoid to the EAM before the sound has diminished. The patient is then asked which is the loudest sound.

The test results can be confusing, because a pathological test result is called a negative test! This is contrary to almost all other tests in medicine where a positive result is an abnormal result and a negative result is normal.

• **Positive test:** air conduction is better than bone conduction.
• **Negative test:** bone conduction is better than air conduction.

▶ *False negative Rinne's test*

This happens when the sound is actually being heard by the other ear. Sound conducted by bone is absorbed and travels across the skull, so when the tuning fork is placed on the left side it will be heard almost as well by the right inner ear as the left . To stop this effect the other ear can be masked.

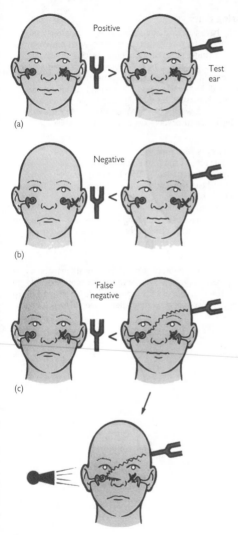

Fig. 2.6. Diagram of Rinne's tests

Free field hearing tests

Patients will usually have a formal audiogram when they attend an ENT outpatients appointment. However, there are some situations when you may need to make a rough guess at a patient's hearing threshold. This might happen because there are no formal audiometric facilities available, or if you suspect a patient may be exaggerating a hearing loss.

During this test, your own voice is used as a sound stimulus, while the patient's non-test ear is masked by rubbing your finger over the tragus. This produces some sound, which helps to 'mask' that ear. Practise is essential as the positioning for this procedure can be awkward. See Fig. 2.7.

Procedure

- Shield the patient's eyes with your hand.
- Tragal rub with your other hand to the non-test ear.
- Whisper a number at approximately 60cm from the test ear.
- If the patient cannot hear, use a normal volume spoken voice, followed by a shout if necessary.
- Repeat with opposite ear.

Patients should be 50% accurate at repeating your words to pass the test. If they hear your whisper at a distance of 60cm, then their hearing is better than 30dB.

▶ Examining tip

You can perform a cruder version of this test in a covert manner. When the patient sits in front of you, a whispered question as you hold the patient's notes in front of your mouth, can produce an interesting response, not always corresponding to the patient's seemingly poor audiogram!

Fig. 2.7. Positioning for free field testing

Examination of the nose

The most difficult part of this examination is learning to hold the thudicum's speculum. This is a bit like a nose clip used in swimming but in reverse—it holds the nose open rather than closed.

Basic position

The patient should be sitting in a swivel chair opposite the seated examiner. It is useful to have the patient's chair slightly higher than the examiner's chair. A good light source is essential: either a bull light positioned over the patient's left shoulder reflected onto the nose via a head mirror or use a headlight. Examination is systematic as always.

External nose

- Check for scars.
- Look at the skin type and thickness.
- Observe and palpate the nasal bones, upper lateral, and lower lateral cartilages.
- Look for symmetry and abnormal seating of the cartilages with the patient in the right and left lateral position and straight on.
- Tilt the head back to view the columella and alar cartilages in a similar way.

Internal nose

- Check the patency of each nasal airway.
- Occlude one nostril with a thumb and then ask the patient to sniff in through the nose.
- Repeat on the opposite side.
- In children a metal tongue depressor held under the nose will show exhaled air; if there is a blockage, it will not steam up.
- Perform Cottle's test if there is obstruction, to improve airflow (see Fig. 2.8.).
- Inspect the nose internally using the thudicum speculum. An otoscope with a large speculum can be used for children.
- Assess the straightness and integrity of the septum.
- Assess the size of the turbinates.
- Note the mucosal appearance.
- Use the endoscope to assess the posterior part of the nose.
- Feel for lymph nodes.

Postnasal space examination (Fig. 2.9.)

- Inspect the posterior choanae and postnasal space with an endoscope or with a mirror.
- Anaesthetize the oropharynx with co-phenylcaine.
- Hold a Luc's tongue depressor in the right hand and use it to depress the patient's tongue.
- In the other hand use a small mirror run along the top of the tongue depressor to enter the oropharynx behind the soft palate.
- The reflected light should illuminate the postnasal space to visualize the posterior choanae and the ends of the inferior turbinates. Any adenoidal tissue will also be seen.

Fig. 2.8. Cottle's Test diagram (Lift the skin upwards and laterally to see if there is an imrovement in nasal patency)

Fig. 2.9. Diagram of visualization of Post nasal space (PNS)

Rigid nasendoscopy

This is regarded as the standard technique for assessing the nose. It may be performed with the patient seated or with them laid supine on an examination couch. The advantage of having the patient lying down is that they cannot back away!

Procedure

- Before starting, warn the patient that the nasal spray tastes dreadful, that their throat will be numb and that hot food or drink should be not be consumed for an hour to avoid burns.
- Prepare the patient's nose with co-phenylcaine spray—usually five sprays to each nostril. The anaesthetic and vasoconstrictive effect of the spray takes six minutes to work. So it is essential to wait six minutes before starting the procedure. A diluted solution of the co-phenylcaine can be given to children.
- Use a 4mm 0° and 30° endoscope. A 2.7mm scope can be helpful in a narrow nose.
- Use the standard three pass technique as shown in Fig. 2.10.

Fig. 2.10. Three pass technique diagram

1. View along floor of nose to postnasal space

2. View into middle meatus

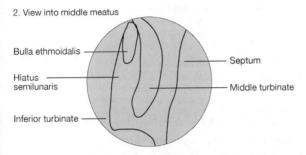

3. View into frontal recess

Fig. 2.11. Views on endoscopy seen during the passes in right nasal cavity

Examination of the mouth, larynx, and pharynx

Examination of the oral cavity

A good light source is essential. Ask the patient to remove all dentures in order to avoid important pathology being hidden. Ask the patient to open their mouth wide; limitation of jaw opening (trismus) may occur as a result of acute inflammation or tumour infiltration of the muscles of mastication. In an orderly way inspect the tongue, looking first that it upper surface then the lateral edges and it's under surface. Pay particular attention to the lateral edges of the tongue especially posteriorly, it may be necessary to use the tongue depressor to push the tongue medially in order to adequately examine this area. Any abnormality seen should also be examined with a gloved finger, since tumours of the tongue are usually hard and the depth of invasion can be difficult to assess by inspection alone. Now turn your attention to the floor of the mouth, the lower teeth and gums. Use a tongue depressor to distract the cheek and look at the parotid duct opening, opposite the second upper molar tooth. Inspect both hard and soft palate. Inspect in turn each of the tonsils as well as the posterior pharyngeal wall. Test the movements of the palate by asking the patient to say 'aahh' and the integrity of the hypoglossal nerve by asking for the tongue to be stuck out. The best way to assess the submandibular gland is via bimanual palpation with one hand placed on the neck and a gloved finger of the other in the floor of the mouth.

Examination of the pharynx and larynx

A lot of information can be gained by simply listening to the patient's voice. A week, breathy voice with a poor cough may suggest vocal cord palsy. A harsh hoarse voice is suggestive of a vocal cord lesion. With experience one can also recognize the characteristic voice of vocal cord nodules and Reinkes' oedema, however the definitive diagnosis depends upon inspection of the vocal cords.

How to perform indirect laryngoscopy

Positioning the patient is very important, they should be placed leaning slightly forward with the head slightly extended. An appropriately sized laryngeal mirror should be selected which is large enough to give a good view but small enough to be placed comfortably at the back of the mouth. The mirrored surface should be gently warmed using either a spirit lamp, or electrical mirror warmer. Ask the patient to open their mouth and put out their tongue. Gently wrap their tongue in a gauze and hold it between finger and thumb. Now, introduce the warmed mirror into the mouth, gently pushing the soft palate and uvula upwards and away from you. Ask the patient to concentrate on their breathing, sometimes asking them to pant helps them to focus further and also improves your view. Ask the patient to say 'eeee' and note the movements of the vocal cords. In some patients, where there is a strong gag reflex, some local anaesthetic spray (e.g. xylocaine) may be helpful.

Fig. 2.12. Indirect laryngoscopy

Flexible nasal endoscopy and stroboscopy

ENT surgeons will commonly in use a flexible nasendoscope in order to examine the upper aero digestive tract. This is easy to perform in the outpatient clinic usually with the aid of some topical decongestant and anaesthetic. The highly manoeuvrable flexible scope is passed through the nose giving the opportunity to inspect the middle and inferior turbinates, nasal septum, and osteomeatal complex. The endoscope is then advanced to the post nasal space where the Eustachian tube orifices and adenoids can be seen. By advancing over the superior aspect of the soft palate the endoscopist can see the tongue base, vallecula, laryngeal inlet and pyriform fossae. Visualization of these areas can be improved by asking the patient to stick out their tongue and also performing a Valsavoer whilst the examiner pinches the patients nose to prevent their escape. Asking the patient to speak the movements of the vocal cords can also be assessed.

Fine movements of the vocal cords and 'mucosal wave' require stroboscopic examination. Here, a microphone is placed on the patients neck and the frequency of vocal cord vibration is matched to the frequency of a strobe light flashing. The resulting images shown in effect a slow motion movie picture of the vocal cords. Video stroboscopy is most commonly performed in the specialist voice clinic.

Examination of the neck

Start by inspecting the neck from the front. Look for any scars or masses, deformity or asymmetry which may be visible. Ask the patient to swallow and pay particular attention to the lower central neck looking for a thyroid mass which should rise on swallowing. Now move to behind the patient and lay hands on the patient having enquired if they have any pain or tender areas. Again a systematic examination will ensure that no area is missed. See Fig. 2.13 which illustrates a suggested method of examination.

Examination of a neck lump

If you do find a lump or abnormality ensure you can adequately describe it and how it is related to anatomy of the neck i.e. site, size, consistency, surface, fixity, single?, pulsitile? The position of a neck lump will give clues as to the likely cause. The facing diagram gives a list of the common differential diagnoses dependent upon the site of the lump.

Examination of the thyroid

Thyroid lumps are common and often appear in exams at all levels. Full examination of the neck, as above is required, however some additional points are important to demonstrate. Start by shaking the patients hand and looking at their face. Note a cold or hot and sweaty hand which may indicate hypo/hyper thyroidism, similarly look at the skin and hair quality. Look for loss of the outer third of the eyebrow, which may occur in hypo function. Look at the neck from the front and ask the patient to swallow noting any thyroid lump which will rise during swallowing. Ask the patient to cough, listening for a weak cough and breathy voice which may occur in a recurrent laryngeal nerve palsy due to malignant infiltration of the nerve. Now move to behind the patient and feel the midline from the chin to the sternal notch. Feel for any midline lumps, especially thyroglossal cysts which will elevate on protrusion of the tongue so distinguishing them from isthmus thyroid lumps. Remember that the normal thyroid gland is impalpable. Feel each of the lobes in turn as well as the isthmus, asking the patient to swallow once more and checking that any palpable lump rises during swallowing.

Examination of salivary glands

Palpation of the parotid gland should be included within the routine examination of the neck. Remember that most parotid lumps are found just behind the angle of the mandible and that the tail of the parotid gland can extend down into the neck as far as the hyoid. Tumours of the deep lobe of the parotid may present as a mass arising in the mouth and pushing the tonsil medially (just like a quinsy!). Examination of the parotid gland includes testing the function of the facial nerve and visualization/palpation of the duct.

Submandibular gland masses are best felt via bimanual palpation. Remember to also inspect/palpate the length of the submandibular duct as it runs along the floor of the mouth and opens at a punctum next to the frenulum of the tongue.

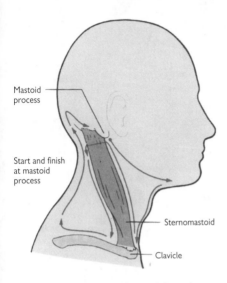

Fig. 2.13. Systematic examination of the neck

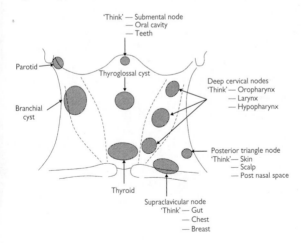

Fig. 2.14. Diagram of neck lumps by position and likely diagnosis

Common methods of presentation

Hoarse voice

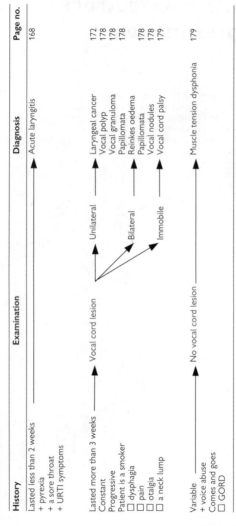

History	Examination	Diagnosis	Page no.
Lasted less than 2 weeks + pyrexia + a sore throat + URTI symptoms	⟶	Acute laryngitis	168
Lasted more than 3 weeks Constant Progressive Patient is a smoker ☐ dysphagia ☐ pain ☐ otalgia ☐ a neck lump	Vocal cord lesion → Unilateral	Laryngeal cancer Vocal polyp Vocal granuloma Papillomata	172 178 178 178
	→ Bilateral	Reinkes oedema Papillomata Vocal nodules	178 178
	→ Immobile	Vocal cord palsy	179
Variable + voice abuse Comes and goes ☐ GORD	No vocal cord lesion ⟶	Muscle tension dysphonia	179

Epistaxis (nosebleed)

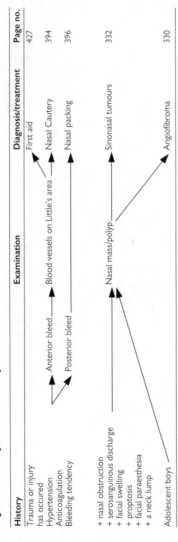

History	Examination	Diagnosis/treatment	Page no.
Trauma or injury has occured		First aid	427
Hypertension	Anterior bleed → Blood vessels on Little's area	Nasal Cautery	394
Anticoagulation			
Bleeding tendency	Posterior bleed	Nasal packing	396
+ nasal obstruction + serosanguinous discharge + facial swelling + proptosis + facial paraesthesia + a neck lump	Nasal mass/polyp	Sinonasal tumours	332
Adolescent boys		Angiofibroma	330

Dysphagia (swallowing difficulty)

History	Examination	Diagnosis	Page no.
Constant	± a neck lump	Carcinoma	204
Progressive	Endoscopy—lesion seen	Post cricoid web	198
Solids worse than liquids	Endoscopy—pooling of saliva	Achalasia	200
Pain			
Otalgia			
Neck lump			
Constant			
Progressive		Pharyngeal pouch	202
Regurgitation			
Halitosis			
Liquids worse than solids	+ neurology/cranial nerve palsies	Neurological dysphagia	196
Intermittent			
Saliva worse than solids or liquids			
Variable			
With or without variable voice problems	Normal	Globus	194
Heartburn		GORD	
Feeling of a lump in the throat			
Mucus in the throat			

A feeling of a lump in the throat

History	Examination	Diagnosis	Page no.
Constant			
Same site			
Worse with solids	Lesion seen on examination ⟶	Carcinoma of pharynx	106
Unilateral	Palpable neck lump	Carcinoma of oesophagus	204
± pain			
± otalgia			
± neck lump			
± hoarse voice			
Patient is a smoker			
Variable site			
Comes and goes			
Worse with saliva	⟶ Examination normal ⟶	Globus	
No true dysphagia			
Central in the neck			
Variable voice problems			
Anxiety			
Patient has a cancer phobia			
Heart burn/GORD			

A lump in the neck

All of the below may apply to children, but the majority of neck masses in children are benign and most are reactive lymph nodes. Parotid lumps in children are more frequently malignant than in adults.

History	Examination	Diagnosis	Page no.
Short history (weeks/months)	Laterally placed	Malignant lymphadenopathy	220
Lump is enlarging	Firm/hard	ENT primary	
Unilateral nasal obstruction	Single/multiple		
Otalgia			
Sore throat			
Patient is a smoker			
Hoarse voice			
Swallowing problems			
Weight loss	Multiple	Malignant lymphoma	220
Night sweats	Rubbery	Glandular fever/toxoplasma	218
Anorexia	Groin/axillary nodes		
Fever		Tuberculosis	218
Foreign travel			

Previous/recent URTI ——— Multiple/single ———→ Reactive lymphadenopathy 218

Long history (months/years) ——— Single & lateral ———→ Branchial cyst 214
No associated symptoms

Single & midline ———→ Thyroid lump 228
Rises on swallowing ———→ Thyroglossal cyst 214
Rises on tongue protrusion ———→ Dermoid cyst 214
No relation to swallowing ———→ Lymph node 218/220

Parotid region
No facial weakness ———→ Benign parotid tumour 148
Facial weakness & pain ———→ Malignant parotid tumour 148

Submandibular region ———→ Submandibular gland tumour 148

Changes with eating ——— Parotid ———→ Parotid stone/parotitis 150/152
Submandibular ———→ Submandibular stone/sialadenitis 150/152

Mouth or tongue ulcer

History	Examination	Diagnosis	Page no.
Trauma or injury Poor fitting denture Sharp tooth Pain	Lateral tongue Buccal mucosa	→ Traumatic ulcer	92
Patient is a smoker Alcohol Betel nut chewer Progressive Pain Neck mass Otalgia	Lateral tongue Floor of mouth Tonsil Firm/hard ulcer Neck nodes	→ Malignant ulcer (SCC)	94
Normal immune function Recurrent	Multiple ulcers Tongue tip/lateral border	→ Aphthous ulcers	92
Dietary insufficiency	Angular stomatitis Skin lesions	→ Dietary/blood disorders	92

Stridor

History	Examination	Diagnosis	Page no.
Neonate			
Feeding problems	Positional	Laryngomalacia	166
Failure to thrive		Tracheomalacia	166
Abnormal cry		Vocal cord lesion/palsy	167
	Biphasic stridor	Subglottic stenosis	166
Child			
Preceding URTI	Drooling	Croup	170
Rapid onset	Pyrexia	Epiglottitis	169
Malaise	Toxic		
Voice muffled/changed			
Short history	Inspiratory/mixed stridor	Foreign body	182
Previously well child	Expiratory wheeze		
Short lived coughing fit			

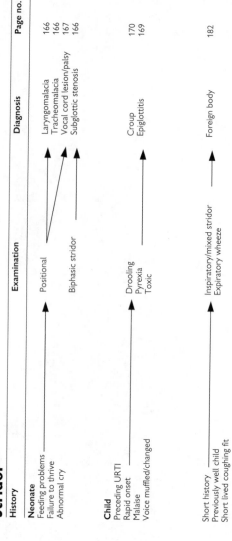

Adult
Normal voice
Recent surgery (thyroid/chest) ⎯⎯⎯⎯⎯⎯ Inspiratory stridor ⎯⎯⎯⎯⎯⎯▶ Bilateral cord palsy   167

Preceding URTI
Malaise
Swallowing difficulty
Sore throat

Inspiratory stridor
Pyrexia ⎯⎯▶ Supraglottitis   169
Drooling

Long standing hoarse voice
Pain
Patient is a smoker

Inspiratory stridor ⎯⎯⎯⎯⎯⎯▶ Laryngeal carcinoma   172
Neck node

Facial nerve palsy

History	Examination	Diagnosis	Page no.
Recent trauma	Haemotympanum head injury Trauma to ear canal/drum CSF from ear/nose	Fractured Temporal bone	320
Rapid onset Other weakness	Forehead unaffected Abnormal neurological exam	CVA	
Rapid onset Isolated weakness Otalgia	Forehead affected Vesicles in ear	Bell's palsy Ramsay Hunt	422 422
Gradual onset Other weakness	Abnormal neurological exam	MS Motor neurone disease	
Gradual onset Facial pain	Parotid lump	Parotid carcinoma	148
Hearing loss Balance disturbance	Sensorineural hearing loss ataxia	CPA tumour	326
Ear discharge	Conductive hearing loss	Cholesteatoma	270

Nasal obstruction

Careful examination of the nasal anatomy will reveal what is responsible for nasal obstruction. Always remember that several anatomical problems can co-exist. Symptoms can vary, especially for mucosal problems, so ascertain the severity of the problem when you examine the patient's nose.

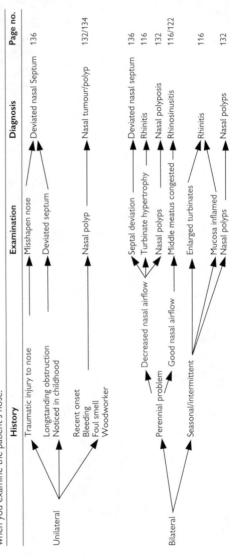

History	Examination	Diagnosis	Page no.
Traumatic injury to nose	Misshapen nose	Deviated nasal Septum	136
Longstanding obstruction	Deviated septum		
Noticed in childhood			
Recent onset	Nasal polyp	Nasal tumour/polyp	132/134
Bleeding			
Foul smell			
Woodworker			
	Septal deviation	Deviated nasal septum	136
Decreased nasal airflow	Turbinate hypertrophy	Rhinitis	116
	Nasal polyps	Nasal polyposis	132
Perennial problem	Middle meatus congested	Rhinosinusitis	116/122
Good nasal airflow	Enlarged turbinates	Rhinitis	116
Seasonal/intermittent	Mucosa inflamed		
	Nasal polyps	Nasal polyps	132

Unilateral

Bilateral

The discharging ear

The timing of the onset of discharge in relation to any pain often helps with diagnosis. Otitis externa in particular can be secondary to infection spreading from the middle ear. Microsuction, or dry mopping, is often necessary to visualise the tympanic membrane. A final diagnosis is sometimes not possible until the ear has been cleaned and the local infection has been treated. It is important to visualise the ear drum after treatment in order to exclude serious pathology at the level of the tympanic membrane.

History	Examination	Diagnosis	Page no.
No pain	EAC appears normal and the TM appears to have attic retraction/keratin →	Cholesteatoma	270
	EAC appears normal and the TM is perforated or has grommets →	CSOM/infected grommet	268
Pain before discharge	Normal EAC with a bulging TM →	Acute otitis media	262
Pain after discharge	Granulations in floor of EAC with a normal TM →	Necrotising otitis externa	250
	Narrow oedematous EAC when the TM is normal or not seen →	Otitis externa	248

Dizziness and vertigo

The most important aspect here is the patient's history. Take great care to elicit the character of the dizziness and its time course to establish if this is dizziness or true vertigo.

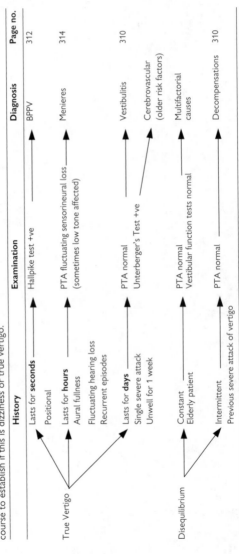

History	Examination	Diagnosis	Page no.
Lasts for **seconds** → Positional	Hallpike test +ve →	BPPV	312
Lasts for **hours** Aural fullness Fluctuating hearing loss Recurrent episodes →	PTA fluctuating sensorineural loss (sometimes low tone affected) →	Menieres	314
Lasts for **days** Single severe attack Unwell for 1 week →	PTA normal Unterberger's Test +ve →	Vestibulitis	310
	→	Cerebrovascular (older risk factors)	
Disequilibrium Constant Elderly patient →	PTA normal Vestibular function tests normal →	Multifactorial causes	
Intermittent Previous severe attack of vertigo →	PTA normal →	Decompensations	310

True Vertigo

Otalgia (earache)

Patients who present with otalgia can present a challenging problem. A careful history can help distinguish many conditions. Beware the red reflex—a reflex dilatation of the blood vessels on the handle of the malleus caused by the otoscope speculum touching the bony ear canal. This is often misdiagnosed as early acute otitis media, and the true cause of otalgia is missed. Always consider if the otalgia is referred pain.

History	Examination (using an otoscope)	Diagnosis	Page no.
Severe pain Child/preceding URTI Very painful	Erythema—a bulging drum ⟶ A high temperature Distressed patient	Acute otitis media	262
Severe pain ⟶ Not diabetic Preceding itch Longstanding Surfer/swimmer	Narrow EAC ⟶ Mucopus	Otitis externa	248
Severe pain ⟶ Diabetic Elderly	EAC floor granulated ⟶ Patient unwell Cranial nerve palsies	Necrotising otitis externa	250
Intermittent severe pain At night time Known glue ear	Middle ear effusion ⟶	Glue ear	266
Severe pain Anterior to tragus Worse with eating	Normal TM ⟶ Tender over TMJ Malaligned bite	TMJ dysfunction	
Moderate/severe pain	Normal TM ⟶ Tumour head and neck region	Referred pain	106

Hearing loss

A diagnosis of hearing loss in children and adults depends on combining the information from the patient's history, the examination and any special investigations. An audiogram, or a tympanogram with tuning fork tests will help to distinguish conductive from sensorineural hearing loss and will determine if the problem is bilateral or affects only one ear.
Sudden hearing loss is an emergency.

	History	Examination (otoscopy)	Type of loss (unusual features)	Diagnosis	Page no.
	Sudden onset after URTI	Middle ear effusion	Conductive	Effusion	266
	Sudden onset after trauma	Disrupted TM annulus	Conductive Type Ad tympanogram	Ossicular discontinuity	278
Unilateral	**Gradual** onset Hong Kong/Southern Chinese Neck nodes, epistaxis	Middle ear effusion	Conductive	Nasopharyngeal Carcinoma	328
	Gradual onset Family history Female/pregnancy	Flamingo pink blush or normal TM	Conductive Carhart's Notch on audiogram	Otosclerosis	276
	Sudden onset	Normal TM	Sensorineural	Vascular/Autoimmune	298/318
	Gradual onset Tinnitus	Normal TM	Sensorineural High frequency	Acoustic Neuroma	326

Bilateral

Gradual onset Child ⟶ Middle ear effusion ⟶ Conductive Type B tympanogram ⟶ Glue ear — 266

Sudden onset ⟶ Normal TM ⟶ Sensorineural ⟶ Autoimmune — 298

Gradual onset Elderly ⟶ Normal TM ⟶ Sensorineural ⟶ Presbyacusis — 290

Gradual onset Noise exposure ⟶ Normal TM ⟶ Sensorineural Audiogram notch at 4KHz ⟶ NIHL — 292

Tinnitus

It is important to distinguish between objective tinnitus (which the examiner can hear) and subjective tinnitus (which only the patient can hear). The character of the tinnitus is also important. A thorough otoneurological examination—of the ears, cranial nerves and central nervous system—is essential. Auscultate the ear, eye and carotids.

Remember that tinnitus can be caused by medication or other drugs.

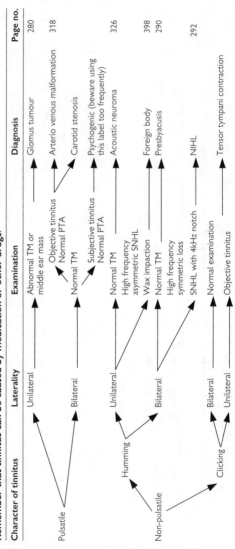

Character of tinnitus	Laterality	Examination	Diagnosis	Page no.
Pulsatile	Unilateral	Abnormal TM or middle ear mass	Glomus tumour	280
		Objective tinnitus Normal PTA	Arterio venous malformation	318
	Bilateral	Normal TM	Carotid stenosis	
		Subjective tinnitus Normal PTA	Psychogenic (beware using this label too frequently)	
Non-pulsatile / Humming	Unilateral	Normal TM	Acoustic neuroma	326
		High frequency asymmetric SNHL		
	Bilateral	Wax impaction	Foreign body	398
		Normal TM	Presbyacusis	290
		High frequency symmetric loss		
		SNHL with 4kHz notch	NIHL	292
Clicking	Bilateral	Normal examination		
	Unilateral	Objective tinnitus	Tensor tympani contraction	

Facial pain

Patients with this problem may present to a variety of specialties for an opinion e.g. ENT, neurology or maxillofacial surgery. It is important to have a broad mind to avoid a misdiagnosis. Never be afraid to ask for another specialist's opinion.

History	Examination	Diagnosis	Page no.
Severe acute pain Pain periorbital/cheeks Provoked by URTI Nasal obstruction Temperature	Pus/polyps in middle meatus	Acute sinusitis	124
Chronic fullness Worse bending over Nasal obstruction	Middle meatus occluded/narrowed	Chronic sinusitis	130
Severe pain Localised to specific site No nasal obstruction No rhinitic symptoms	Normal nasal examination Normal nasendoscopy	Atypical facial pain	
Intermittent pain Worse on eating Radiates to ear	Normal nasal examination Normal nasendoscopy Tendernes over TMJ	TMJ dysfunction	

Investigations in ENT

Children's hearing assessment

Assessing the hearing of babies and children can be difficult, because most hearing tests involve the active co-operation of the participant. To get round this problem, a number of tests have been specially designed for children and different tests are used at different ages.

Neonatal screening

In the past, neonatal screening for hearing problems was for high risk infants only. The success of pilot studies means that now all babies get neonatal screening. The otoacoustic emissions test is used. This phenomenon measures the active sounds produced by the outer hair cells which are recorded in response to tone clicks applied to the ear. The test is accurate, rapid, and easy to perform.

Distraction testing

This test is usually done by health visitors, as part of the routine health screening of infants at nine months of age. Two testers are required for this examination. The child sits on the parent or carer's lap, and one of the examiners sits in front of the child to occupy its attention. The other tester stands behind the child and uses sounds of particular frequency and volume to stimulate the child to turn its head. Turning is a positive response.

Visual reinforcement audiometry

This test is similar to distraction testing, but it uses speakers or headphones to deliver the unilateral sound. If the child turns round correctly then a light or a toy turns on to reward their turning.

Conditioned response audiometry

The child is conditioned to perform a task in response to a sound. For example, putting a toy man into a toy boat.

McCormick toy testing

This test uses 12 paired toys or objects with similar sounding names for example, a cup and a duck. The child points to or picks up the correct toy. The intensity of the sound of the command can be changed. The child's hearing threshold is determined by an 80% response.

Pure tone audiogram

This test can sometimes be performed by children as young as three years old. PTA using bone conduction can be uncomfortable for younger children (see p.74 for details).

Tympanometry

This test measures pressure in the middle ear and is useful and accurate in detecting glue ear in children (see p.76 for details).

Pure tone audiometry (PTA)

This is the most common method used for assessing hearing. The examination will ideally take place in a soundproof booth. To avoid cheating, the patient should not be able to see the audiometer controls.

The examiner and the patient are in contact via a microphone and a headset. The patient wears headphones and is given a handheld button to press when they hear a sound during the test. The better hearing ear is tested first.

The test begins using air conducted sounds. Initially, sound is played through the headphones at a level above the hearing threshold. The sound is decreased in 10dB increments until it is no longer heard. The sound intensity is then increased in 5dB increments until a 50% response rate is obtained.

- The frequency order of testing is 1kHz, 2kHz, 4kHz, 8kHz, 500Hz, 250Hz and then repeated at 1kHz.
- The re-test at 1kHz should be within 10dB of the initial result.
- The test-retest error is approximately 5dB.

The test is then repeated using bone conduction if necessary. The bone conductor is tightly applied to the mastoid area where the skin is tethered to the bone more securely and better contact is obtained.

Masking

Like tuning fork testing, there is a potential source of error in the pure tone audiogram. This is because sound can be perceived in the non-test ear if it is conducted through bone or through the air. The main differences are:

- 10dB for bone conduction.
- 40dB for air conduction. When thresholds show a difference of >40dB then masking should be used.

This is the amount of sound intensity travelling to the opposite ear when a sound is presented to one ear.

Masking is noise which is applied to the non-test ear to prevent it from picking up sounds presented to the test ear. The audiological rules of masking are complex to understand at first. Essentially masking is required when:

- Air conduction audiometry shows a greater than 40dB difference in the two ears.
- The difference in air conduction threshold between the test ear and the bone conduction in the non-test ear is >40dB.
- An unmasked air bone gap in the test ear is greater than 10dB (a sensorineural loss may be hidden).

Tympanometry

Tympanometry is a way of measuring the pressure in the middle ear. It was developed and popularized by Jerger[1] as a way of establishing the cause of conductive deafness. He classified the different patterns described opposite.

Method

During the test a probe is placed in the external auditory meatus to give a tight seal to the external ear canal (EAC). This probe can vary the pressure in the EAC whilst firing a 225Hz sound signal at the tympanic membrane (TM) or ear drum. The probe then measures the amount of sound reflected from the TM and calculates how much of the sound energy is admitted. Most sound is admitted when the pressure in the EAC matches that of the middle ear space. Thus the instrument measures the compliance of the tympanic membrane. By calculating the amount of air needed to change the EAC pressure the machine also calculates an approximate EAC volume.

Normal Ear

Type A—Peak at atmospheric pressure or maximal compliance.

Ossicular chain problems

Type As—the normal tympanogram can be flattened as a fixed ossicular chain reduces compliance.

Type Ad—the disarticulated ossicular chain causes the compliance to increase.

Middle ear effusion/glue ear

Type B—when there is fluid in the middle ear the ear drum's compliance alters giving a flat rate.

Type C—negative middle ear pressure may occur prior to or after an episode of glue ear.

Perforation

Type B—if there is a perforation in the tympanic membrane, the compliance will remain unchanged. But EAC volume will be increased as the tympanometer is changing the pressure of the EAC and middle ear space.

1. Jerger, J. (1970). Clinical experience with impedance audiometry. *Arch. Otolaryngol.* **92**, 311–24.

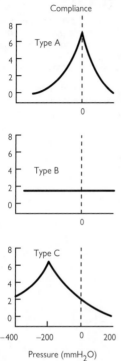

Fig. 4.1. Types of tympanogram

Electronystagmography (ENG)

Electronystagmography (ENG) is a balance test and it measures the chorioretinal electrical potential difference. Electrodes placed near the eyes can pick up electrical changes caused by eye movements. ENG allows testing of the vestibulo-ocular reflex (VOR). The VOR allows clear vision during head movements by producing compensatory eye movements.

The ENG test is usually done in a dimly lit room with a light bar to provide visual calibration. The patient sits on an examination couch.

Uses of ENG

ENG enables an assessment of the following:
- Disorders in SCC and otolith organs.
- Integrity of brainstem-cerebellar pathways.
- Integrity of central vestibulo-ocular pathways.

Subtests

If a patient needs more detailed investigations, they may be sent for more tests which may include:
- Oculomotor control test
  - Saccades
  - Tracking/Smooth pursuit
  - Optokinetic Test
  - Gaze Test.
- Positional testing
  - Headshake
  - Dix–Hallpike Test (see p.312).
- Caloric tests
  - Warm and cold irrigations
  - Ice calorics
  - Fixation tests.

Calorics

This balance test involves irrigating warm or cold water into the ear. This stimulates the inner ear balance mechanisms and will make the patient dizzy. The degree of stimulation can be measured by observing the nystagmus that is produced. This test is performed on both ears and any difference gives an indication of pathology in the balance system. It is used to confirm an inner ear cause of a balance problem.

Procedure

- Irrigation with warm water at 44°C and cool 30°C the EAC for 30 seconds with 200ml of fluid.
- Alternatively warm air at 50°C and cool at 24°C for 60 seconds at 9L/min flow rate.
- Temperature difference stimulates eddie currents in lateral SCC. Nystagmus induced according to COWS (cold opposite warm the same).
- Responses compared according to formula below.

Unilateral weakness (>25% significance)

$$\frac{(RC + RW) - (LC + LW) \times 100}{RC + LC + RW + LW} = \text{unilateral weakness}$$

Directional preponderance (>25–30% significance)

$$\frac{(RC + RW) - (LC + RW) \times 100}{RC + LC + RW + LW} = \text{directional preponderance}$$

where: RC = <u>R</u>ight <u>C</u>old;
RW = <u>R</u>ight <u>W</u>arm;
LC = <u>L</u>eft <u>C</u>old;
LW = <u>L</u>eft <u>W</u>arm.

CT scan

Computed tomography (CT) provides excellent information for defining differences between bony and soft tissue. In ENT it is used for looking for problems affecting the temporal bone and the inner ear.

Procedure

The patient lies supine on the scanner bed. The scan uses X-rays applied in a circumferential manner to acquire information. Information is produced in the form of pixel cubes. These can be joined to produce images in multiple planes. There is a significant radiation dose with this technique.

Uses

- Evaluation of bony anatomy for endoscopic sinus surgery.
- Evaluation of mandibular involvement in floor of mouth tumours.
- Assessment of middle ear in suspected mastoiditis.
- Evaluation of traumatic head injury and temporal bone fracture.

MRI scan

This technique provides excellent soft tissue definition with no radiation risk. In ENT it is used for looking at the nerves to and from the inner ear.

Procedure

The patient is placed lying down, inside a circular magnet. The magnetic field aligns all the hydrogen atoms, mainly body water. An electromagnetic pulse is directed towards the patient, which knocks the hydrogen atoms out of alignment. Once the pulse wave has subsided the hydrogen atoms spring back into alignment. This process causes energy to be released, which is detected by the scanner.

The timing of recording, and the information collected can be analysed separately to give different information. Software algorithms produce the 3D image information. Contrast can enhance the information.

Common protocols

- T1 weighted scans (fat bright).
- T2 weighted scans (water bright).
- STIR sequence (short tau inversion recovery) produces fat suppressed images.
- MRA angiographic information from scan sequence.

Uses

- Identifying acoustic neuroma—MRI is the gold standard.
- Checking the spread of a tumour.
- Assessing the involvement of vascular structures in head and neck malignancy.
- Assessing the intracranial spread for sinonasal tumours.

Skin prick testing

This test enables you to detect if a patient is allergic to various substances. It has a rapid result, allowing you to see the allergic response. Skin prick testing is used in patients with rhinitis, to guide therapy and to aid advice on which allergens to avoid.

Procedure

- Before starting this test, it is important to ensure that resuscitation facilities are nearby, with adrenaline.
- The procedure for testing should be explained to the patient. The test solutions are then placed on the patient's forearm. These include a positive control substance (histamine) and a negative control substance (excipient solution). A small amount of solution is innoculated intradermally by using a lancet pricked into the patient's skin.
- A positive response is measured after 30 minutes, as a wheal >2mm.

The mouth, tonsils, and adenoids

Anatomy

The nose and throat

The nose and throat can be divided into the following anatomical areas (see Fig. 5.1.):

- Oral cavity—extends from the lips to the anterior pillar of the tonsil.
- Oropharynx—extends from the anterior pillar to the posterior pharyngeal wall. It contains the tonsils and the base of the tongue.
- Nasopharynx—located above the soft palate and contains the adenoids. The Eustachian tubes open into it laterally and it communicates with the nasal cavity anteriorly.

The tongue

The anterior third and posterior two thirds of the tongue have different embryological origins, and different nerve supplies.

- *Motor supply* to the tongue is via the hypoglossal nerve.
- *Sensation* to the anterior two thirds of the tongue is via the lingual nerve. The posterior third is supplied by the glossopharyngeal nerve.
- *Taste* fibres pass with the facial nerve to the middle ear. From here they separate—as the chorda tympani—and pass forwards. As they exit the middle ear they merge with the mandibular division of the trigeminal nerve to eventually run with the lingual nerve.

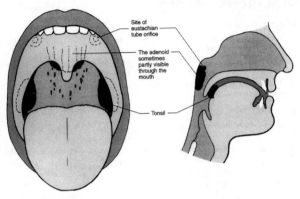

Fig. 5.1. Oral cavity AP and oropharynx/nasopharynx lateral

Oral ulcers—benign

Traumatic ulcers

Acute traumatic ulcers are common, they heal quickly and patients rarely seek any medical attention. Chronic traumatic ulcers are seen more often. These can arise from ill-fitting dentures, sharp or rotten teeth. These usually occur on the lateral aspect of the tongue, or on the inside of the cheek. The only treatment required is a dental review or a refitting of the denture.

Aphthous ulcers

These are the common mouth ulcers that most people will suffer from at some time in their lives. They are small and painful and usually appear in crops. They most often affect the lateral border or the tip of the tongue, but they may occur anywhere in the oral cavity. It is unclear what causes them, but hormonal changes, poor oral hygiene, trauma, poor diet and stress have all been suggested as factors. Usually, these ulcers present little more than a minor irritation for 24–48 hours. However, occasionally they are severe and recurrent. Treatment in this case should consist of simple analgesia, local anaesthetic gels or steroid pastels. Rarely, a single giant aphthous ulcer may develop. This can look alarming or may even appear malignant. In this case, a biopsy may be necessary.

Infective ulcers

Herpes simplex may cause mouth ulcers which look similar to aphthous ulcers. However the patient will often have additional symptoms of mild pyrexia and malaise. Acyclovir is effective if given in the early stages. Herpes zoster may affect the oral cavity but is usually seen in immuno-compromised and debilitated patients.

The 'snail track' ulcers of syphilis are rarely seen. Oral ulceration along with candidiasis, tonsillitis, Kaposi's sarcoma and hairy Leukoplakia are all features of AIDS infection.

Dietary and blood disorders

Deficiencies in iron, folate, and vitamin B12 can cause oral ulceration, since these agents are required for normal mucosal development. Mouth ulcers also occur as a result of leukaemia, polycythaemia and agranulocytosis. Signs of scurvy and pellagra include a sore mouth and ulceration.

Torus palatinus

This is a benign osteoma on the hard palate. Its surface may become ulcerated, usually as a result of trauma from an overlying denture. In this case the lesion may look and feel malignant. These lesions need only be removed if they interfere with the fitting of a dental plate.

Oral ulcers—malignant

Squamous cell carcinoma

This is the commonest malignant lesion found in the mouth. Risk factors include smoking, drinking alcohol (in particular spirits), chewing betel nuts and having sharp teeth.

Symptoms and signs

It usually starts as an ulcer, often on the lateral border of the tongue, the floor of the mouth, or the gum. These ulcers progress and are painful, often with referred pain to the ear. Malignant ulcers of the tongue may be superficial or deeply infiltrating, but in either case they usually feel hard.

Investigations

More information can usually be gathered from palpation than from inspection. It is vital to adequately examine the neck for lymph node metastasis, paying particular attention to the submandibular and submental triangles as well as those nodes deep to the sternomastoid running along the internal jugular vein. SCC of the oral cavity will most commonly metastasize to the nodes in levels 1, 2 and 3 (see p.210). A MRI scan or a spiral CT scan is most often employed to assess the neck. Ultrasound guided FNA is a highly sensitive and specific tool in assessing the neck in skilled hands.

Management

Any ulcer which fails to heal within two weeks should be biopsied in order to exclude malignancy. Many patients who develop oral cavity SCC have widespread mucosal field change as a result of their smoking and drinking. They are at a high risk of developing another upper aerodigestive tract cancer at the same time or at some time in the future. All patients presenting with SCC should have a panendoscopy under general anaesthetic in order to exclude any additional primary tumour. The panendoscopy will also allow proper assessment of the primary tumour.

Treatment

Options include both external beam and interstitial radiotherapy as well as surgical en-bloc resection with all the affected hard and soft tissues. The surgically created defect will require reconstruction to produce an acceptable functional and cosmetic result for the patient.

White patches in the mouth

There are many possible causes of white patches in the mouth. These include:

Candida

Candida tends to occur in debilitated and immunocompromised patients. White specks coalesce to form patches, or a white membrane, which when lifted reveals a red raw mucosal surface. It sometimes occurs on the soft palate and can complicate the use of steroid inhalers in asthma patients. Candida is usually diagnosed by looking at it, but if any doubt remains, scrapings of the lesion should be taken and sent for microbiological examination.

Leukoplakia

Any white patch in the mouth can be called leukoplakia. But it usually refers to hyperkeratosis of the oral mucosa. This happens to patients who share the same risk factors as those who develop SCC: smoking, alcohol, strong spices and prolonged irritation from sharp teeth or poorly fitting false teeth. This lesion is premalignant and 3% will undergo malignant change within five years of diagnosis. A biopsy and regular reviews are essential. A particular form of leukoplakia known as hairy leukoplakia occurs in AIDS patients, the condition is so named because of its histological appearance.

Lichen planus

This condition usually occurs on the inside of the cheek and has a white lace-like appearance. It may be extremely painful but usually responds to topical steroid preparations. The aetiology remains unclear.

Mucus retention cysts

These usually form a smooth pale round swelling which may occur anywhere in the oral cavity, base of tongue or the tonsils. These swellings arise from a blockage in one of the many mucus glands found throughout the mucosa of the upper aerodigestive tract. Reassurance is usually all that is required. If there is any diagnostic uncertainty, or if they become large enough to cause symptoms as a result of their size, then excision/marsupialization may be required.

Miscellaneous mouth conditions

Geographic tongue

This is a common condition where depapillation of the tongue surface occurs as red patches with a white border. The sites vary and seem to move around the tongue. The cause is unknown but it often runs in families. Reassurance is the only treatment required.

Angioedema

This allergic reaction causes generalised swelling of the tongue. Seafood, peanuts and drugs such as lisinopril can all have this effect. The swelling may progress rapidly and obstruct the airway. Medical treatment consists of intravenous steroids, piriton and nebulized adrenaline. The airway may need to be secured either by endotracheal intubation or tracheostomy.

Median rhomboid glossitis

This appears as a raised smooth patch in the centre of the dorsum of the tongue. It has been linked with reflux and candida infection. In most cases simple reassurance is all that is required.

Tongue tie

This is a birth defect in which the frenulum is short. Babies usually grow out of it before the age of two—speech defects do not occur as a result of this condition. Reassurance is usually all that is required. Occasionally parents may request surgical division.

Macroglossia

Enlargement of the tongue can be seen in acromegaly, Downs syndrome, multiple endocrine adenoma syndrome, hypothyroidism and amyloidosis.

Burning tongue syndrome

The anterior and lateral aspects of the tongue are most commonly affected and it tends to occur in young women. This is an unsatisfying condition to treat because its cause is unknown and simple analgesics are the only available medications which seem to help.

Hairy leukoplakia

This condition appears as white patches on the lateral border of the tongue, in patients with AIDS.

Black hairy tongue

This aptly named condition occurs due to overgrowth of the filiform papillae of the tongue and generally occurs in smokers. Treatment consists of brushing the tongue with a soft toothbrush.

Ranula

This is a retention cyst which forms in the floor of the mouth under the tongue. It develops from the submandibular or sublingual glands. It is treated by marsupialisation.

Cystic hygroma

This is a benign tumour of the lymph vessels (lymphangioma) which consists of large, dilated lymphatic channels. They usually present at, or soon after birth and can grow to massive proportions. They may cause life-threatening compression of the airway. They may be injected with sclerosant or surgically exercised.

Tonsillitis

Tonsillitis, or infection of the tonsils is commonly seen in ENT and in general practice. Common bacterial pathogens are β-haemolytic streptococcus, pneumococcus and haemophilus influenzae. Sometimes this occurs following an initial viral infection. Treatment consists of appropriate antibiotics (e.g. penicillin), regular simple analgesia, oral fluids and bed rest.

Signs of acute tonsillitis
- Sore throat
- Enlargement of the tonsils
- Exudate on the tonsils
- Difficulty in swallowing
- Pyrexia
- Malaise
- Bad breath
- Ear ache.

Complications of tonsillitis

Airway obstruction: This is very rare, but may occur in tonsillitis due to glandular fever. The patient may experience severe snoring and acute sleep apnoea. This may require rapid intervention e.g. insertion of nasopharyngeal airway or intubation.

Quinsy (paratonsillar abscess): This appears as a swelling of the soft palate and tissues lateral to the tonsil, with displacement of the uvula towards the opposite side. The patient is usually toxic with fetor, trismus and drooling. Needle aspiration or incision and drainage is required, along with antibiotics which are usually administered intravenously. See Fig. 19.8 and *How to drain a quinsy*, p.410.

Parapharyngeal abscess: This is a serious complication of tonsillitis and usually presents as a diffuse swelling in the neck. Admission is required and surgical drainage is often necessary via a neck incision. The patient will usually have an ultrasound scan first, to confirm the site and position of the abscess.

Management

Patients with complicated tonsillitis, and those who are unable to take enough fluid orally, will need to be admitted to hospital for rehydration, analgesia, and intravenous antibiotics. Ampicillin should be avoided if there is any question of glandular fever, because of the florid skin rash which will occur.

Treatment
See p.104 for tonsillectomy.

Indications for tonsillectomy
Absolute indications for surgery
- Suspected malignancy
- Children with OSA (obstructive sleep apnoea)
- As part of another procedure such as UPP for snoring.

Relative indications for surgery
- Recurrent acute tonsillitis
- 3 attacks per year for 3 years or
- 5 attacks in any one year
- More than one quinsy.

Big tonsils which are asymptomatic need not be removed.

Glandular fever

Glandular Fever is also known as infectious mononucleosis or Epstein–Barr virus infection. It is common in teenagers and young adults. Patients with glandular fever may present a similar picture to patients with acute bacterial tonsillitis, but with a slightly longer history of symptoms. Diagnosis relies upon a positive monospot or Paul–Bunnell blood test, but early in the course of the disease this test can still show up negative.

Signs and symptoms
- Sore throat
- Pyrexia
- Cervical lymphadenopathy
- White slough on tonsils
- Petechial haemorrhages on the palate
- Marked widespread lymphadenopathy
- Hepatosplenomegaly.

Treatment

This is a self limiting condition for which there is no cure as such. Treatment is largely supportive with painkillers, although patients may appreciate a short course of corticosteroids to decrease swelling. IV fluids may be necessary if they cannot drink enough.

Complications

Patients should be advised to refrain from contact sports for six weeks because of the risk of a ruptured spleen. This can lead to life threatening internal bleeding.

Tonsillectomy

This is one of the most commonly performed operations. Patients usually stay in hospital for one night, so that bleeding may be recognized and treated appropriately. Tonsils are removed by dissection under general anaesthetic. Haemostasis is achieved with diathermy or ties.

Post-op

Tonsillectomy is very painful and regular simple analgesia is always required afterwards. Patients should be advised that referred pain to the ear is common. Until the tonsillar fossae are completely healed, eating is very uncomfortable. The traditional jelly and ice cream has now been replaced with crisps, biscuits, and toast, since chewing and swallowing after tonsillectomy is very important for recovery and in helping to prevent infection.

In the immediate postoperative period the tonsillar fossae become coated with a white exudate, which can be mistaken as a sign of infection.

Complications

Postoperative haemorrhage is a serious complication for between 5–15% of patients after a tonsillectomy.

A reactive haemorrhage can occur in the first few hours after the operation, this will frequently necessitate a return trip to the operating theatre.

A secondary haemorrhage can occur any time within two weeks of the operation. See ENT emergencies, Chapter 20, p.430.

Tonsillar tumours

Benign tumours are very rare. But tonsillar stones (tonsiliths) with sur-rounding ulceration, mucus retention cysts, herpes simplex or giant aphthous ulcers, may mimic the more common malignant tumours of the tonsil. These tumours are becoming increasingly common, and unusually, are now being found in younger patients and in non-smokers.

Squamous cell carcinoma (SCC)

This is the commonest tumour of the tonsil. It tends to occur in middle-aged and elderly people, but in recent years tonsillar SCC has become more frequent in patients under the age of 40. Many of these patients are also unusual candidates for SCC because they are non-smokers and non-drinkers.

Signs and symptoms
- Pain in the throat
- Referred otalgia
- Ulcer on the tonsil
- Lump in the neck.

As the tumour grows it may affect the patient's ability to swallow and it may lead to an alteration in the voice—this is known as 'hot potato speech'.

Diagnosis is usually confirmed with a biopsy taken at the time of the staging panendoscopy. Fine needle aspiration of any neck mass is also necessary. Imaging usually entails CT and/or a MRI scan. It is important to exclude any bronchogenic synchronous tumour with a chest X-ray and/or a chest CT scan and bronchoscopy where necessary.

Treatment
Decisions about treatment should be made in a multidisciplinary clinic, taking into account the size and stage of the primary tumour, the pres-ence of nodal metastases, the patient's general medical status and the patient's wishes.
Treatment options include:
- Radiotherapy alone
- Chemoradiotherapy
- Trans oral laser surgery
- En-bloc surgical excision—this removes the primary and the affected nodes from the neck. It will often be necessary to reconstruct the surgical defect to allow for adequate speech and swallowing afterwards. This will often take the form of free tissue transfer such as a radial forearm free flap.

Lymphoma
This is the second most common tonsil tumour.

Signs and symptoms
- Enlargement of one of the tonsils
- Lymphadenopathy in the neck—may be large
- Mucosal ulceration—less common than in SCC.

Investigations
- Fine needle aspiration cytology may suggest lymphoma, but it rarely confirms the diagnosis. It is often necessary to perform an excision biopsy of one of the nodes.
- Staging is necessary with CT scanning of the neck chest, abdomen, and pelvis. Further surgical intervention is not required other than to secure a threatened airway.

Treatment
Usually consists of chemotherapy and/or radiotherapy.

Adenoidal enlargement

The adenoid is a collection of loose lymphoid tissue found in the space at the back of the nose. The Eustachian tubes open immediately lateral to the adenoids. Enlargement of the adenoids is very common, especially in children. It may happen as a result of repeated upper respiratory tract infections which occur in children due to their poorly developed immune systems.

Signs and symptoms

- Nasal obstruction
- Nasal quality to the voice
- Mouth breathing which may interfere with eating
- A runny nose
- Snoring
- Obstructive sleep apnoea syndrome (OSAS)
- Blockage of the eustachian tube.

A diagnosis of adenoidal enlargement is usually suspected from the history. Using a mirror or an endoscopic nasal examination will confirm the diagnosis.

The glue ear which arises as a result of poor eustachian tube function may cause hearing impairment (see p.266). Adenoiditis or infection of the adenoid, may allow ascending infections to reach the middle ear via the eustachian tube.

Treatment

An adenoidectomy is performed under a general anaesthetic. The adenoids are usually removed using suction diathermy or curettage.

Complications

Haemorrhage (primary, reactionary, and secondary): These are serious complications of an adenoidectomy, but this is less common than with a tonsillectomy. The procedure is frequently carried out safely as a day case.

Nasal regurgitation: The soft palate acts as a flap valve and separates the nasal and the oral cavity. If the adenoid is removed in patients who have even a minor palatal abnormality, it can have major effects on speech and swallowing. Palatal incompetence can occur in these patients resulting in nasal regurgitation of liquids and nasal escape during speech. Assessment of the palate should form part of the routine ENT examination before such an operation, in order to avoid this complication.

The nose and sinuses

Structure and function of the nose

Structure

The structure of the nose is made up of four parts:

- The surface anatomy—see Fig. 6.1. for the surface landmarks.
- The nasal skeleton—composed of the two nasal bones, the paired upper lateral and lower lateral cartilages and the nasal septum, covered in subcutaneous tissue and skin (see Fig. 6.2.).
- The internal anatomy—includes the septum of the nose which forms the medial wall of the nasal cavity. The turbinates on the lateral wall are also called conchae (the Latin term for scroll) which describes their appearance neatly (see Fig. 6.3.).
- The osteomeatal complex—a key functional area of the nose. Understanding its anatomy is essential in understanding the aetiology of sinus disease (see Fig. 6.4.).

Knowing the anatomical terms for parts of the nose helps you to describe the site of lesions accurately, and to document the findings of examinations accurately.

Function

The nose is the main route for inspired air, and its structure is related to this function. As the air passes over the large surface area of the turbinates, the inspired gases are warmed and humidified. Mucus on the mucosa of the nose removes large dust particles from the air as it is breathed in (as anyone who has blown their nose after a trip on the London underground knows!).

The voice resonates in the sinuses and nose and this provides character to the speech. Patients with very obstructed nasal passages have what is often described as a nasal quality to their speech.

Pneumatization of the sinuses—they are air filled spaces—reduces the weight of the skull.

Fig. 6.1. Diagram of the surface markings of the nose

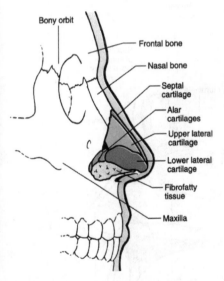

Fig. 6.2. Diagram of the nasal skeleton

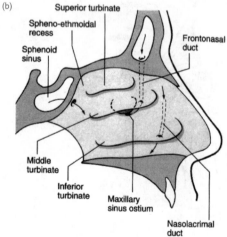

Fig. 6.3. Diagram of the internal structure of the nose

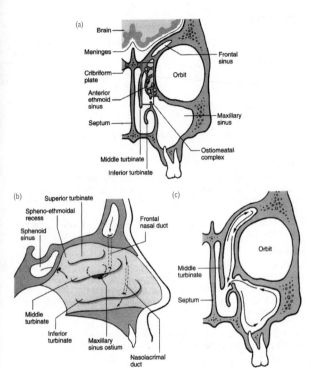

Fig. 6.4. The osteomeatal complex

Rhinitis

Rhinitis is an inflammation of the nasal lining. Rhinitis may be diagnosed if a patient has two out of three of the following symptoms for more than one hour every day for over two weeks:

Symptoms
- Blocked nose
- Running nose—including postnasal drip
- Sneezing.

This condition is very common. Approximately one in six adults suffer from rhinitis.

Causes

There are a multitude of factors which cause rhinitis. It may be caused by several different factors, so it is important to treat each different cause. The symptoms of rhinitis may also be part of systemic disease (see Table 6.1).

   The commonest forms of rhinitis are allergic and infective. Classification of the disease and its rarer forms are shown in Table 6.1.

History

It is important to take a full history to determine the cause of rhinitis. This includes asking the patient about any history of atopy or asthma, and any seasonal variation in the symptoms. Documenting the main symptoms—blockage, running, and sneezing—and noting which one is predominant will help in treatment selection.

   The patient should be asked what medications are being used and about their smoking history—almost every smoker has a degree of rhinitis. The patient should be asked about any previous treatment for rhinitis, including its duration and effectiveness.

Investigations
- **Anterior rhinoscopy**—looking for enlarged turbinates (a blue tinge often indicates an allergic rhinitis) or nasal polyps.
- **Rigid nasendoscopy**—examining the middle meatus for mucopus or polyps.
- **Skin prick tests**—tiny amounts of test substances are placed on the skin and a pin prick is made—a positive result leads to a small raised, red, itchy patch.
- **RAST tests**—a blood test which indicates if patients are allergic to a range of test substances.
- **Peak flow**—many patients with rhinitis also have asthma—their peak flow test may be reduced.

Table 6.1 Classification of rhinitis

Common		Rare	
Allergic	Infect	Other	Part of systemic disease
Seasonal	Acute	Idiopathic	Primary mucus defect
Perennial	Chronic	NARES (non-allergic rhinitis with eosinophilia)	• Cystic fibrosis
Occupational			• Young's disease
		Drug-induced	Primary ciliary dyskinesis
		B-blockers	• Kartageners syndrome
		Oral contraceptives	Immunological
		Aspirin	• SLE
		NSAIDS	• Rheumatoid arthritis
		Local decongestants	AIDS
		Autonomic	Antibody deficiency
		Atrophic	Granulomatous disease
		Neoplastic	• Wegener's/sarcoidosis
			Hormonal
			• Hypothyroidism
			• Pregnancy

Medical treatment of rhinitis

Treatment of rhinitis is related to the underlying aetiology of the condition. Medical treatment is given if the patient feels their symptoms are bad enough.

Allergen avoidance

If the patient's rhinitis is caused by an allergy, skin prick testing can identify allergens to be avoided. It gives a visual feedback to the patient to confirm the diagnosis. Following a positive skin prick test, allergen avoidance information can be given to the patient both verbally and on information sheets.

Pharmacological treatments

Each of the different medications have different effects on symptoms (see Table 6.2).

- Steroids—should ideally be delivered topically to the nasal mucosa using sprays or drops. When using drops it is important to use the correct position i.e. head down. Oral steroids can be very effective but their systemic effects limit their long term use. A short course can be ideal for an important summer event such as an exam or a wedding.
- Antihistamines—non sedating antihistamines are effective against sneezing, itch and watery rhinorrhoea. Used systemically they can be effective for other atopic problems such as watery eyes. They are not useful for symptoms of blockage.
- Nasal decongestants—are only useful in the short term at the start of other therapy or for flying. Prolonged use can produce intractable rhinorrhoea of rhinitis medicamentosa.
- Ipratropium bromide—this is an intranasal preparation and is effective for watery vasomotor type rhinitis.
- Sodium cromoglycate—this is a mast cell stabilizer and is useful for allergic rhinitis.

Table 6.2 Medications and their symptom control

	Sneezing	Discharge	Blockage	Anosmia
Cromoglycate	++	+	+	–
Decongestant	–	–	+++	–
Antihistamine	+++	++	+/–	–
Ipratropium	–	++	–	–
Topical steroids	+++	++	++	+
Oral steroids	++	++	+++	++

N.B. Degree of benefit where +++ is maximum and – is minimum.

Surgical treatment of nasal obstruction

The role of surgery is limited in the treatment of rhinitis. Surgery to improve nasal function may be a useful adjunct to other treatments. Even if a surgically correctable problem is found it is worth a trial of medical therapy alone in the first instance. There is often a high rate of symptom resolution. It is also worth obtaining a CT scan of the paranasal sinuses if surgery is considered in order to review the need for sinus surgery.

Turbinate reduction

The turbinates often hypertrophy in all types of rhinitis but particularly in allergic rhinitis. Their hypertrophy often obstructs the airway to such a degree that it is impossible to deliver topical medication. Reduction can be achieved by several means:

- Surface linear cautery—burning the surface
- Submucous diathermy—burning under the surface
- Cryotherapy—freezing
- Outfracture—pushing out of the airway
- Submucosal conchopexy—changing the shape of the turbinate
- Trimming or excising the turbinate.

These techniques are effective in improving the airway for 18 months but additional medical therapy is needed to prevent recurrence of the hypertrophied mucosa. The technique of trimming has a better long term result, but has the potential for severe postoperative haemorrhage. Surgeons undertaking this type of surgery are known as turbinate terrorists!

Septal surgery

A deviated septum may need to be corrected to improve nasal function and help medication delivery.

Functional endoscopic sinus surgery

This surgery is aimed at the osteomeatal complex—it aims to remove blockage in the critical area and restore the normal function and drainage of the sinuses. It could benefit patients with sinusitis who do not respond to medical treatments.

Sinusitis

Sinusitis is a common inflammation of the sinuses. It is now regarded as a continuation of the spectrum of rhinitis.

The work of Messerklinger has shown that effective sinus drainage occurs through the area known as the osteomeatal complex (see Fig. 6.4. p.115). Obstruction in this area due to anatomical or mucosal problems impairs sinus drainage and leads to obstructed outflow. This can occur as an acute phenomenon (see p.124) or as a chronic condition (see p.128).

Acute sinusitis

It is thought that everyone will suffer from an episode of sinusitis at some time in their life. It is caused by an acute bacterial infection which often develops after a preceding viral illness, such as a cold.

Signs and symptoms

- Preceding URTI
- Nasal obstruction
- Severe facial pain over the sinuses particularly the maxillae/cheeks
- Pain which is worse on bending down or coughing.

A swelling on the face is usually caused by a dental abscess rather than by sinus disease. Tenderness over the sinuses is an overemphasized sign.

Investigations

- An anterior rhinoscopy—to examine the inside of the nose
- A rigid nasendoscopy—often shows pus in middle meatus or oedematous mucosa.

Treatment

In previously healthy adults, medication alone is usually effective.

- Antibiotics may be given—Augmentin 625mg po tds for 1 week
- Decongestant—Xylometolozine 0.5% drops 2 drops tds for 1 week
- Anti-inflammatory Betnesol drops—2 drops bd both nostrils.

If sinus symptoms do not resolve, consider sinus washout or endoscopic sinus surgery after CT to confirm the diagnosis.

In immunocompromised patients, consider a sinus washout to obtain microbiology for more effective antimicrobial treatment. Also, seek advice from local microbiologists for other appropriate therapy.

Tip: A pledget soaked in 5% cocaine solution placed in the middle meatus under endoscopic guidance may relieve the obstructed osteomeatal complex due to its intense vasoconstriction.

Recurrent acute sinusitis

Patients presenting with a history of recurrent sinusitis are often difficult to diagnose. This is because in the absence of an acute infection there may be no abnormal physical signs. Even CT scans may be entirely normal. If the history is good then functional endoscopic sinus surgery (FESS) is appropriate if the number of episodes of infection is sufficient to cause disruption to the person's lifestyle.

To avoid misdiagnosis, patients can be given an open appointment to turn up when their symptoms are severe. Endoscopic examination at this time may reveal pus in the middle meatus. When a patient is symptomatic a CT scan can also be helpful, but this depends on a cooperative radiology department who will allow rapid access.

▶ **Differential diagnosis of sinusitis**

- Migraine—typical or non-classical migraine symptoms may mimic sinus symptoms
- Dental problems—Abscess or temporomandibular joint disorders
- Trigeminal neuralgia
- Neuralgias of uncertain origin
- Atypical facial pain.

Remember that the CT paranasal sinuses may be normal unless the patient is symptomatic.

Beware of operating on patients where there is no good evidence of sinus disease on a CT scan or on endoscopic examination—the results of surgery in this group are disappointing.

Chronic sinusitis

Chronic sinusitis is an inflammation of the sinuses lasting more than six weeks. Diagnosing chronic sinusitis, like diagnosing acute sinusitis, may be difficult, as other causes of facial pain may mimic it.

Signs and symptoms
- Pressure in the face—which gets worse on bending over
- Pain when flying—in particular when descending
- A feeling of nasal obstruction—can be objective or subjective
- Rhinitis—runny or blocked nose and sneezing.

Investigations
- Nasal examination—to check the patency of the airway
- Anterior rhinoscopy—to examine the septum and nasal cavity
- Posterior rhinoscopy with rigid endoscope—to examine the middle meatus and look for nasal polyps.

Treatment
80% of patients respond to medical therapy. This will involve one or more of the following medication for at least three months:
- Intranasal steroid—for mild inflammation/oedema in the nose such as Flixonase 2 sprays od both nostrils. For gross oedema a higher concentration of steroids is needed—use Betamethasone drops 2 drops bd both nostrils
- Oral antihistamine such as Cetirizine hydrochloride 10mg od po.
If medical treatment fails, the following treatments may be considered:
- A CT scan—to provide a surgical road map
- FESS—extent dictated by disease process at surgery
- Septoplasty—may be necessary in addition to above.

Complications of sinusitis

Mucociliary damage

Long standing or chronic sinusitis can lead to mucociliary failure. This means that the sinus cannot drain properly, even if it is anatomically ventilated. Cigarette smoke will also paralyse cilia action, so smoking should be avoided by those with sinusitis.

Orbital complications

An unresolved episode of acute ethmoid or pansinusitis may lead to orbital complications as shown in Fig. 6.5. The management of this problem is dealt with in the emergencies section (see p.414). The Chandler classification of orbital complications is shown in Fig. 6.5.

Intracranial complications

Infection can spread from the frontal sinuses causing problems as shown in Fig. 6.6.

Potts puffy tumour

Ongoing frontal sinusitis can lead to osteomyelitis of the frontal bone. A soft boggy swelling then appears on the skin of the forehead. It was given this colourful name by Percival Pott.

1. Preseptal oedema   2. Postseptal oedema   3. Subperiosteal abscess

4. Interconal abscess   5. Cavernous sinus
                            involvement

Fig. 6.5. Chandler classification of orbital complications

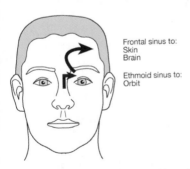

Frontal sinus to:
Skin
Brain

Ethmoid sinus to:
Orbit

Fig. 6.6. Pathways of spread for intracranial complications

Nasal polyps

Simple nasal polyps are part of the spectrum of rhinosinusitis as the lining of the nose becomes inflamed and thicker. These polyps are oedematous sinus mucosa, which prolapse to fill the nasal cavity to a variable extent. They are common, and their cause is unknown.

Signs and symptoms

- Variable symptoms—with the season or with URTI
- Rhinitis—blocked or runny nose and sneezing
- Sinusitis—due to osteomeatal obstruction
- Nasal obstruction
- Appearance of the polyps at the anterior nares.

Investigations

- Anterior rhinoscopy—Inferior turbinates are often incorrectly diagnosed as polyps, a rhinoscopy can help avoid this misdiagnosis (see Fig. 6.7.).
- Rigid nasendoscopy—examining the nose with an endoscope.
- Polyp size can be graded (see Fig. 6.8.).

Treatment

- For small nasal polyps—give Betamethasone drops. 2 drops bd for 2 weeks followed by Flixonase 2 sprays od both nostrils for 3 months.
- For large nasal polyps—give oral steroids 30mg od for 1 week followed by Flixonase 2 sprays bd for 3 months.

If medical treatment fails, the following treatments should be considered:

- Surgical removal for obstructive polyps—if the patient is sufficiently symptomatic.
- A CT scan to provide a road map prior to surgery.
- FESS—using a microdebrider for atraumatic polypectomy.
- Postoperative intranasal steroids to prevent recurrence.

Samters triad associated polyp

This is the association of:

- Aspirin sensitivity—making patients wheezy when they take asprin
- Late onset asthma
- Nasal polyps.

It is caused by a defect in leukotriene metabolism. Polyps in this condition are florid and recur frequently.

Treatment

- Diet—refer patient to a dietician for advice on a low salicylate diet. This is very bland and difficult to maintain.
- Intranasal steroids—patients often elect to use long term Betamethasone drops despite their risk of systemic side effects.
- Repeat surgery as for nasal polyps above—the microdebrider is the atraumatic instrument of choice.
- Leukotriene antagonists e.g. Monteleukast aim to reduce the polyps—results may vary.

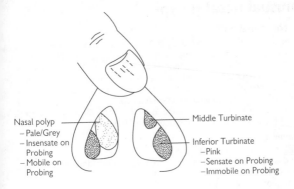

Fig. 6.7. Diagram of nasal polyp showing features compared with inferior turbinate

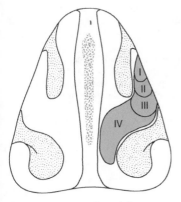

Fig. 6.8. Polyp size can be graded

Unusual nasal polyps

Antrochoanal polyps

These polyps originate from the maxillary sinus and often present as a unilateral pendulous mass in the nasopharynx (see Fig. 6.9.). The uncinate process directs the polyp posteriorly as it emerges from the maxillary sinus. They are uncommon and their cause is not known.

Macroscopically, the polyp is formed from a nasal component which is similar in appearance to a common nasal polyp.

The maxillary antral component is a thin fluid filled cyst. A small fibrous band joins the two as it passes out of the sinus.

Treatment

- CT scan—to confirm the diagnosis.
- Endoscopic removal of the polyps from its point of attachment in the maxillary sinus.
- Caldwell–Luc approach for recurrent problem—an open sinus operation accessing the sinus via a cut in the mouth under the top lip.

Childhood polyps

Polyps presenting in childhood are very unusual. They are usually associated with an underlying mucociliary abnormality such as cystic fibrosis or Kartagener's syndrome.

Investigations

- Consider a sweat test—the diagnostic test for cystic fibrosis.
- Send samples to the lab to check that it is not a tumour.
- Fresh sample of nasal lining for special tests of ciliary function.
- Sample for electron microscopy—to check the cillary structure.

Treatments

- Medical treatment with steroids.
- Surgical removal.

Fig. 6.9. Antrochoanal polyp and its anatomical relations

a = maxillary sinus attachment; b = maxillary ostium; c = osteomeatal complex;
d = posterior choana; e = nasopharynx.

Septal problems

The nasal septum provides an important mechanical support for the external nasal skeleton. Problems with the nasal septum can lead to both a cosmetic and functional disturbance of the nose. The nose may look bent to one side and/or the nasal airway may be restricted.

Septal deviation

The causes of septal deviation can be either congenital or traumatic. A traumatic septal deviation could be the result of a broken nose. Congenital septal deviation can occur after birth trauma to the nose, or the differential growth of the nasal septum compared to the rest of the skull.

Almost all nasal septae are deviated to some extent. Most people do not experience any problems, but some find their airway has become restricted.

Acoustic rhinomanometry and computer flow modeling has shown that deviations at the area of the nasal valve cause most functional impairment to airflow. This area is situated about 1cm posterior to the nares. It is bounded superiorly by the overlap of the upper and lower lateral cartilages. Laterally is the origin of the anterior part of the inferior turbinate. Inferiorly, the floor of the nose and medially, the nasal septum. Changes in the relative position of any of these structures causes a change in the cross-sectional area of the nasal valve.

Investigations
- Anterior rhinoscopy—to exclude other problems e.g. rhinitis.
- Cottle's test (see p.29)—to exclude alar collapse.
- Nasendoscopy—to exclude sinusitis.

Treatment
- Three months trial of an intranasal steroid.
- Surgery—septoplasty or a sub-mucous resection (SMR) is an operation on the nasal septum to improve nasal breathing.

Septal perforation

There are several reasons why a patient's septum may be perforated. These include:
- Trauma or accident.
- Post septal surgery.
- Nose picking.
- Granulomatous disease—must be excluded before treating perforation (see p.140).
  - Wegener's
  - Sarcoidosis
  - TB
  - Syphilis
- Cocaine addiction.

Signs and symptoms
- Whistling—if there is a small anterior perforation.
- Bleeding from the nose.
- Crusting of the nose at the site of the perforation.

Treatment
- Apply Vaseline to the edge of the perforation.
- Treat epistaxis expectantly.
- Septal button—this is a plastic prosthesis fitted into the hole in the septum. Only half of patients find it tolerable and continue using it long term.
- Surgical septal repair—the results of surgery are variable even in experienced hands.

Granulomatous conditions

These are an uncommon group of diseases which are classified together because of their histological appearance—they all form granulomas. These conditions include:
- **Wegener's granulomatosis**—this is a multisystem disease characterised by perivascular granuloma formation—it most often affects the respiratory system and the kidneys.
- **Sarcoidosis**—this is another granulomatous condition; its cause is unknown.
- **Syphilis**—a sexually transmitted disease which can affect the nose.

Signs and symptoms
- The patient may present with nasal granulomas as part of generalised condition e.g. sarcoid with chest problems.
- Patients may have isolated nasal symptoms such as septal perforation (posterior in syphilis) or crusting on the nasal septum.

Investigations
- FBC
- U&Es
- ESR
- Syphilis serology
- ANCA
- CXR
- Nasal biopsy.

Treatment
- Involve the medical team who deal with the condition in hospital such as chest or renal teams.
- Give immunosuppressants—both steroids and non steroid are used.

Sinonasal malignancy

Sinonasal malignancy is dealt with in Chapter 15, p.332.

The salivary glands

Structure and function of the salivary glands

There are three main pairs of salivary glands—the parotid, the submandibular and the sublingual. In addition, there are a number of other tiny minor salivary glands scattered throughout the mucosa of the mouth and throat. They produce the saliva which is needed for digestion and lubricating the food bolus.

The parotid gland

This gland lies on the side of the face or upper neck behind the angle of the mandible and in front of the ear. The gland is pyramid shaped and covered in thick fibrous tissue. It produces watery, serous saliva. The parotid duct opens into the mouth opposite the second upper molar tooth.

The external carotid artery, retro-mandibular vein and lymph nodes all lie within the parotid gland.

The facial nerve traverses the skull base and exits at the stylomastoid foramen. It then passes through the parotid gland splitting into its 5 main divisions—temporal, zygomatic, buccal, mandibular, cervical—as it does so.

The submandibular gland

This gland lies just below the jaw in front of the angle of the mandible. It produces saliva. The submandibular duct runs from the deep lobe and ends as a papillae, at the front of the floor of the mouth (see Fig. 7.1.).

The lingual nerve—which gives sensation to the anterior two thirds of the tongue—and the hypoglossal nerve—which provides the motor to intrinsic muscles of the tongue—lie in close apposition to the deep surface of the gland.

The marginal mandibular branch of the facial nerve runs just deep to the platysma close under the skin which overlies the gland. Surgeons must be aware of these nerves in order to prevent iatrogenic damage.

A number of lymph nodes also lie close to or within the submandibular gland.

The sublingual gland

This is the smallest of the major salivary glands. It is found, or felt in the floor of the mouth, running along the submandibular duct, into which it opens via 10–15 tiny ducts.

Parasympathetic secretor motor supply to the salivary glands

This is rather complicated and is best shown diagrammatically (Fig. 7.2.).

Fig. 7.1. Relations of parotid and SMG

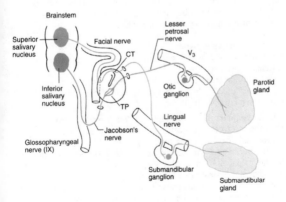

Fig. 7.2. Parasympathetic secretomotor nerve supply

Salivary gland tumours

80% of all salivary gland tumours occur in the parotid gland.
80% of these are benign pleomorphic or mixed adenomas.
50% of submandibular gland tumours are malignant.
80% of minor salivary gland tumours are malignant.

Benign tumours

Pleomorphic adenomas

Parotid pleomorphic adenomas are the most common salivary tumour. They are benign, but if they are present for many years they may turn malignant. They appear most often as an asymptomatic lump behind the angle of the mandible—this may displace the ear lobe upwards slightly. If the patient has weakness of the facial nerve, this suggests a malignant infiltration and the diagnosis must be questioned.

Diagnosis is usually made via fine needle aspirate, and treatment is surgical. In order to prevent the adenomas recurring, the surgeon should remove a cuff of normal parotid tissue around the lump, and ensure that no tumour is spilt during excision. The surgeon will take great care to identify and preserve the facial nerve during parotid surgery.

Warthins tumour or adenolymphoma

This is the next most common benign tumour of the salivary glands. It is common in elderly men. It occurs most often in the parotid gland, often in its tail—the part of the parotid that extends into the neck. This is the only tumour which is recognised as occurring bilaterally, and its cause is unknown. Treatment is surgical.

Other benign swellings in the salivary glands include lipoma, cysts, oncocytoma and monomorphic adenoma.

Malignant tumours

Malignant salivary gland tumours are much less common than benign ones, but the symptoms can be similar—usually a lump in the neck. The following symptoms may suggest a malignant tumour:

• Pain
• Facial or other nerve weakness
• Skin involvement such as ulceration or fixation of the overlying skin
• Bloodstained discharge into the mouth
• Local lymph node enlargement suggesting metastasis.

There are minor salivary glands in the mucosa of the nose, mouth and throat. Neoplastic transformation here is often malignant.

Adenoidcystic tumours (have nothing to do with the adenoids!)

These are the most common malignant salivary gland tumours. They are slow growing and have a strong tendency to spread along the nerves—this is called perineural infiltration. They can spread several centimeters beyond the palpable lump in this way. Treatment is excision of the tumour and postoperative radiotherapy.

The short term or 5 year prognosis tends to be good, and patients with a recurrent tumour and even lung metastases may live for years. But the long term or 25 year prognosis is less good and in most cases patients will eventually die of this disease.

Mucoepidermoid carcinomas
These are unusual tumours in that they have a range of aggressiveness from low to high. High grade tumors require excision and post-operative radiotherapy, whereas low grade tumors will usually only need surgery.

Sialadenitis

This is an acute infection of the submandibular or parotid gland. Sialadenitis usually occurs in elderly or debilitated patients, who may be dehydrated and have poor oral hygiene. Drugs, such as the oral contraceptive pill, thiouracil and alcohol may cause mild sialadenitis.

Signs and symptoms

The symptoms are usually a painful swelling of the gland and pyrexia. Pressure over the affected gland may lead to pus leaking from the duct.

Treatment

Treatment involves rehydration, antibiotics and attention to oral hygiene. Sialogogues, such as lemon drops which stimulate saliva production, are helpful. Surgical drainage may be required if an intra glandular abscess complicates this infection,

Chronic salivary gland inflammation or recurrent acute attacks of sialadenitis may arise as a result of stones or stricture within the gland or duct. Stones arise as accumulations of calcium and other salts found in saliva, deposits on foreign material, and food debris within the ducts. Strictures most often occur after an episode of inflammation in the duct. Pain and swelling when eating are common. This usually occurs in the submandibular gland, and surgical excision may be required.

Sialolithiasis

Sialolithiasis, or salivary stones, is common, and usually affects the sub-mandibular gland since the secretions are richer in calcium and thicker.

Signs and symptoms

Symptoms may include pain and swelling in the affected gland during or after meals. The gland will become tense and tender. Inspection of the floor of the mouth may reveal the thickened inflamed submandibular duct, and the stone maybe palpable within the duct. If there is any uncertainty about the diagnosis, a plain X-ray or a sialogram (an X-ray of the duct system using dye) should be used.

Treatment

Conservative treatment with rehydration, analgesia, and sialogogues may be all that is required. Sometimes a small stone will spontaneously pass out of the duct into the mouth and the symptoms will settle. Larger stones may need to be removed. This can be performed trans-orally if the stone is palpable in the floor of mouth. If the stone is placed close to the gland, the whole gland may need to be removed by an open operation via the neck.

Other inflammatory conditions

- **Sjögren's syndrome**—an autoimmune disease. It causes a dry mouth, dry eyes and in many cases diffuse enlargement of the parotid gland. The diagnosis can be confirmed by biopsying a minor salivary gland found in the mucosa of the oral cavity.
- **Systemic viral infections**—such as mumps and HIV may cause inflammation of the parotid or submandibular glands.
- **Granulomatous conditions**—such as tuberculosis and sarcoidosis may affect the salivary glands.

Pseudosalivary swellings

These swellings may mimic salivary gland enlargement, such as:
• Intra-glandular lymph nodes.
• Hypertrophy of the masseter muscle—may mimic parotid enlargement.
• Parapharyngeal space masses—may present as an intra oral mass in a similar way to a deep lobe of parotid mass.
• Lesions/cysts of the mandible or teeth—may look like a submandibular gland mass.
• Winging of the mandible—may mimic parotid swelling.

Salivary gland surgery

See figures showing incisions (Fig. 7.3.), the facial nerve and its relations to the parotid (Fig. 7.4.), and the submandibular gland and anatomy (Fig. 7.5.).

The facial nerve passes through the parotid gland—this is a risk in parotid surgery. Surgeons will often use the facial nerve monitor to help them identify the facial nerve.

Other surgical pointers to the position of the facial nerve are listed below:

- The facial nerve exits from the stylomastoid foramen which lies at the root of tympanomastoid suture. This is palpable during parotid surgery.
- The facial nerve lies approximately 1cm deep and 1cm inferior to a small V shaped piece of cartilage known as the tragal pointer.
- The facial nerve bisects the angle made between the mastoid process and the posterior belly of the digastric muscle.

Complications of parotid gland surgery

- Paraesthesia or numbness of the ear lobe is common, because the greater auricular nerve may need to be divided to gain access to the parotid gland.
- Haematoma.
- Salivary fistula—when saliva leaks out through the incision.
- Temporary facial nerve weakness—occurs in about 10% of cases.
- Permanent facial nerve weakness—occurs in less than 1% of cases.
- Frey's syndrome—sweating and redness of the skin overlying the parotid gland when eating. It occurs when post synaptic secretomotor nerve fibres are severed during surgery, and they re-grow abnormally, innervating the sweat glands of the skin.

Complications of submandibular gland surgery

- Haematoma—the most common complication.
- Weakness of the marginal mandibular nerve—this can usually be avoided by a low horizontal incision being made 2cm below the angle of the mandible. The surgical dissection should be carried out deep to the capsule of the gland i.e. in a plane deep to the nerve.
- Lingual and hypoglossal nerve damage—these nerves lie close to the deep surface of the gland and are potentially at risk during the surgery—in reality damage is extremely rare.

Fig. 7.3. (a) Incision for parotid surgery; (b) incision for submandibular surgery

Marginal
mandibular
division of VII th
nerve at risk in
submandibular
gland surgery

Fig. 7.4. Diagram of facial nerve and relations to the salivary glands

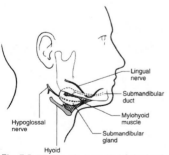

Lingual
nerve

Submandibular
duct

Mylohyoid
muscle

Hypoglossal
nerve

Submandibular
gland

Hyoid

Fig. 7.5. Diagram of submandibular gland and anatomy

The larynx

Structure and function of the larynx

Structure

The larynx is a tube made up of cartilage and bone, held together by membranes, ligaments and muscles. Above, the larynx connects with the pharynx and oral cavity, below it connects with the trachea and major airways (Fig. 8.1). Behind the larynx is the opening of the oesophagus.

Food and drink are guided from the mouth to the oesophagus, while air passes via the trachea to the lungs. Food passes over the back of the tongue and runs down two channels called the piriform fossae. These lie slightly behind and to the side of the larynx. They join behind the cricoid cartilage and form the oesophagus (see Fig. 8.2.).

Function

The main function of the larynx is to protect the lower airways from contamination by fluids, liquids and saliva. The way this happens is as follows: the larynx rises during swallowing, bringing the laryngeal inlet closer to the tongue base and allowing the food bolus to pass on either side. The epiglottis folds down to cover the larynx. The vocal cords and false cords, (see Fig. 8.3.) come together.

Fig. 8.1. Vocal tract

Fig. 8.2. External view of larynx

Fig. 8.3. Internal side view of larynx

The vocal cords

Structure

The vocal cords, also called the vocal folds, and collectively called the glottis, are suspended in the airway. They divide the larynx in two—the supraglottis lies above the vocal cords and the subglottis lies below.

The cords are made of a stiff central muscle and ligament, and a soft loose cover. They are fixed to the thyroid cartilage at the front and to the arytenoid cartilages at the back. These cartilages can slide away from and towards each other, opening and closing the laryngeal inlet.

Innervation: The sensation of the supraglottis is carried by the internal branch of the superior laryngeal nerve. The external branch carries motor fibres to the cricothyroid muscle. This muscle is important in adjusting the tension of the vocal cord. The vagus nerve gives rise to the recurrent laryngeal nerve and this in turn carries sensation to the subglottis and is motor to all the other muscles of the larynx. The left recurrent laryngeal nerve has an unusually long course and loops down into the chest, lying close to the hilum of the lung. It is prone to infiltration by tumors of this region. (See Fig. 8.8., p.180, Neurological laryngeal conditions.)

Lymph drainage: The vocal cords are a watershed for lymphatic drainage. Above, the supraglottis drains to the pre-epiglottic and upper deep cervical nodes, whilst below, drainage is to the lower deep cervical and pre-tracheal nodes. The cords have very poor lymph drainage, so tumors limited to vocal cords have a low risk of lymphatic spread. Tumors of the lymphatic rich supra or sub-glottis frequently present with lymph node metastases and consequently will have a worse prognosis (see Fig. 8.4., p.165).

Function

The vocal cords are the source of the sound vibration, which we adapt with our mouth, tongue, lips and teeth to produce speech. As air passes up between the cords the Bernoulli effect draws the mucosa of the cords together. They meet for a fraction of a second and then the pressure rises below the cords, blowing them apart again. This vibration of the cords and the distortion of the mucosa that results from it is known as the mucosal wave. This causes the voice.

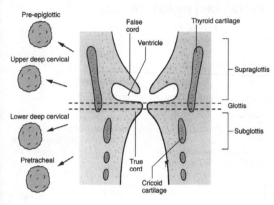

Fig. 8.4. Lymph drainage of larynx

Congenital laryngeal lesions

Babies are more prone to breathing difficulties because their larynx differs from an adults in the following ways:
- The airway is smaller both relatively and absolutely.
- The laryngeal mucosa is less tightly bound down and as a result may swell dramatically.
- The cartilaginous support for the airway is less rigid than in an adult—this makes it more prone to collapse, especially during inspiration.

Laryngomalacia

Signs of this condition show themselves shortly after birth with inspiratory stridor and feeding difficulties. When breathing in, these babies experience an excessive collapse and indrawing of the supraglottic airways, leading to breathing difficulties.

Usually this condition is mild and self limiting. When it is severe an aryepiglottoplasty may be performed. This involves dividing the excessively tight aryepiglottic folds, which allows the epiglottis to spring upwards and open up the airway.

Subglottic stenosis

This abnormality is caused by an excessively narrow cricoid cartilage. It is either a birth defect, or it arises as a result of intubation and prolonged ventilation. Subglottic cysts and haemangiomas may present with similar symptoms.

The main sign of this condition is stridor at any age from birth to 2 years. Diagnosis is made by inspecting and measuring the diameter of the subglottis under general anaesthetic. Mild cases may be treated conservatively, but more severe stenoses require surgical invervention and laryngo-tracheal reconstruction. See Table 8.1 of stenosis opposite.

Laryngeal web

This condition occurs when the vocal cords fuse together and the airway is reduced. Fusion can be minimal, with little effect on the airway; or complete fusion can occur which is incompatible with life.

The main signs of this condition are respiratory difficulties, stridor and a hoarse cry. Severe cases will require immediate surgical intervention either via a tracheostomy (when an artificial breathing hole is made in the neck below the cords to bypass the obstruction) or by endoscopic division of the web.

Laryngeal cleft

This condition occurs when the posterior larynx has failed to fuse. At its most severe this will also extend down to involve the posterior wall of the trachea.

The main signs are respiratory problems associated with feeding, as a result of aspiration into the trachea. Mild cases can be difficult to diagnose. Where there are symptoms, surgical repair may be needed.

Vocal cord palsy

The recurrent laryngeal nerves are long in children and adults, reaching from the skull base down into the chest and back up again to the larynx. Because of their length, they are prone to damage anywhere along their course. Unilateral palsy will cause a weak breathy cry and feeding difficulties as a result of aspiration, and bilateral palsy will present as marked stridor.

Table 8.1 Congenital laryngeal lesions: Cotton grading of tracheal stenosis

Grade 1	≤50% obstruction
Grade 2	51–70% obstruction
Grade 3	71–99% obstruction
Grade 4	No lumen

Infections of the larynx

Acute laryngitis

Inflammation of the larynx may occur in isolation or as part of a general infective process affecting the whole of the respiratory tract. It is very common, often presenting as a sore throat and loss of voice with a cold.

Signs and symptoms
- Hoarse voice
- Pain on speaking and swallowing
- Malaise
- Slight pyrexia
- Examination of the vocal cords will show them to be reddened and swollen.

Treatment

Most patients with acute laryngitis either self medicate or are treated in the primary care setting with supportive therapy such as voice rest, simple analgesia, steam inhalations and simple cough suppressants.

Voice rest is especially important for any professional voice user. Patients should be advised of this, and of the risk of haemorrhage into the vocal cord, which can produce permanent adverse effects on the voice.

Chronic laryngitis

Chronic laryngitis is a common inflammation of the larynx caused by many different factors. It often begins after an upper respiratory tract infection. Smoking, vocal abuse, chronic lung disease, sinusitis, post nasal drip, reflux, alcohol fumes and environmental pollutants may all conspire together to maintain the inflammation.

Signs and symptoms
- A hoarse voice.
- A tickle in the throat or a feeling of mucus in the throat.
- A patient who is constantly clearing their throat or coughing—this causes still more inflammation of the cords and establishes a vicious circle.
- A laryngoscopy which reveals thickened, red, oedematous vocal cords.

The patient should be referred for a laryngeal examination if their symptoms fail to settle within 4 weeks. If any concern remains after this examination, the patient should be admitted for an examination and a biopsy, under general anaesthesic, to exclude laryngeal malignancy.

Treatment

The agents that are causing the chronic laryngitis should be removed. The patient may require the skills of a speech therapist. Patients will also respond well to explanation and reassurance that they do not have a more serious condition.

Reinke's oedema

This is a specific form of chronic laryngitis found in smokers. The vocal cords become extremely oedematous and filled with a thin jelly-like fluid. The oedema fails to resolve due to poor lymph drainage of the vocal cord. Stopping smoking and speech therapy are helpful in removing the causes of this condition. In many cases microlaryngeal surgery is required to incise the cord and suck out the oedema. It is important to avoid any damage to the free edge of the vocal cord when performing this operation, as it can permanently affect the mucosal wave and hence the voice.

Epiglotitis and supraglottitis

This is an inflammation of the epiglottis or supraglottic tissues that affects children and adults. Epiglotitis is now rare in children in the UK (as a result of the HIB vaccination). It is seen more often in adults, where it tends to affect the whole of the supraglottic tissues (and is called supraglottitis). Most ENT departments see one case per month in the winter. The causative agent is usually *H. influenzae*.

Signs and symptoms

- Difficulty in swallowing leading to drooling of saliva.
- Change in the voice, described as a muffled or 'hot potato voice' or change in the child's cry.
- Dramatic swelling of the supraglottic tissues.
- Pools of saliva seen collected around the larynx on endoscopy.

This condition should not be underestimated. It may start with features similar to any other respiratory tract infection, but it can rapidly progress to total airway obstruction within hours of onset. Consider this diagnosis early on, and get expert help.

Management

- Admit the patient and keep them upright. Lying the patient flat could obstruct their airway.
- Do not attempt to examine the mouth, as this may obstruct the patient's breathing.
- No X-rays—they do not add much to the diagnosis and remove the patient from immediate expert assistance should they need it
- Call for senior help—an ENT surgeon and an anaesthetist.

Treatment

If epiglotitis or supraglottitis is suspected, stop further investigations. Escort the patient calmly and quickly to an operating theatre where an experienced paediatric anaesthetist and scrubbed consultant ENT surgeon are standing by with the appropriate equipment (laryngoscope, ventilating bronchoscope and tracheostomy set).

Where possible the patient should be intubated and treated with the appropriate antibiotics. However, oral intubation may be difficult and the ENT surgeon may be asked to secure the airway surgically.

Croup

This infection is common in children. It affects the whole of the upper respiratory tract (URT), hence the more descriptive name, acute laryngo-tracheo-bronchitis. It is usually viral in origin, but a bacterial infection with *H. influenzae* is sometimes seen. The speed of onset of croup is slower than in epiglottitis, but it can be extremely serious and even life threatening.

Signs and symptoms

- Mild preceeding upper respiratory tract infection
- Rising pyrexia
- Stridor
- Malaise.

Treatment

- Admission to hospital may be necessary in all but the most minor cases
- Intravenous antibiotics
- ± nebulised adrenaline
- Ventilatory support where required.

Cancer of the larynx

The vast majority of laryngeal cancers are squamous cell carcinomas. Smoking is the risk factor for laryngeal cancer, although smoking and drinking in combination puts the patient at even more risk. It is the most common neck and head malignancy.

Since the whole of the upper aerodigestive tract has been exposed to the same risk factor (that is, smoke), there is a widespread field change throughout this mucosa. These patients therefore have an increased risk of developing another cancer in the mouth, pharynx, larynx or oesophagus. 5% of patients with one head and neck cancer will present with a second primary tumour elsewhere in the head or neck. This may be silent and cause no symptoms at all!

Signs and symptoms

The patient's symptoms will depend upon which site(s) within the larynx is affected. A tumour on the vocal cord will cause a hoarse voice, and a patient in this situation will usually present early. However, a tumour in the supra-glottis may present few symptoms until much later and a patient may present with advanced disease. All patients with a lump in the neck must be referred for an ENT examination.

Signs of advanced laryngeal cancer are:
- Pain—often referred to the ear.
- Voice change—the voice is muffled rather than hoarse, unless the tumour also extends to involve the true vocal cords.
- Breathing difficulties and stridor.
- Difficulty swallowing or inhaling.
- Lymph node enlargement in the neck—this is often the only presenting feature.

Investigations

Although a clinical diagnosis can often be made after examination of the larynx, a biopsy is essential. This is because conditions such as laryngeal papillomas, granulomas and polyps may mimic laryngeal cancer. All patients should also have an examination of the whole of the upper aerodigestive tract (panendoscopy) to check for a second primary tumour.

All patients must have at least a CXR. A CT scan of the chest is routine practice in many centres. CT/MRI scanning of the neck is also mandatory, particularly looking for thyroid cartilage erosion and enlarged lymph nodes in the deep cervical chain.

Staging

TNM staging is applied to head and neck cancers in a similar way to other sites.

- The T stage is determined by the anatomical site/sites affected.
- The N stage refers to the local nodal spread.
- The M stage is determined by the presence or absence of distant metastases (see Boxes 8.1–8.3).

Box 8.1 T staging of laryngeal cancer

TX: Tumour cannot be assessed.

Tis: Carcinoma in situ.

T1a: Tumour limited to one cord and not affecting the anterior commisure.

T1b: Tumour limited to the cord but involving the anterior (or posterior) commisure.

T2: Tumour spreading upwards or downwards from the cord to involve the supraglottis or subglottis with normal vocal cord mobility.

T3: Tumour which fixes the vocal cord either by involvement of the recurrent laryngeal nerve or by infiltration of the cricoarytenoid joint or simply as a result of the bulk of the tumour.

T4: Tumour escaping from the larynx to involve another site or erosion of the cartilaginous framework of the larynx.

Box 8.2 N staging for the head and neck

N1: A single ipsilateral node, <3cm in size.

N2a: A single ipsilateral node >3cm but <6cm in size.

N2b: More than one ipsilateral node <6cm in size.

N2c: A contralateral node or bilateral nodes <6cm in size.

N3: Any node >6cm in size.

Box 8.3 M staging for the head and neck

M0: No distant metastases.

M1: Distant metastases.

Treatment of laryngeal cancer

Treatment is either surgery or external beam radiotherapy. Early laryngeal tumours are satisfying to treat, since more than 90% can be cured.

If a patient is too unfit to undergo radical treatment, palliative radiotherapy or chemotherapy may be used to shrink the tumour. This can reduce symptoms and improve the patient's quality of life.

Although practice does vary slightly between different units and countries, in general, treatment is as follows:

- Small tumours (stage T1 and T2) are treated with radiotherapy—surgery is used only if they recur afterwards.
- Big tumours (stage T4) are treated with radical excision—a partial or total laryngectomy.
- The treatment of T3 tumours is controversial—some opt for primary surgery and others advocate radiotherapy, holding surgery in reserve for radiation failures.

Each patient should be assessed individually and treatment decisions must be made in an multi disciplinary team setting, with the knowledge and consent of the patient.

Surgery for laryngeal cancer

The decision as to which type of surgery is performed is largely dependant on the size and extent of the tumour. Surgery may be performed endoluminally—with endoscopes from the inside—usually with the aid of a laser. Or, the radical excision of part of, or the entire larynx may be needed. In general, smaller tumours (T1 and T2) are more easily treated with endoscopic laser surgery, and larger T3 and 4 tumours are offered radical excisional surgery. (see Laryngectomy p.175)

Radical radiotherapy for laryngeal cancer

A total dose of 50–70 Gy is given over 4–6 weeks, Monday to Friday.

Each treatment only lasts a few minutes but the patient has to wear a custom made Perspex mask, rather like a neck brace. This holds the patient in exactly the same position each day, ensuring that the radiotherapy fields are directed accurately onto the tumour and immediate area. This spares the uninvolved areas of the head and neck.

Towards the end of treatment the patient will suffer with painful mucositis. Swallowing can become difficult, and the patient may need to be admitted for enteral feeding and analgesia.

> **Box 8.4 Key learning points—Radiotherapy for laryngeal cancer**
>
> - Treatment intent maybe palliative or curative
> - Chemotherapy is only used as an addition to radiotherapy (or surgical) treatment
> - Small tumours do very well
> - Radiotherapy is usually given for small tumours
> - Large tumours are usually treated with a laryngectomy
> - Post operative radiotherapy is often given in advanced disease with poor histology.

Laryngectomy

Several different types of partial laryngectomy have been described. These are collectively known as 'less than total' and are beyond the scope of this book.

A *total laryngectomy* was first described at the beginning of the last century, but it remains a reliable and effective treatment. During a total laryngectomy the larynx is removed and the trachea is brought to the skin as an end stoma in the neck. The pharynx is opened and repaired to reconstitute the swallowing mechanism. (See Fig. 8.5.). A neck dissection is often performed in combination with this procedure. This is because patients with advanced or recurrent laryngeal disease are at considerable risk of having nodal metastases, which may be palpable or hidden.

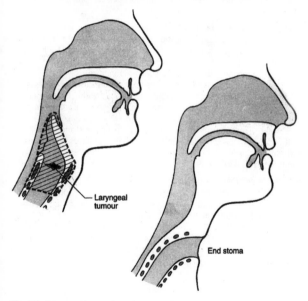

Fig. 8.5. Diagram of pre and post laryngectomy anatomy

Voice restoration after laryngectomy (see also p.384)

Oesophageal speech (See Fig. 8.6a)

In those who can achieve it, oesophageal speech offers near normal verbal communication. The basic principle is that air is swallowed into the stomach and then regurgitated into the pharynx. This causes vibration of the pharyngo-oesophageal segment (PE segment) similar to a belch. This can be modified with the lips and teeth into intelligible speech.

The main problem is that not all patients can manage to achieve this type of speech, and even if they do, only small amounts of air can be swallowed. This means that the resultant speech can only be made up of short phrases at best.

Tracheo-oesophageal puncture (See Fig. 8.6b)

This is when artificial communication is created between the back wall of the trachea and the front wall of the pharynx/oesophagus. This is usually done at the time of the initial surgery (primary puncture) but can be performed at anytime thereafter (secondary puncture).

A one-way valve is inserted into this tract which allows the passage of air from the trachea to the oesophagus, vibrating the PE segment as above. In order to activate the valve, the patient must occlude their stoma and try to breathe out. This may be done with a finger, or by using a second manually operated valve which sits over the stoma as part of a heat and moisture exchanger (HME). The HME also filters the inhaled air and prevents excess water vapour being lost from the respiratory tract—in effect this replaces some of the functions of the nose.

Artificial larynx (Servox)

Some patients cannot achieve either of the above forms of speech, and require an external vibrating source. The vibrating end of this device is held firmly onto the patient's neck, floor of their mouth or cheek, and this causes these tissues to vibrate. As a result, the air within the pharynx and oral cavity vibrates and sound is produced. The voice produced does sound rather unnatural but this is a simple and effective means of communication (see Fig. 8.7.).

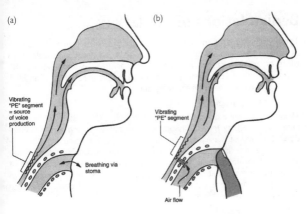

Fig. 8.6. Diagram of TEP voice

Fig. 8.7. Diagram of servox

Benign lesions of the larynx

These are lesions of the vocal cords which are not cancer. Signs of a benign lesion—such as a hoarse voice—can be indistinguishable from those of laryngeal cancer. It is therefore imperative that any patient with a change in their voice lasting more that 4 weeks is referred to an ENT surgeon to exclude a laryngeal malignancy.

Vocal cord polyp/cyst

These lesions are indistinguishable histologically. They usually arise spontaneously, but they may be associated with previous laryngeal inflammation. The symptoms are a sore throat and/or a hoarse voice.

The cysts are intra-cordal, whereas polyps are pedunculated and may be difficult to see because they sometimes hang down on their stalk to sit below the cords. Treatment is with microsurgical excision, taking care to avoid iatrogenic damage to the free edge of the vocal cord, and hence the mucosal wave and voice.

Vocal cord granuloma

This lesion is usually unilateral and affects the posterior aspect of the vocal cord. As a result, it can have quite a minimal effect on the voice. Vocal cord granuloma arises as a result of inflammation of the arytenoid cartilage (perichondritis). It is most often seen as a result of intubation trauma or excessive coughing. The patient usually complains of pain in their larynx. Reflux is a commonly associated feature.

The lesion requires a biopsy as SCC can present with similar features. Treatment may include surgical excision, speech therapy and the treatment of acid reflux.

Singer's nodules

These nodules—also known as screamers' nodules—occur as a result of prolonged voice abuse or misuse. They are common in children, amateur actors and singers—they give a characteristic huskiness to the voice.

They are always bilateral and occur at the junction of the anterior third and posterior two thirds of the vocal cords. Early or 'soft' nodules will resolve with speech therapy and good vocal habits, but long established 'hard' nodules may require surgery.

Papillomas

These non cancerous growths are most commonly seen in children but may also occur in adults. Papillomas arise as a result of human papilloma virus (HPV). The route of transmission is thought to be through inhalation. There may also be some defect in the host immune system, as some individuals are affected and others are not. Spontaneuous resolution tends to occur in children around puberty, but this is less common in adults.

In its most severe form, papilloma may result in significant airway obstruction in the larynx, trachea and major bronchii. If the patient's airway is obstructed, surgical debulking of the papilloma is required. Removal of every last papilloma in not advised, since this will cause scarring of the vocal cords and they often recur. A tracheostomy may be required, but even then papillomas may grow around the stoma.

Malignant transformation may occur in adults especially with subtypes 7 and 11. Systemic treatment with interferon is effective, but rebound growth may be dramatic when it is stopped.

Muscle tension dysphonia

This is a common problem seen in general and ENT practice. Symptom is a hoarse voice which tires easily and may vary in pitch. Patients sometimes say their voice 'cracks' or 'gives out' and the quality of the voice varies from day to day and moment to moment. Occasionally the patient may present with aphonia.

These problems are caused by laryngeal muscular tension abnormalities. They are associated with voice misuse, psychological stress and psychiatric disease.

Globus type symptoms are frequent. These include a feeling of a lump in the throat, a feeling of mucus in the throat and frequent throat clearing. The treatment is reassurance and explanation, with speech therapy for patients who do not respond well.

Vocal cord palsy

Palsy or paralysis of the vocal cords will mean that the patient may have a weak breathy voice rather than the harsh hoarse voice of laryngeal cancer. They will have a poor, ineffective cough and aspiration is common. See Box 8.5, p.180.

The recurrent laryngeal nerve (RLN) is a branch of the vagus nerve and has a long course (see Fig. 8.8. p.180). This makes it susceptible to damage in a variety of sites.

Investigation

Remember the rule of thirds below:
- 1/3 idiopathic
- 1/3 surgery
- 1/3 neoplasia

Where there is no history of recent surgery, order:
- CXR—if it is negative proceed to—
- CT scan—skull base to hilum
- ± USS thyroid
- ± oesphagoscopy

If the above are negative then post viral neuropathy is the most likely cause. The causes of vocal cord immobility (fixation rather than palsy) include rheumatoid arthritis, laryngeal trauma, prolonged intubation and carcinoma affecting the cricoarytenoid joint. An endoscopy, together with palpation of the joint is necessary to confirm this abnormality.

Treatment

Where there is a small gap between the cords, speech therapy may be all that is needed to strengthen the mobile cord and aid compensation. When there is a larger gap, the paralysed cord can be medialised, either by an injection technique or via a thyroplasty. (See Fig. 8.10., p.181 and Fig. 8.11., p.181). Poor function of the cords may lead to aspiration and chest infections. Dietary modifications, tube feeding and even a tracheostomy may be required to protect the airway from soiling.

Neurological laryngeal conditions

Any condition which affects the brainstem (CVA, trauma or tumour) will affect the function of the vagus nerve and as such the recurrent laryngeal nerve. With these conditions, the voice problems may be less a cause for concern than the lack of protection of the airway, which can lead to life threatening aspiration. Any systemic neurological or neuromuscular condition such as multiple sclerosis or muscular dystrophy may also affect the voice. But it is rare for these conditions to present first to an ENT surgeon as voice problems.

Box 8.5 Learning points—vocal cord palsy

- Unilateral vocal cord palsy leads to vocal cord lateralisation and a weak voice but a good airway.
- Bilateral vocal cord palsy leads to vocal cord medialisation and airway problems but a good voice.

Fig. 8.8. Diagram of RLN anatomy and sites of damage

Fig. 8.9. Diagram of palsy positions

Fig. 8.10. Diagram of injection

Fig. 8.11. Diagram of thyroplasty

Stridor

Stridor is a high pitched noise caused by a restricted airway. It is most common in children, due to the anatomical differences between the paediatric and the adult larynx (see p.166).

The timing of the stridor in respiration tells you the site of the obstruction or restriction:

- Laryngeal stridor = inspiratory
- Tracheal stridor = expiratory—a wheeze
- Subglottic stridor = biphasic—occurs when breathing in or out

A small reduction in the diameter of the airway leads to a dramatic increase in the airway resistance and hence the work of breathing (Poiseuille's law states that airway resistance varies with the 4th power of radius).

Causes of stridor

Congenital
- Laryngomalacia
- Vocal cord web
- Bilateral vocal cord palsy
- Subglottic stenosis.

Acquired
- Trauma
- Foreign body
- Epiglottitis/supraglottitis
- Croup
- Carcinoma
- Airway compression e.g. thyroid.

Assessment

Stridor is an ominous sign. Even if the patient appears to be coping, be sure that they are closely observed and that facilities to secure the airway are readily at hand. Patients may suddenly decompensate with devastating consequences.

- Take a rapid history
- Measure O_2 saturation
- Take temperature
- Check respiratory rate.

In children, pyrexia, drooling, dysphagia and a rapid progression of the illness, suggests epiglottitis. Take the patient to a place of safety such as a resuscitation room or operating theatre, and call for a senior ENT surgeon and experienced anaesthetist.

A similar history in adults suggests supraglottitis. This diagnosis can usually be confirmed by a careful nasolaryngoscopy.

See also 'The emergency airway', p.184.

The emergency airway

Remember to keep calm!
The following questions should be answered first
- Will admission and observation be sufficient for the time being or do you need to intervene to secure the airway?
- If intervention is required do you need to do something now, or do you have time to wait for senior help to arrive?

Assessment

Assessment should follow three stages: Look, listen, and observation.

Look
- What is the patient's colour—are they blue?
- Is there any intercostal recession or tracheal tug?
- What is the patient's respiratory rate?

Listen
- Can the patient talk in sentences, phrases, words or not at all?
- Do they have stridor? Is it inspiratory, expiratory or mixed?
- What history can the patient give?

Observation
- Is the patient's respiratory rate climbing?
- Is the patient feverish?
- What is the patient's O_2 saturation? Is it falling?

Interventions

Consider the following options:
- Give the patient oxygen via a face mask or nasal prongs.
- ± broad spectrum antibiotics, such as Augmentin (check they are not allergic).
- Nebulized adrenaline (1ml of 1:1000 with 1ml saline).
- Heliox—this is a mixture of helium and oxygen that is less dense than air. It is easier to breathe, and it buys you time. during which you can take steps to stabilize the airway.

Endotracheal intubation
This should be the first line of intervention where possible. If it proves difficult or impossible, move on quickly.

Cricothyroidotomy (See Fig. 8.13.)
Any hollow tube can be inserted through the cricothyroid membrane into the airway. The Biro is famous for having being used in this way, but a wide bore cannula, 'mini-trac', or trans-tracheal ventilation needle are probably more appropriate! If you are unsure of your landmarks, fill a syringe with a little saline and use a needle to probe for the airway, with suction applied. A steady stream of bubbles will appear when the airway is entered.

Tracheostomy

A surgical hole is made in the trachea below the cords. In an emergency, a longitudinal incision is made in the midline of the neck and deepened to the trachea, dividing the thyroid. Brisk bleeding is to be expected. The blade is plunged into the airway and twisted sideways to hold the tracheal fenestration open. A cuffed tracheostomy or ET tube is inserted into the airway and the bleeding thyroid is dealt with afterwards.

Hyoid

Thyroid cartilage

Cricoid cartilage

Trachea

Cricothyroid membrane

Position for insertion of emergency airway

Fig. 8.13. Cricothyroidotomy

Tracheostomy care and trache tubes

Tracheostomy operation

In an elective tracheostomy, the incision is usually placed horizontally. The strap muscles are separated in the midline, and the thyroid isthmus is carefully divided and over sewn. The trachea is opened at the 3rd or 4th tracheal ring, and a window of tracheal cartilage is removed. A tracheostomy tube of the right size (three quarters of the diameter of the trachea) is inserted and the cuff is inflated.

Tracheostomy tubes (See Figs. 8.14. and 8.15.)

The choice of tubes may seem bewildering, the basic principles are as follows:

Trache tubes with inner tubes

The inner tube is slightly longer than the outer, and crusting tends to occur at the distal end and on the inner tube. The inner tube can easily be removed, cleaned and replaced without removing the outer tube. Any patient who is likely to require a tracheostomy for more than 1 week is probably best fitted with a trache tube with inner.

Cuffed and non-cuffed tubes

The cuff, as in an endotrachial tube, is high volume and low pressure. This prevents damage to the tracheal wall. The cuff prevents fluid and saliva leaking around the tube and into the lungs. In addition, it makes an airtight seal between the tube and the trachea, so allowing for positive pressure ventilation. Most tubes are cuffed, but when a tracheostomy is in place long term, a non-cuffed tube may be used to prevent damage to the trachea.

Metal tubes

Metal tubes are non-cuffed and are used only for patients with permanent tracheostomies. They have the advantage of being inert and 'speaking valves' can be inserted.

Fenestrated tubes

Most tubes are non fenestrated. The advantage of a fenestrated tube (one with a hole in its side wall) is that air can pass through the fenestration, through the vocal cords and enable the patient to talk. The disadvantage is that saliva and liquids may penetrate through the fenestration, into the lower respiratory tree.

Post tracheostomy care

In the first few days after a tracheostomy operation, special care needs to be taken. The patient should be nursed by staff familiar with tracheostomy care. The patient should be given a pad and pencil with which to communicate.

Precautions

- The tube should be secured with tapes, and knotted at the side of the neck until a tract is well established.
- The tapes should be tied with the neck slightly flexed.

- The cuff should not be over-inflated, in order to prevent ischemic damage to the tracheal wall. Use a pressure gauge to check the cuff's pressure.
- The patient must be given humidification for at least the first 48 hours to reduce tracheal crusting.
- Regular suctioning of the airway to clear secretions may be needed.
- A spare tracheostomy tube and an introducer should be kept by the patient's bed in case of accidental displacement of the tube.
- Tracheal dilators should also be close by for the same reason.

Fig. 8.14. Diagram of tracheostomy tubes. (a) Cuffed fenestrated tube; (b) non cuffed nonfenestrated tube; (c) paediatric tube

Fig. 8.15. Diagram of tracheostomy tube position (note fenestration)

The oesophagus

Introduction

The oesophagus is a muscular tube connecting the pharynx to the stomach. In adults it is 25cm long. It starts at the level of C6, the cricoid cartilage and it ends at the gastro-oesophageal junction, or the diaphragm. The cricopharyngeus muscle acts as an upper oesophageal sphincter.

Congenital oesophageal conditions

These rare conditions may account for some cases of infant death, feeding problems or failure to thrive. They are frequently associated with other abnormalities of the larynx and/or the trachea. Complex surgery may be required and treatment should be given in specialist paediatric centres (see Fig. 9.1.).

Oesophageal foreign bodies

See p.428, ENT emergencies.

Stenosis   Tracheo-oesophageal fistula   Atresia with abnormal connection to trachea

Fig. 9.1. Congenital oesophageal lesions

Globus

Globus pharyngeus/syndrome/hystercus are all terms which have been used to describe a common symptom complex of a 'feeling of a lump in the throat (FOSIT) with no obvious cause'. It is probably caused by excess muscle tension in the pharyngeal musculature.

Features include

- Feeling of a lump in the throat
- Mucus collection in the throat which is rarely cleared
- Symptoms come and go
- Symptoms are usually in the midline
- The sensation is most noted when swallowing saliva rather than food or drink.
- Worse when stressed
- Worse when tired
- More common in women
- Associated with GORD.

Pharyngeal malignancy may present with similar symptoms so beware especially

- Unilateral globus
- Globus and Otalgia
- Globus and a neck lump
- Persistent/progressive symptoms.

Reassurance is usually all that is required to treat globus but barium swallow or endoscopy may be required to exclude malignant disease.

Gastro-oesophageal reflux disease (GORD) and hiatus hernia

Gastro-oesophageal reflux disease or GORD is a common condition. It is caused by changes in the oesophagus and the upper aero-digestive tract due to stomach acid reflux. It is often associated with an incompetent lower oesophageal sphincter or hiatus hernia.

Doctors and patients may not recognise that GORD, a stomach problem, could be responsible for their throat symptoms.

Classical symptoms of GORD
- Heartburn
- Discomfort behind the sternum
- Nausea
- Waterbrash—bitter fluid regurgitation
- Odynophagia—discomfort with hot or cold drinks.

ENT symptoms of GORD
- Mucus in the throat
- A feeling of a lump in the throat
- Hoarse voice
- Sore throat on waking.

Investigations
Patients with a history of reflux symptoms such as indigestion, heartburn and burping, may be treated with a therapeutic trial of a proton pump inhibitor (PPI) for 1 month.

If the GORD recurs, or if the treatment fails completely, patients should be referred for further investigation with an upper GI endoscopy, barium swallow ± 24 hour pH monitoring.

Conservative treatment
Patients should be advised on the following:
- Making dietary changes such as avoiding spicy food, fizzy drinks, and alcohol
- Trying to lose weight, if obesity is a problem
- To avoid going to bed within 3 hours of eating
- Stopping smoking
- Propping up the head of the bed on a couple of bricks or blocks.

Medical treatment
- Antacids such as Gaviscon
- H_2 antagonists such as Ranitidine
- Proton pump inhibitors such as Lansoprazole.

Surgical treatment
Patients who are resistant to treatment may require anti reflux surgery, which can be performed laproscopically.

Neurological causes of swallowing problems

The mechanics of the upper aero-digestive tract are complex. Food, drink and saliva are directed towards the oesophagus, via the pyriform fossae, while air passes to the lower respiratory tract via the larynx.

The swallowing mechanism is a complex process involving both sensory and motor functions. It is initiated voluntarily but progresses as a dynamic reflex. A neurological condition which affect a patient's motor or sensory function may also cause problems with swallowing.

Common neurological causes of swallowing problems

- CVA (stroke)
- Bulbar palsy
- Motor neurone disease
- Multiple sclerosis
- Tumours of the brain stem
- Cranial nerve lesions e.g. vagal neuroma
- Systemic neurological conditions e.g. myasthenia gravis.

Investigations

Assessment will involve taking a detailed swallowing history and asking the patient about any coughing or choking attacks, indicating aspiration.

A general neurological examination, and a specific cranial nerve examination, should be done. A CXR may show lower lobe collapse or consolidation if aspiration is present. A video swallow gives detailed information about the function of the oesophagus (such as delay, pooling, inco-ordination, spasm etc). A barium swallow test may be of limited value because it will only give static pictures.

Treatment

Wherever possible, the patient's underlying condition should be treated, but there will be times when treatment aims to control the symptoms. This could involve:

- Swallowing therapy as directed by a speech and language therapist.
- Dietary modification, such as thickened fluids.
- Percutaneous endoscopic gastrostomy (PEG)—a long-term feeding tube.
- Cricopharyngeal myotomy—surgical division of the upper oesophageal sphincter muscle.
- Vocal cord medialisation procedures—where a vocal cord paralysis causes aspiration.
- Tracheostomy (see p.185).
- Tracheal diversion or total laryngectomy (see p.175).

Post-cricoid web

This is a rare condition and its cause is unknown. An anterior web forms in the lumen at the junction of the pharynx and oesophagus, behind the cricoid cartilage.

Patterson Brown–Kelly (UK) and Plumber–Wilson (USA) both describe this condition—their names are frequently used in association with the syndrome.

A post-cricoid web is linked with iron deficiency anaemia, and it has the potential to become malignant. Because of this chance of malignancy, an endoscopy and a biopsy is recommended. It may also cause dysphagia, and can be seen on a barium swallow.

The web may be dilated and/or disrupted with the help of an endoscope.

Achalasia

This is a rare condition where there is hypertonia in the lower oesophageal sphincter muscle. No increase in pressure is found at endoscopy. Achalasia appears to be due to an abnormality of the parasympathetic nerve supply within the muscles of the oesophagus.

Signs and symptoms
- Progressive dysphagia
- Regurgitation
- Weight loss.

Investigations
A barium swallow may suggest achalasia. An endoscopy is needed to exclude an oesophageal tumour, as this can produce similar X-ray appearance and symptoms.

Treatment
- Inhaled amyl nitrate prior to meals—causes relaxation of the sphincter
- Repeated dilatation—stretches the sphincter
- Cardioplasty—surgical enlargement of the sphincter
- Bypass procedures—surgical bypass of the obstruction.

Pharyngeal pouch

This is a type of hernia or pulsion diverticulum, which affects the junction of the pharynx and oesophagus. Elderly males are most often affected.

It is believed to arise as a result of incoordination of the swallowing mechanism leading to an increased intra-luminal pressure above the closed upper oesophageal sphincter. As a result of this pressure, the pharyngeal mucosa herniates through an anatomical area of weakness, known as Killian's dehiscence—this lies between the two heads of the inferior constrictor muscle (see Fig. 9.2.).

Signs and symptoms

- Dysphagia
- Regurgitation of undigested food
- Halitosis
- Gurgling noises in the neck
- A lump in the neck
- Aspiration
- Pneumonia.

Investigations

A barium swallow will indicate the diagnosis. A rigid endoscopy must follow to exclude the rare finding of a carcinoma within the pouch. This is sometimes the result of long term stasis of its contents.

Treatment

Treatment is only necessary if the patient is symptomatic. Endoscopic stapling of the wall which divides the pouch from the oesophagus is the current treatment of choice. Excision, inversion and suspension of the pouch have been described and are reserved as second line treatments.

Fig. 9.2. Pharyngeal pouch

Oesophageal tumours

Benign oesophageal tumours are rare and arise from the local tissue elements e.g. leiomyoma, adenoma, lipoma.

Malignant oesophagal tumours

The risk factors for a malignant oesophagal tumour include smoking, a high alcohol intake, achalasia, and anaemia. 80% of malignant tumours occur in males over 60 years old. Primary carcinomas are the most common. These carcinomas are squamous and adenocarcinoma. Adeno-carcinoma most frequently occur in the lower third of the oesophagus.

The signs and symptoms of a malignant tumour may include weight loss, pain in the throat and/or epigastrium, and progressive dysphagia.

Investigations

- Barium swallow—may show a narrowing or mucosal abnormality suggesting a malignant tumour.
- Endoscopy and biopsy—will confirm the diagnosis.
- CT scan of the chest and abdomen—to assess the extra-mucosal extent and metastatic spread.

Treatment

- The best chance of a cure is with surgical excision where possible. This may be given with pre-op chemotherapy, and post-op radiotherapy.
- After the excision, the resulting oesophageal defect will be reconstructed, either with either a stomach pull up, free jejunal grafting, or a myocutaneous flap (see Fig. 9.3.).

Where a cure is not possible, palliation may be achieved via:

- Radiotherapy
- Laser debulking of the mass
- Endoscopic stenting
- PEG tube for long-term feeding.

Stomach
pull-up

Jejunal
free graft

Tubed
myocutaneous
free flap

Fig. 9.3. Reconstruction

The neck

Anatomy of the neck

Surface anatomy

Many of the important structures in the neck can be seen or felt on examination These are:

- The mastoid process (a)
- The clavicular heads (b)
- The sternomastoid muscle (c)
- Trachea (d)
- Cricoid cartilage (e)
- Cricothyroid membrane (f)
- Thyroid prominence (g)
- Hyoid bone (h)
- Carotid bifurcation (i)
- Thyroid gland (j)
- Parotid gland (k)
- Submandibular gland (l)
- Jugulodigastric lymph node (m).

Use Fig. 10.1. opposite to identify the above structures on yourself. It is particularly important to quickly identify the cricothyroid membrane in order to be able to perform an emergency cricothyroidotomy (see p.184).

Triangles of the neck

The anterior and posterior triangles of the neck are often referred to in clinical practice and are useful descriptive terms. These triangles maybe subdivided as shown in Fig. 10.2a., but the usefulness of the subdivisions is questionable. (This is not to say that an enthusiastic examiner would not be prepared to quiz you on them!)

Deep anatomy

The neck is divided into anatomical compartments by strong fascial layers (see Fig. 10.2b.).

- *The posterior compartment*—contains the skeletal muscles of the cervical spine
- *The anterior compartment*—contains additional fascial envelopes containing these important structures:
  - The pretracheal fascia encloses the thyroid gland and binds it to the trachea
  - The carotid sheath encloses the carotid, internal jugular and vagus nerve.

Between these fascial planes lie the parapharyngeal space and the retropharyngeal space. These spaces are clinically relevant because they may become involved in and allow the spread of deep seated infections or malignancy.

(a)

(b)

Fig. 10.1. Surface anatomy of the neck

Lymph node levels

The classification of lymph node levels in the neck are commonly referred to in clinical practice and it is important to have an understanding of them. (See Fig. 10.3)

Most lymph drainage from the aero-digestive tract is through the deep cervical chain which runs along the internal jugular vein deep to the sternomastoid muscle. It has been discovered that particular anatomical sites drain reliably to particular groups of lymph nodes.

A nodal level system has been devised in order to simplify the discussion of lymph nodes and to ensure that we are all talking the same language. Essentially this is a naming system which gives a number or level to groups of lymph nodes in a particular area. See Fig. 10.3., which is a diagram of the lymph node levels in the neck.

This nodal level system is of particular importance when considering the lymphatic spread of ENT cancers. The first group of nodes which a cancer involves is called the first echelon nodal level. For example, the first echelon nodes for tonsil cancer are level 3, from here other nodal levels may be affected, usually levels 2 and 4.

Cancers in other sites may metastasize in different patterns, for example the first echelon nodes from nasopharyngeal cancer tends to be level 5. This concept and model has led to the development of selective neck dissections i.e., supra-oma-hyoid neck dissections (see p.221).

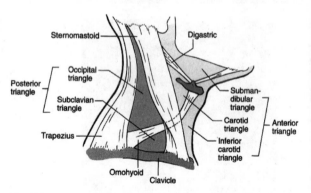

Fig. 10.2a. Triangles of the neck

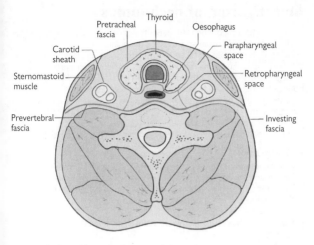

Fig. 10.2b. Fascial layers and spaces of the neck

Fig. 10.3. Lymph node levels in the neck

Investigation of neck lumps

Neck lumps are common. All patients with a neck lump must have an ENT examination in order to exclude a malignancy.

A full history should be taken including duration, change in size, smoking history, pain (including referred otalgia), and any inter-current illness.

A neck lump should be thoroughly examined and the following aspects noted: site, size, shape, texture (smooth or lobulated), position (midline or lateral), solid or cystic, single or multiple, tender, attached to deep structures, movement on swallowing, movement on tongue protrusion, pulsatile (see p.37, Fig. 2.14.).

In addition to the above, a full ENT examination should be given.

Investigations

- **Fine needle aspiration cytology (FNAC)**: is the single most important diagnostic test. It is like a blood test but involves taking cells from the lump rather than blood from a vein, There is no danger of seeding malignant cells if the appropriate method is used (see p.412, How to perform an FNA).
- *Blood tests*: Where the history suggests an inflammatory mass consider:
  - FBC
  - ESR/CRP
  - Paul–Bunnell/monospot/IM screen
  - Toxoplasma
  - HIV test.
- **Biopsy**: May be needed if a diagnosis cannot be made. Wherever possible this should be excisional rather than incisional. All but the most trivial neck masses should be biopsied under general anaesthetic.
- **Endoscopy**: Cancers of the silent sites of the head and neck may give little or no symptoms themselves but may metastasize to the neck, presenting as a neck mass. Examination of these sites is vital, usually under general anaesthetic i.e. a panendoscopy, which looks at all the food and breathing passages . The silent sites are:
  - Nasopharynx
  - Tongue base
  - Tonsil
  - Vallecula
  - Pirifom fossa
  - Post-cricoid region.
- **Radiology**
  - CXR—for malignancy, TB, HIV.
  - USS—for thyroid, salivary glands. This test is may be useful in children as it is non-invasive and easy, and it can distinguish between a solid or a cystic lump.
  - Spiral CT—rapid acquisition is useful for mobile structures like the larynx and for those patients who find lying flat difficult.
  - MRI—provides excellent soft tissue definition but is degraded by patient movement.

Congenital neck remnants

Thyroglossal cysts and fistulae

The thyroid gland develops at the base of the tongue and descends through the tissues of the neck to its final position overlying the trachea. It leaves a tract which runs from the foramen caecum of the tongue to the thyroid gland. This tract curves around the body of the hyoid bone. Thyroglossal cysts and fistulae arise from congenital abnormalities of this process. They are common in teenagers and in young adults.

Signs and symptoms

These may present as a midline or paramedian swelling or a discharging sinus. The cyst will rise on tongue protrusion, due to its attachment to the tongue base. (See Fig. 10.4. and Fig. 11.1, p.227.)

Treatment

Before surgical excision of the lesion, ensure that there is a normal functioning thyroid gland in its usual position in the neck. Surgical excision, known as Sistrunk's operation, involves removing the lesion plus that tissue block between the lesion and the hyoid, plus the mid portion of the hyoid bone and any associated tract passing to the foramen caecum of the tongue. If there is a risk of recurrence, less radical procedures may be used.

Branchial cysts

These common, benign neck cysts usually appear before the age of 30. They occur at the junction of the upper third and lower two thirds of the sternomastoid muscle. They often arise following an URTI. They are thought to be caused by degeneration of epithelial inclusions in a lymph node.

Branchial cysts are usually asymptomatic, but they may become painful due to a secondary infection. A FNAC test yields a pus-like aspirate that is rich in cholesterol crystals. The treatment is surgical excision.

In patients over 50 years old, branchial cysts may be confused with metastatic deposits of SCC, which have undergone cystic degeneration. In this group, a FNAC suggesting a branchial cyst should be treated with suspicion.

Branchial fistulae

These arise as a defect in the fusion of branchial clefts. They present as a discharging skin sinus somewhere along the anterior border of the sternomastoid. There is an associated tract, which runs from the skin to the oropharynx, usually ending at the anterior pillar of the tonsil. This tract will pass between the external and internal carotid arteries, in close proximity to cranial nerves X, XI and XII. Surgical excision of the complete tract, including the tonsil may be necessary.

Dermoid Cysts

These cysts lie anywhere between the chin and the suprasternal notch. They arise from defects in fusion of the midline and are an example of 'inclusion cysts'. They present as painless midline swellings and do not move on swallowing or tongue protrusion. Treatment is via surgical excision.

Cystic hygroma

These are rare, benign lymphangiomas found in neonates and infants. They insinuate themselves between the tissues of the neck and may reach a massive size. They may cause compressive airway symptoms.

Treatment involves securing the airway where necessary, surgical excision (which can be staged), or injection with sclerosant.

Fig. 10.4. Thyroglossal cysts rise on tongue protrusion

Neck infections

Parapharyngeal abscess

This is a deep seated infection of the parapharyngeal space (see p.208). It often results from a primary infection in the tonsil or is an extension from a parapharyngeal abscess (or quinsy) (see p.100). It is more common in children than in adults.

Signs and symptoms

Include pyrexia, neck swelling deep to sternomastoid muscle and a patient who seems unwell. There may be trismus, or a reduced range of neck movements. The tonsil and the lateral pharyngeal wall may be pushed medially. Airway compromise is a late and ominous sign.

If the diagnosis is in doubt, a CT scan will often distinguish between lymphadenitis and an abscess.

Treatment

This will involve a high dose of IV broad-spectrum antibiotics (Augmentin), in addition to surgical drainage via a lateral neck approach.

Retropharyngeal abscess

This is a very rare infection of the retropharyngeal space. It is much more common in children and infants than in adults.

Signs and symptoms

An unwell patient, with pyrexia, often with preceding URTI or swallowing difficulty. There may be shortness of breath or stridor, or torticollis—due to prevertebral muscle irritation.

Treatment

A high dose of IV broad-spectrum antibiotics (Augmentin). Where necessary the airway will be secured and surgical incision and drainage may be performed via the mouth.

Ludwig's angina

This is a rare infection of the submandibular space, it usually occurs as a result of dental infection. It is more common in adults than in children.

Signs and symptoms

These include pyrexia, drooling, trismus, airway compromise due to backward displacement of the tongue. There may be firm thickening of the tissues of the floor of mouth—best appreciated on bi-manual palpation

Treatment

High doses of IV broad-spectrum antibiotics (Augmentin). Secure the airway (try a naso-pharyngeal airway first since this will often suffice, but where necessary consider a tracheostomy). Surgical incision is often unsatisfying since little pus may drain away.

Lymph node enlargement

- The majority of neck nodes in children are benign
- The majority of neck nodes in adults are malignant
- Neck nodes may be involved secondarily in an infection of any part of the ENT systems.

(See p.210 Lymph nodes.)

Infective lymphadenopathy

This secondary lymphadenopathy is extremely common in children. An example is jugulo-digastric node enlargement during or following tonsillitis. A single node or a group of nodes may be enlarged. There may be tenderness and symptoms related to the primary infection.

Specific infections presenting with lymph node enlargement (primary lymphadenopathy) include:

- Glandular fever
- TB
- Toxoplasmosis
- Brucellosis
- Cat-scratch fever
- HIV.

The diagnosis in these cases will often be made following the appropriate screening blood test and CXR. FNAC and even excision biopsy may be needed to exclude malignancy.

Neoplastic lymphadenopathy

Lymphoma

This is a primary malignant tumour of the lymphatic tissues.

Signs and symptoms

Multiple nodes of a rubbery consistency. The patient may or may not experience night sweats, weight loss, axillary or groin nodes, and lethargy.

Investigations

FNAC may be suspicious but an excision biopsy is often required to confirm the diagnosis and allow for sub typing. A CXR and/or a chest CT scan may be done, or, for staging, a CT scan of the abdomen or pelvis. Bone marrow may be needed for staging.

Treatment

May involve chemotherapy and/or radiotherapy. The patient may need a lymphoma multi-disciplinary team review.

Squamous cell carcinoma

This is a primary muco-cutaneous malignancy which commonly spreads to local lymph nodes. It can affect single or multiple nodes.

Signs and symptoms

The patient may have ENT-related symptoms such as a sore throat, a hoarse voice or otalgia. The nodes may have a firm or hard consistency. The patient may have a history of smoking.

Investigations

These may include FNAC, ENT examination looking for ENT primary carcinoma, a CT or MRI scan of the neck, a CT scan of the chest and/or CXR (metatases), a liver USS (metastases), a panendoscopy and biopsy.

Where no ENT primary is seen on examination, a rigorous search should be done for a silent tumor. This will usually involve imaging as above with ipsilateral tonsillectomy, biopsy of the tongue base, post nasal space and piriform fossa as a minimum. (See Silent areas of ENT, p.212).

Treatment

This depends on the stage, the size and the site of the primary (see also Box 10.1). Options for treatment include:

Radiotherapy: this involves 4–6 weeks of daily treatment with a total dose of 50–60Gy.

Radical neck dissection: this involves removing the affected nodes as well as all the other nodal groups and lymph-bearing structures on that side of the neck. This includes the lymph nodes at level 1, 2, 3, 4, and 5, the internal jugular vein (IJV), the sternomastoid muscle, and the accessory nerve submandibular gland.

Modified radical neck dissection: this takes all the nodal levels (1, 2, 3, 4, 5) but preserves one or all of the IJV, the Sternomastoid and the accessory nerve.

Selective neck dissection: Instead of all the nodal groups being removed, those groups thought to be at most risk are selectively dissected and removed. All other structures are preserved.

Box 10.1 N staging of the neck	
N1	A single node <3cm
N2a	A single node >3cm but <6cm
N2b	>1 ipsilateral node <6cm
N2c	Bilateral or contralateral nodes <6cm
N3	Any node >6cm

Neck Hernias

Pharyngeal pouch

See p.202.

Laryngocoele

This is caused by expansion of the saccule of the larynx. The saccule is a blind-ending sac arising from the anterior end of the laryngeal ventricle (p.163, Fig. 8.3.). A laryngocoele is an air-filled herniation of this structure. This can expand, and either remains within the laryngeal framework (internal laryngocoele), or part of it may extend outside the larynx (external laryngocoele). It escapes through a point of weakness in the thyrohyoid membrane.

There is a rare association with a laryngeal cancer of the saccule, and all patients should have this area examined and biopsied.

There is little evidence to support the supposition that this condition is more frequent in trumpet players and glass blowers.

Signs and symptoms

- Lump in the neck which may vary in size
- Hoarseness
- A feeling of something in the throat (FOSIT)
- Swallowing difficulties
- Airway problems

If the laryngocoele become infected and full of pus (laryngo-pyo-coele) then it may rapidly increase in size and cause additional pain.

The thyroid

Embryology and anatomy of the thyroid

Thyroid problems are frequent topics in both undergraduate and post graduate exams. It is therefore well worth investing some time in understanding the thyroid.

Embryology of the thyroid

The thyroid begins its development at the foramen caecum at the base of the tongue. The foramen caecum lies at the junction of the anterior two thirds and the posterior third of the tongue in the midline. (see Fig. 11.1.)

The thyroid descends through the tissues of the neck and comes to rest overlying the trachea. This descent leaves a tract behind it—this can be the source of pathology in later life (e.g. thyroglossal cysts—see Chapter 10, p.214).

Anatomy of the thyroid

The thyroid gland is surrounded by pre-tracheal fascia and is bound tightly to the trachea and to the larynx. This means the gland moves upwards during swallowing. The recurrent laryngeal nerves (branches of the vagus) lie very close to the posterior aspect of the thyroid lobes. These nerves have ascended from the mediastinum in the tracheo-oesophageal grooves and they are at risk in thyroid operations. They may become involved in thyroid malignancy—in cases of malignancy a patient will sometimes present with a weak and breathy hoarse voice.

The thyroid gland has a very rich blood supply—trauma or surgery to the gland can lead to impressive haemorrhage into the neck.

The parathyroid glands—important in calcium metabolism—lie embedded on the posterior aspect of the thyroid lobes.

> ### Box 11.1 Key points—thyroid related swellings
>
> - Thyroid masses move on swallowing
> - Thyroglossal cysts move on tongue protrusion (see p.214).

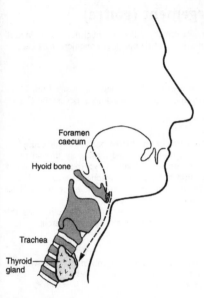

Fig. 11.1. Embryology of the thyroid gland

Thyroid enlargement (goitre)

Goitre simply means an enlargement of the thyroid gland. It is not in itself a diagnosis. Both physiological and pathological conditions may cause a goitre.

Simple goitre

This is a diffuse enlargement of the thyroid and may result from iodine deficiency. Diffuse enlargement of the gland also occurs in Graves' disease.

Multinodular goitre

This benign goitre is the commonest thyroid problem. It is caused by episodic periods of thyroid hypo-function and subsequent thyroid stimulating hormone hyper secretion which leads to hyperplasia of the gland. This is followed by involution of the gland. Prolonged periods of hyperplasia and involution are thought to be responsible for the nodular enlargement of the gland found in a multi nodular goitre.

A finding of a single nodular enlargement of the thyroid raises the question of malignancy. This should be managed as described (see Fig. 11.2.).

Treatment

A partial thyroidectomy may be necessary but only in a patient with one or all of the following signs:
• Pressure symptoms in the neck
• Dysphagia
• Airway compression
• Cosmetic deformity.

Graves' disease

This is an auto-immune condition where antibodies are produced which mimic the effect of TSH. A hyperthyroid state develops and there is often a smooth goitre. The patient's eye signs may be most impressive, (the actor Marti Feldman had this condition). See p.232 for eye signs in Graves' disease.

Treatment

Hormonal manipulation with carbimazole. Surgery to correct the proptosis may be achieved via a trans-nasal orbital decompression. Here, the medial wall of the bony orbit is removed to allow the orbital contents to herniate into the nasal cavity.

Hashimoto's thyroiditis

This is an auto-immune condition where patients go through both hyper and hypo-thyroidism during their disease course and many patients develop a goitre. Thyroxine replacements may be necessary. Patients with this condition have an increased risk of developing a thyroid lymphoma.

Fig. 11.2. Management of a thyroid lump

Thyroid neoplasia

Thyroid tumours may arise from either the follicular cells or the supporting cells found in the normal gland. They are quite common and each of these tumours has its own particular characteristics (see Fig. 11.3.). Papillary and follicular adenocarcinomas are frequently referred to as differentiated thyroid tumours.

Follicular cell neoplasms
- Papillary adenocarcinoma
- Follicular adenocarcinoma
- Anaplastic adenocarcinoma

Supporting cell neoplasms
- Medullary carcinoma

Papillary adenocarcinoma

These usually affect adults age 40–50 years. There are usually multiple tumours within the gland. 60% of affected patients have involved neck nodes.

If the disease is limited to the gland, 90% of patients will survive 10 years or more. If the disease has spread to involve the neck nodes, 60% of patients will survive 10 years or more.

Treatment: Involves a near total thyroidectomy. Plus a neck dissection where there are involved nodes. Post operative radio-iodine may be given to ablate any viable thyroid tissue or tumour left behind after the surgery. After surgery, patients will need life-long thyroid replacement at TSH suppressing doses.

Follicular adenocarcinoma

It usually affects adults age 50–60 years. There is a well defined capsule enclosing the tumour and it spreads via the bloodstream. Up to 30% of patients will have distant metastases at presentation and hence to prognosis is less good than in papillary adenocarcinoma.

Treatment: As above for papillary adenocarcinoma.

Anaplastic thyroid carcinoma

This condition occurs in adults over 70 years of age, and is more common in women. It involves rapid enlargement of the thyroid gland and pain. The patient will have airway, voice or swallowing problems due to direct involvement of the trachea, larynx or oesophagus.

The prognosis is very poor. 92% of patients with this condition will die within 1 year, even with treatment.

Medullary carcinoma

This arises from the parafollicular C cells (or calcitonin secreting cells). The patient's level of serum calicitonin is raised and their serum calcium level remains normal. Neck metastases are present in up to 30% of patients.

Treatment: Involves a near total thyroidectomy and radiotherapy.

Benign thyroid adenoma

These can be functioning or non functioning:

Functioning adenomas

They produce thyroxine and will take up iodine and technetium. They appear bright or 'hot' on isotope scanning. Symptoms of thyrotoxicosis may develop. They are rarely malignant.

Treatment is usually medical via thyroid suppressing drugs, but may be treated surgically via excision. Radiotherapy and ablation may be required.

Non-functioning adenomas

These adenomas do not take up iodine. They appear 'cold' on isotope scanning. 10–20% will be malignant. Treatment will be via a surgical excision.

Fig. 11.3. Distribution of thyroid tumours

Thyroid investigations

Before performing any special investigations look for signs of abnormal thyroid function. Classic signs are given Table 11.1:

Table 11.1 Classic signs of abnormal thyroid function

Hyperthyroidism	Hypothyroidism
Irritability	Mental slowness
Heat intolerance	Cold intolerance
Insomnia	Hypersomnolence
Sweatiness	Dry skin
Amenorrhoea	Menorrhagia
Weight loss	Weight gain
Diarrhoea	Constipation
Palpitations	Bradycardia
Hyper-reflexia	Slow relaxing reflexes
Tremor	Loss of outer third of eyebrow
Atrial fibrillation.	Hoarse voice.

Graves' disease gives rise to particular 'eye signs'. These include:
• Lid lag
• Exopthalmos
• Ophthalmoplegia
• Lid retraction
• Proptosis
• Chemosis.

Blood tests

Thyroid function tests (TFTs)

T4 (thyroxine) and T3 (tri-iodo-thyronine) are both bound to plasma proteins in the blood, but a proportion of both remains unbound and is physiologically active. Bear this in mind when interpreting these results in conditions where the free-to-bound ratio may be disturbed e.g. nephrotic syndrome or pregnancy.

Thyroid stimulating hormone (TSH) controls the production of thyroid hormones via a negative feedback mechanism. TSH is usually raised in hypothyroidism and reduced in hyperthyroidism.

Thyroglobulin

This is the carrier protein for T4. Its levels can be measured directly in the blood. It is most frequently used as a tumour marker for the differentiated thyroid carcinomas.

Calcitonin

This is produced by the medullary C cells of the thyroid. Levels are raised in medullary thyroid carcinomas.

CEA—carcinoembryonic antigen

This is a tumour marker of medullary carcinoma of the thyroid.

Thyroid autoantibodies

Specific thyroid autoantibodies can be identified in Graves' disease and Hashimoto's thyroiditis.

Radioisotope scanning

Radio labelled iodine (^{123}I) or technetium (^{99}Tc) is given to the patient orally. Then radiology is used to assess its subsequent uptake into metabolically active thyroid tissue. A thyroid nodule may take up the marker—it will appear bright or 'hot', or it will fail to accumulate the marker—and it will appear 'cold'.

- 80% of thyroid nodules are 'cold'
- 10–20% of 'cold' nodules are malignant
- 'Hot' nodules are almost always benign.

Ultrasound (USS)

This is an excellent investigation to demonstrate the thyroid. It will readily distinguish solid and cystic masses inside the thyroid. Often, a USS will show that what appears clinically as a single nodule is in fact part of a multinodular goitre.

MRI/CT scan

These scans may be helpful in determining the extent of a retrosternal swelling. They may confirm airway distortion or compression from a large goitre or they may demonstrate nodal metastases.

FNAC (fine needle aspiration cytology)

This test will differentiate solid from cystic masses and may diagnose malignancy. A residual mass noted after cyst aspiration should be tested again by FNA to exclude malignancy. It is difficult to distinguish between follicular adenoma and follicular carcinoma. This difference relies on demonstrating capsular invasion which is impossible on cytological features alone. Formal histology is usually required to confirm this diagnosis.

Treatment of thyroid conditions

Management of a thyroid lump

This is best shown diagrammatically, see the flow chart in Fig. 11.2., p.229.

Hormonal manipulation

Thyroxine: Patients experiencing hypothyroid states and after thyroidectomy may need to take thyroxine for life. Doses of thyroxine sufficient to suppress the TSH production are given in well differentiated thyroid cancers in order to reduce tumour growth since these tumours are also TSH driven.

Carbimazole or propylthirouracil: May be given in hyperthyroidism since these inhibit the formation of T3 and T4.

Radioactive ablation

Most well differentiated thyroid tumours will trap iodine. This ability can be put to therapeutic effect by administering radioactive iodine. The patient is first rendered hypothyroid by thyroidectomy. The tumour cells then become hungry for iodine and as such will avidly take up the radioactive iodine to their own cytotoxic demise! Radio-iodine therapy can also be used to control a persistent hyperthyroid state.

Thyroid surgery

Thyroid surgery is generally safe and well tolerated by patients.

Hemithyroidectomy: This involves the removal of one thyroid lobe. It is indicated in benign thyroid conditions and as an excisional biopsy procedure where malignancy is suspected but not confirmed.

Total thyroidectomy: This is indicated in thyroid malignancy. Because it increases the risks to the recurrent laryngeal nerves and to the parathyroid glands, some surgeons will perform a near total thyroidectomy, leaving a small amount of thyroid tissue behind in the area of the recurrent laryngeal nerve.

Risks and complications of thyroid surgery

These are some of the most common and important risks of thyroid surgery:

Vocal cord palsy

This is due to recurrent laryngeal nerve damage. Patients will present with a weak and breathy voice. All patients should undergo a vocal cord check pre-operatively to document cord mobility before the procedure.

Bilateral vocal cord palsy

This will lead to medialisation of the vocal cords resulting in life threatening airway obstruction. Facilities for re-intubation and tracheostomy must be readily available.

Haematoma

Haematoma after thyroid surgery is another potentially serious complication. This is because the vascular nature of the thyroid can lead to a rapid accumulation of blood in the neck, resulting in compression of the airway. For this reason, all thyroidectomy patients should have stitch/clip removers at the bedside. If a patient's neck begins to swell rapidly after thyroid surgery, the wound should be re-opened (on the ward if necessary), the clot evacuated and the airway restored. Once the airway has been secured, the bleeding point can be found and controlled.

Hypocalcaemia

This should be anticipated whenever a total thyroidectomy has been performed. Daily calcium levels should be checked and the patient should be observed for the signs of hypocalcaemia such as:
• Tingling in the hands and feet
• Perioral parasthesia
• Muscle cramps
• Carpopedal spasm—muscle spasms affecting the hands and feet
• Chvostek's sign—facial spasm seen on tapping over the facial nerve in the region of the parotid
• Tetany—generalized muscle spasm
• Laryngospasm—give IV calcium gluconate immediately.
As soon as hypocalcaemia is suspected give the patient IV calcium gluconate and start oral replacement therapy.

The external ear

Structure and function

A working knowledge of the anatomy of the ear helps in documentation, correspondence and in describing sites of lesions and trauma over the telephone. The main anatomical points are shown in Figs. 12.1. and 12.2.

The external part of the ear consists of two parts:
• The pinna
• The external auditory canal (EAC).

The pinna collects sound waves and directs them into the external auditory canal. Its shape helps to localize sound direction and amplification. The EAC helps in transmitting sound waves to the eardrum or tympanic membrane.

The EAC has two parts:
• An outer cartilaginous part.
  • In adults, the cartilaginous canal slopes forward and downward.
  • In neonates and infants, the canal slopes forward.
  • The outer canal contains hairs and ceruminous glands that produce wax.
• An inner bony part.

(a)

(b)

Darwins tubercle (variable)

Triangular fossa

Antihelical fold

Tragus

Helical fold

External ear canal

Conchal bowl

Antitragus

Lobule

Fig. 12.1. Diagram of the Pinna

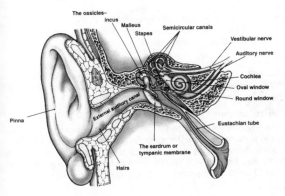

The ossicles—incus

Malleus

Stapes

Semicircular canals

Vestibular nerve

Auditory nerve

Cochlea

Oval window

Round window

Pinna

External auditory canal

Eustachian tube

The eardrum or tympanic membrane

Hairs

Fig. 12.2. Diagram of the EAC

Congenital abnormalities

Minor abnormalities of the ear are common, but often they do not come to medical attention.

Malformed pinna

The pinna develops from the six hillocks of His. Maldevelopment or failure to fuse, can produce obvious abnormalities of the ear. Malformed pinna are described as microtia or anotia. They may or may not be associated with middle or inner ear abnormalities. The various classifications are shown in Fig. 12.3.

Investigations

This includes documenting the defect, examining the EAC, and doing a hearing assessment. A CT scan to assess middle ear/ossicles/cochlea anatomy may also be done.

Treatment

• Where there are minor anatomical abnormalities, no treatment is given or hearing support is given as required.
• Where there is a major deformity or anotia, removal of the pinna may be considered. Consider a Bone Anchored Hearing Aid (BAHA) and abutments to attach an artificial pinna.

Skin tags

Skin tags are often detected at a neonatal baby check. They are often incidental. Investigations involve checking for normal EAC and screening hearing.

Preauricular sinus

This is a small dimple anterior to the tragus. It is usually detected at a baby check and is caused by the incomplete fusion of the hillocks of His. This preauricular dimple may be the external opening of a network of channels under the skin. Patients who present late may have a discharge from the punctum. Occasionally, repeated infections may require drainage.

Treatment

Where there is simple discharge treat with oral antibiotics such as Augmentin. Where there are repeated infections antibiotics may be given and surgical removal may be necessary (Fig. 12.4.).

Fig. 12.3. Diagram of Microtia grade III. Grading of Microtia: I Normal ear;
II All pinna elements present but malformed; III Rudementary bar only; IV Anotia

Fig. 12.4. Diagram of preauricular sinus

Infection of the pinna

This would present as a painful, hot, red ear.

Investigations

- Identify the cause of the infection. Is this a spreading infection from the EAC or is it a primary infection of the pinna?
- Identify whether it is an infection of the skin or does it involve cartilage? If the cartilage is infected there is severe tenderness on touching the pinna.
- Take a history and exclude trauma or an insect bite. Remember non-accidental injury in children. Diabetic or immunocompromised patients may have severe cellulitis of the pinna.

Treatment

- Where there is a localized infection—remove any cause such as piercing or an insect's sting. Give oral antibiotics such as Augmentin 625mg tds 1 week PO.
- Where there is cellulitis of the pinna—remove the cause and treat with IV antibiotics such as Cefuroxime 1.5g 8 hourly and Metronidazole 500mg tds IV 8 hourly until cellulitis resolves; for at least 24 hours followed by oral antibiotics for 1 week in total.
- Where there is perichondritis—remove the cause or treat otis externa if present. Treat with IV antibiotics such as Cefuroxime 1.5g 8hourly Metronidazole 500mg tds IV 8 hourly until cellulitis resolves; for at least 24 hours followed by oral antibiotics for 1 week in total.

Box 12.1 Piercings

- Trends in fashion dictate that piercings are often multiple and not in the lobule of the ear. Lobule piercings have less likelihood of infection as there is no cartilage in the lobule.
- Other piercings transfix the cartilage framework of the pinna. This can lead to infection and cellulitis of the pinna.

Trauma to the pinna

Assess the patient, bearing in mind that a blow to the ear is a head injury. Discover the force and mechanism of the injury. The site of the injury should be carefully documented with the help of a diagram or a photograph.

Any blunt trauma to the ear may cause a hearing loss or a traumatic perforation of the eardrum. Always examine the EAC drum and perform a simple bedside hearing assessment as follows:

- Examine the pinna and note the findings
- Examine the EAC
- Examine the tympanic membrane
- Perform tuning fork tests
- Perform free field testing of hearing
- Check patient's tetanus status.

Lacerations of the skin

These are simply repaired, using non absorbable sutures such as 5.0 Prolene. Apply local anaesthetic to the area, clean the wound, and use interrupted sutures. Pay careful attention to everting the edges and ensuring good opposition of the skin edges. Check the patient's tetanus status.

Lacerations involving the cartilage

- Clean wounds can be simply sutured in layers to include the cartilage.
- The cartilage is very painful to suture and a general anaesthetic (GA) may be required.
- Dirty wounds may need surgical debridement under GA before closure.
- All wounds require antibiotic cover such as Augmentin 625mg tds PO.

Haematoma of the pinna

This is a collection of blood between the perichondrium and the cartilage which leads to pressure necrosis of the cartilage. Subsequent deformity, infection and fibrosis with cartilage loss, leads to the typical 'cauliflower ear' of the rugby player.

Aspiration of the haematoma is difficult due to the thickness of the clot. It is better to incise the haematoma and suture, using bolsters to prevent reaccumulation (see Fig. 12.5 and p.408).

Treatment

- Local anaesthetic or GA
- Incision over haematoma
- Dental roll bolsters tied in place
- Removal of dressing after 5 days
- Oral antibiotics e.g. Augmentin 625mg tds 1 week PO.

Fig. 12.5. Haematoma of pinna

Otitis externa

This common condition forms a large percentage of both the emergency and the routine workload of an ENT Department. Its presentation is varied and it produces a spectrum of disorders which are classified below.

Risk factors
- Swimmers and surfers
- Daily hairwashers
- Diabetics
- Psoriais sufferers
- People with an abnormal migration of keratin.

Clinical grading
- Is the pinna normal? if there is cellulitis, admission may be needed— severe OE
- What is the appearance of EAC after cleaning under microscope?
- Is the EAC normal diameter?—mild OE
- Is the EAC narrow but the tympanic membrane (TM) is still visible?— moderate OE
- Is the EAC narrow but the TM is not visible due to oedema?— severe OE
- Is there a furuncle in the EAC?
- Are there granulations in the floor of the EAC?—this may be necrotizing OE (see p.250)
- Test the patient's facial nerve function.

Treatment
All patients should keep ears water-free during treatment.

Mild OE
Presentation: scaly skin with some erythema.
- Use either 0.5% Hydrocortisone cream prn to be applied to the EAC.
- Or Betnovate scalp lotion.
- Or Earcalm Spray (contains acetic acid). Lowering of the pH changes the flora of the EAC.
- Regular aural toilet and avoid swimming.

Moderate OE
Presentation: painful, discharging smelly ears. Narrowed EAC with cream cheese-like discharge.
- Microsuction clearance.
- Swab for microscopy if there has been previous antibiotic treatment.
- Otowick if the EAC very narrow.
- Hygroscopic drops e.g. aluminium acetate.
- Change wick in 48 hours.
- Swab if no improvement. Consider combination therapy with antibiotic steroid drops depending on swab result and response to treatment.

Severe OE

Presentation: complete occlusion of the EAC or spreading pinna cellulitis.

- Microsuction clearance.
- Treat as moderate OE.
- If there is severe pain, it may be furunculosis. Lance boil with a needle or fine end of sucker. Add flucloxacillin 500mg qds PO to regime.
- If there is cellulitis, admission for IV antibiotics may be needed.
- Exclude the tympanic membrane during treatment.

❶ Beware of allergy

Patients not responding to the appropriate therapy may be allergic to the constituents of the drops. Patch testing by a local dermatologist may help to elucidate this problem. Betnovate scalp lotion can be useful as it has none of the excipients that can cause allergic reactions.

Necrotizing otitis externa

This is an uncommon, severe, bacterial ear infection where the infection spreads beyond the ear canal and into the surrounding bone. It was formerly known as malignant otitis externa, due to the mortality associated with the condition. It is usually seen in diabetics or immuno-compromised patients. If you see a diabetic patient with otitis externa, consider this condition.

Signs and symptoms

- Otalgia out of proportion to the clinical appearance of the EAC.
- Granulation tissue in the floor of the EAC at the junction of the bony and cartilaginous parts of the canal.
- Microvascular disease predisposes to an osteomyelitis which spreads across the skull base. Cranial nerves VII and IX–XII may be affected. The opposite side of the skull base can be affected.
- Pseudomonas on culture.

Management

- Admit patient for assessment
- Take a full history
- Make a thorough ENT examination
- Check cranial nerves
- Perform an aural toilet
- Perform a biopsy of the ear canal under GA/LA to exclude malignancy (p.254)
- Do a CT scan to examine the appearance of the skull base and to stage the extent of the disease
- Give ciprofloxacin drops 2 drops bd
- Give oral ciprofloxacin 400mg bd PO
- Involve the infectious disease team for expert help
- Continue with drug therapy for 6–12 weeks
- Perform a surgical debridement only if the patient does not respond to treatment or if there is skull base extension.

❶ Beware malignancy

If things fail to settle or if the condition progresses, don't forget there may be a possible malignant cause. An initial negative biopsy may be wrong. Consider further deep biopsy or cortical mastoidectomy for histology.

Malignancy of the pinna

- The pinna is a common site for malignant skin lesions to develop.
- The types of cancer are BCC, SCC and malignant melanoma.

Risk factors

- Sun exposure
- Previous skin cancers
- Chemical exposure
- Xeroderma pigmentosum.

Investigations and treatment

It is sometimes possible to make a diagnosis based on clinical observation. Usually excision biopsy is the treament of choice. Histological examination can confirm the type of malignancy. Further wider excision with or without grafting can be undertaken.

Special reconstructions of the pinna

The unique appearance and structure of the pinna leads to several novel methods of reconstruction after tumour removal. These aim to preserve the structure of the pinna and its cosmetic appearance without compromising curative removal. See Fig. 12.6.

If there is gross cartilage involvement, it may be necessary to remove the pinna entirely.

Fig. 12.6. Diagram of wedge resection

Malignancy of the external auditory canal

This is a rare condition, but it forms an important differential in dealing with infections or masses in the ear. When seen, it usually affects the elderly. SCC is the commonest type of malignancy.

Signs and symptoms
- A growth in the EAC
- An otitis externa
- Facial nerve palsy
- Other cranial nerve palsies such as IX–XII
- Lymph node metastases.

Management
- Treat any infection
- Biopsy the lesion
- CT scan to stage the lesion
- MRI scan to assess intracranial spread.

Treatment options
- Palliative
- Curative
- Radiotherapy
- Surgery.

Prognosis
The outlook for these patients is universally poor, with low 5 year survival rates.

The middle ear

Structure and function

The middle ear is made up of the following structures (see p.241, Fig. 12.2):
- The tympanic membrane
- The ossicular chain
- Nerves of the middle ear
- Muscles of the middle ear
- Mastoid air cell system
- Eustachian tube.

The function of the middle ear is to transduce sound waves, amplify them and pass them to the cochlea. There is also an intrinsic mechanism to protect the ear from loud noise.

Tympanic membrane (Fig 13.1.)

This is composed of three layers. It is divided into the pars flaccida and the pars tensa by the anterior and posterior malleolar folds. These two parts differ in their strength. The pars tensa has collagen fibres arranged radially, and the flaccida has randomly arranged collagen and a high elastin content. The squamous epithelium grows from central drum germinal centres. It then migrates radially and out along the EAC to be shed at the EAM.

The ossicular chain

The malleus, incus and stapes conduct and amplify sound. The difference in contact area between the drum and the malleus compared to the conact area between the stapes and the oval window leads to an amplification. When this is added to the mechanical advantage of the articulated ossicular chain, the total amplification is in the order of 22 times.

Nerves of the middle ear

The facial nerve has an intricate course. The chorda tympani is a branch of the facial nerve. The tympanic plexus has secretomotor fibres to the parotid.

Muscles of the middle ear

The stapedius contracts and damps the movement of stapes. The tensor tympani contracts and stabilises the movement of the malleus. Both these mechanisms protect the ear from loud noise.

Mastoid air cell system

This connects with the middle ear via the antrum. It provides a reservoir of air to balance vast changes in air pressure.

Eustachian tube

This tube provides a mechanism for the equalization of air pressure on either side of the eardrum.

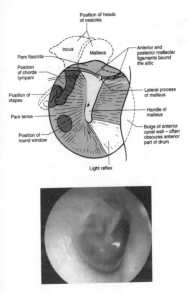

Fig. 13.1. Diagram of tympanic membrane showing quadrants and what lies behind

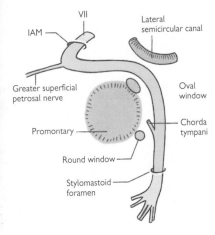

Fig. 13.2. The medial wall of the middle ear

Congenital abnormalities

Congenital abnormalities of the middle ear are rare in isolation. Middle ear abnormalities are more common in association with microtia (see p.242). Abnormalities of the ossicular chain can occur in isolation.

Signs and symptoms

Conductive hearing loss never more than 60dB.
Normal tympanogram/As type/Ad type.

Management

- Diagnosis is usually suggested on CT + confirmed by performing a tympanotomy.
- If the abnormality is in the better hearing ear, use a hearing aid. Surgery carries a higher risk of permanent sensorineural loss.
- If the abnormality is in the worse hearing ear then consider a tympanotomy after a trial of a hearing aid.

Acute otitis media

This is a very common condition (see Fig. 13.3.). Almost everyone will suffer with acute otitis media during their lifetime. Signs and symptoms may include a preceding URTI, severe and progressive otalgia, or a discharge—this is usually associated with a resolution of the otalgia. A diagnosis is made by taking a history, examining the tympanic membrane and taking the patient's temperature.

Treatment for acute otitis media is controversial. Systematic review suggests treatment with analgesia only. However, these reviews may have included a high proportion of viral ear infections where antibiotics would not be expected to be useful.

Management

- Give analgesia in all cases.
- Give oral antibiotics for one week such as Augmentin po.
- Discharge may continue for 1 week.
- When infection has resolved always check the tympanic membrane is normal.

Recurrent infections of the middle ear

These must be differentiated from one persisting infection. Treat any acute infection actively as above. If the patient has more than five infections in six months, then consider alternative treatment.

Treatment

- Medical—consider prophylactic trimethoprim syrup po.
- Surgical—if there is effusion or glue ear consider grommet insertion ± adenoidectomy.
- All treatment needs monitoring—use an infection diary to record episodes of infection pre and post treatment.

❶ Caution

Acute otitis media is often misdiagnosed. Children with nocturnal earache often have glue/eustachian tube dysfunction. The tympanic membrane may be red or injected but there is no discharge and the pain resolves very quickly upon waking.

Fig. 13.3. Diagram of acute otitis media stages

Complications of acute otitis media

Chronic infection

- The infection may persist and become chronic. This may be due to resistant bacteria. Use a broadspectrum antibiotic such as Ciprofloxacin.
- Consider myringotomy for relief of symptoms or to obtain microbiological information.

Facial nerve palsy

- 10% of people have a dehiscent facial nerve—when the bony covering is absent over the nerve. This results in a facial nerve irritation and palsy.
- The patient must be admitted to hospital and given IV antibiotics.
- Consider myringotomy and grommet insertion if the condition fails to resolve in 24hrs.

Acute mastoiditis

This is an infection of the mastoid air cells which will lead to a severe ear ache with tenderness, swelling and redness behind the pinna. The pinna may also be pushed forwards, making it look more prominent.

This is an ENT emergency and requires admission IV antibiotics ± surgical drainage.

Perforation of tympanic membrane

Repeated infections which perforate the tympanic membrane can lead to perforations that do not heal.

Sensorineural hearing loss (SNHL)

Rarely, toxins can spread to the inner ear to produce a sensorineural hearing loss. This is a greater risk with recurrent infection.

Vertigo

Infection near the lateral semicircular canal can produce a para labrynthitis. This can cause a spectrum of vestibular disturbance ranging from mild unsteadiness to disabling vertigo.

Glue ear

Glue ear is caused by a combination of exposure to infection and a non-functioning eustachian tube. Almost 8 out of 10 children will have glue ear at some time during childhood. The incidence of glue ear decreases with age as the immune system develops and the eustachian tube becomes larger.

The signs and symptoms of glue ear can include: decreased hearing, recurrent ear infections, poor speech development, failing performance at school and, sometimes, antisocial behaviour.

Risk factors
- Smoking parents
- Bottle feeding
- Day-care nursery
- Cleft palate
- Atopy.

Investigations

Take a full history, do a full examination including the palate, carry out age appropriate audiometry (see p.72) and tympanometry.

Management

This depends on a balance of:
- **Social factors**—more urgent action is needed if the family is unlikely to re-attend for further appointments.
- **Hearing disability**—how the child is coping with their hearing problem socially and at school is more important than the actual level of hearing loss.
- **Appearance of tympanic membranes**—if there is gross retraction, intervention may be needed to avoid retraction pocket formation.

Treatment

There are three options:
- **Watchful waiting**—this should apply to all patients for three months as glue ear will resolve in 50% of cases.
- **Hearing aid**—there is a window of opportunity at 4–8years old, It is non invasive, but may lead to teasing at school.
- **Insertion of grommets**—short general anaesthetic ± adenoidectomy—see p.356.

Chronic suppurative otitis media without cholesteatoma

- This common condition is associated with eustachian tube dysfunction with or without an infection in the mastoid.
- As with other ear diseases, its prevalence continues despite antibiotics.
- The signs and symptoms of chronic suppurative otitis media include continuous recurrent otorrhoea, perforation in tympanic membrane (usually central), and no cholesteatoma present.

Risk factors
- Smoking patient
- Smoking parents
- Acute otitis media
- Decreased immunity.

Investigations
- Take a full history and do an ENT examination
- Do a microscopy of the eardrum with thorough cleaning, and
- Take a swab for microbiology.

Management
- Give appropriate topical and systemic antibiotics based on the swab result. The condition may settle with antibiotics and water precautions.
- Perform a regular aural toilet.
- Persistent infections may need surgery in the form of myringoplasty and cortical mastoidectomy.

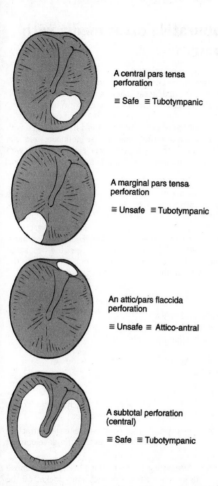

A central pars tensa
perforation

≡ Safe ≡ Tubotympanic

A marginal pars tensa
perforation

≡ Unsafe ≡ Tubotympanic

An attic/pars flaccida
perforation

≡ Unsafe ≡ Attico-antral

A subtotal perforation
(central)

≡ Safe ≡ Tubotympanic

Fig. 13.4. Diagram showing sites of perforations. Safe/unsafe refers to
the risk of developing an associated cholesteatoma

Chronic suppurative otitis media with cholesteatoma

- This is often divided into congenital and acquired:
- **Congenital cholesteatoma** results from an abnormal focus of squamous epithelium in the middle ear space i.e. a dermoid.
- **Acquired cholesteatoma** results from chronic eustachian tube dysfunction.

It was hoped that the incidence of this condition would have changed with the advent of antibiotics. Unfortunately the disease continues and can present at any age. Signs and symptoms include recurrent otitis media with a smelly mucopurulent discharge, hearing loss, facial nerve palsy and vertigo.

Development of a cholesteatoma

The pars flaccida develops a retraction pocket. Prolonged low middle ear pressure allows for propagation of the pocket. The pocket neck becomes small compared to the sac itself. Initially, squamous epithelium migrates with ease through the pocket. As the sac gets bigger the squamous epithelium builds up inside the pocket. Eventually germinal centres are incorporated. Infection supervenes on the impacted squamous epithelium/keratin. Release of lytic enzymes from the cholestaetoma causes destruction of local structures.

Investigations

- Aural toilet
- Microscopy and suction clearance
- Topical antibiotic/steroid drops for 10 days
- Review under the microscope after one month
- Audiometry
- CT scan of the temporal bone to look for pneumatisation of mastoid or erosion of scutum.

Management

This depends on the age and fitness of the patient, which ear is affected, the patient's wishes and their ability to tolerate ear toilet.

Prophylaxis: This is a controversial treatment where early retraction pockets are treated by inserting a grommet to reverse the development of a cholesteatoma.

Early retraction pocket: Attempting to clean the pocket and remove keratin. GA may be required. Maintenance of a cleaned pocket can be undertaken by an aural care nurse.

Established non-cleaning pocket: If the worse hearing ear is the one affected, surgery will be required to remove the risk of intracerebral complications. See Mastoid surgery, p.272.

Follow up

These patients are at risk of recurrence and therefore need careful follow up.

Mastoid surgery

Cortical mastoidectomy

A simple opening of the mastoid and ablation of the individual air cells in order to create one large cavity or drain pus. This was frequently performed in the pre-antibiotic ear to treat acute mastoiditis. This is much less common nowadays and usually performed as part of a more complicated mastoid operation.

Modified radical mastoidectomy (MRM)

See Fig. 13.5. This is performed to remove cholesteatoma from the middle ear and mastoid. The cholesteatoma, head of the malleus and incus are all removed and the connnections between the middle ear cleft and mastoid are enlarged. A 'mastoid cavity' is created by removal of the posterior canal wall, this may require cleaning in the outpatients.

Combined approach tympanoplasty (CAT)

This operation is also performed for cholesteatoma but here the posterior canal wall remains intact and no cavity is formed. The eardrum looks normal after the operation. Benefits of this approach include less outpatient care, better hearing results, and patients are better able to tolerate swimming. However since cholesteatoma can be 'sealed in' behind an intact drum a 'second look' operation is required at 6–12 months to ensure the disease has been eradicated.

Fig. 13.5. (a) An attic cholesteatoma extending backwards into the mastoid. (b) Modified radical mastoidectomy. Here the cholesteatoma has been removed and the mastoid cavity 'exteriorized', i.e. connected to the ear canal by removal of the posterior ear canal wall

Complications of chronic suppurative otitis media

These are related to local and distant effects of cholesteatoma

Local effects

Conductive hearing loss: As the retracted attic segment of the ear drum lies against the long process of the incus, it interferes with its already tenuous blood supply. The incus initially thins then loses its attachment to the stapes. The cholesteatoma can bridge this gap and temporarily improve the conductive loss.

Sensorineural hearing loss: The toxic effect of the local infection can cause a sensorineural hearing loss.

Vertigo: May be due either to a paralabrynthitis causing an irritative vestibulopathy, or it may be the result of erosion into the lateral semicircular canal—called a fistula.

Facial nerve dysfunction: If a dehiscence exists, infection can produce a direct irritation of the nerve. The cholesteatoma may also directly erode the bony covering of the facial nerve.

Mastoiditis: A chronic infection may lead to mastoiditis.

Distant effects

Meningitis: The roof of the middle ear is also the floor of the middle cranial fossa. A thin plate of bone separates the middle ear from the meninges in this area. This can be eroded by an extensive cholesteatoma, with a spread of infection to the meninges.

Cerebral abscess: A spread of infection can lead to abscess formation which can progress to the temporal lobe.

Lateral sinus thrombosis: The lateral sinus is one of the relations of the mastoid air cell systems. Infection can spread to the lateral sinus, causing local thrombosis. This in turn can lead to hydrocephalus.

Bezold's abscess: Infection from the mastoid spreads through the mastoid tip and travels under the sternomastoid, it then points in the neck anterior to the muscle.

Citellis' abscess: Infection spreads medially from the mastoid tip to collect in the digastric fossa.

① Mastoiditis
② Labyrinthitis
③ Extradural abscess
④ Lateral sinus thrombosis
⑤ Temperal lobe abscess
⑥ Meningitis

Fig. 13.6. Routes of spread of infection from middle ear

Otosclerosis

This is an osseous dyscrasia of the temporal bone. It presents as a slow progressive hearing loss, usually beginning in the patient's twenties. There is usually a family history of the condition. The patient may have difficulty hearing when chewing and may have problems with quiet conversations. 69–80 per cent of patients have tinnitus. Dizziness is rarely caused by this condition. There is no history of infection.

In its early stages the lesion is 'spongiotic'. Later, this spongiosis becomes sclerosis, or a combination of these two abnormal bone types. Later, osteocytes at the edge of the lesion extend into the bone, surrounding the central vascular spaces. Stapes fixation occurs when annular ligament or stapes footplate becomes involved. Spread to cochlea produces high tone sensorineural hearing loss.

Incidence

- The female to male ratio is two to one.
- 6.4% of temporal bones have evidence of otosclerosis.
- 0.3% of the population have a clinical manifestation of the disease.
- The condition is bilateral in 70% of patients.
- 50% of patients with otosclerosis have a family history.

Investigations

- Check for a normal mobile intact tympanic membrane.
- Look for 'Schwartzes sign'—flamingo pink blush anterior to the oval window. This means there is increased vascular supply to the otospongiotic focus.
- Perform pure tone audiometry. This shows conductive hearing loss (CHL) typical of a Carhart's notch (see Fig. 13.7.).
- Check for absent stapedial reflex.
- Carry out a CT scan—this may help to exclude other bony abnormalities of the middle ear such as ossicular fixation.

Differential diagnosis

Paget's disease: There is other bony involvement, (e.g. frontal bossing) increased alkaline phosphatase, and mixed hearing loss.

Osteogenesis imperfecta: Also known as Van der Hoeve syndrome, leads to mixed hearing loss with blue sclera. There is frequently a history of multiple bony fractures.

Treatment

The options are:
- No treatment
- Hearing-aid
- Surgery—stapedectomy after 3 month trial of hearing aid

Contraindications to surgery

- Surgery should be performed on a worse hearing ear only.
- Previous sensorineural hearing loss in contralateral ear.
- If there is tympanic membrane perforation, this will necessitate a myringoplasty first.
- Infection.

Cochlear otosclerosis

This is due to the spread of the otosclerotic process to the basal turn of the cochlea. Treatment with sodium fluoride helps to reduce the abnormal bone metabolism and so stabilises hearing loss. Monitor with serial pure tone audiograms.

Fig. 13.7. Pure tone audiometry showing conductive hearing loss typical Cahart's notch

Trauma

Acoustic trauma

Loud noise can produce direct traumatic effects on the middle ear. See Chapter 14, p.292 (NIHL).

Head injury

Direct blows to the head can produce:
- A temporal bone fracture—p.320
- A coexistent haemotympanum—blood in the middle ear
- Ossicular chain disruption
- Rarely, cochlear concussion can produce a SNHL.

Management

Patients with severe trauma may present late to ENT, as they usually have more pressing priorities in their management. Treat the patient's head injury and check for a cervical spine injury. Perform an otoscoopy and look for CSF otorrhoea. Check the facial nerve function.

Hearing assessment

- A tuning fork test will distinguish CHL from SNHL.
- Pure tone audiogram will confirm the tuning fork findings and will quantify any hearing defect.

Treatment

SNHL: Consider steroids. Prednisolone1mg/kg po one week if no contra-indications. Follow with serial audiograms.

CHL: No immediate treatment. Review in OPD six weeks. The haemo-tympanum will have resolved. Re-test the patient's hearing. If CHL persists check the tympanogram to ensure that there is no glue ear and consider tympanotomy with ossicular reconstruction.

Box 13.1 Pens, cotton buds, and lollysticks

If these objects are inserted into the EAC, they rarely reach the ear-drum. They usually impact on the skin of the EAC and tear it, causing bleeding. Careful examination with the otoscope can usually identify this problem.

Traumatic perforations of the TM heal sponataneously. Treat haemo-tympanum and possible ossicular dislocation as above.

Neoplasia

Benign and malignant tumours involving the middle ear space can occur, but these are very rare.

The inner ear

Structure and function of the inner ear

The inner ear can be divided into two parts—the cochlea and the vestibular system (Fig. 14.1.).

The Cochlea

This is the organ of sound transduction. The cochlea is coiled as a helical form, and is encased in hard bone of the petrous temporal bone.

The specialized structure of the cochlea turns sound waves into electrical signals which pass to the brain.

The cochlea has a tonotopic representation – this means that different areas are frequency specific. High frequencies are dealt with at the start or at the base of the cochlea. Low tones are dealt with at the cochlea apex.

See Fig. 14.2. for a cross section of the cochlea.

The neurological pathway to the auditory cortex is best remembered by using the E COLI mnemonic.

E eighth nerve
C cohlear nucleus
O Superior olive
L Lateral lemniscus
I inferior colliculus

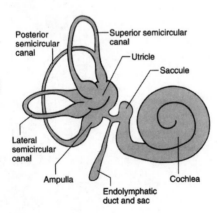

Fig. 14.1. Diagram of the inner ear

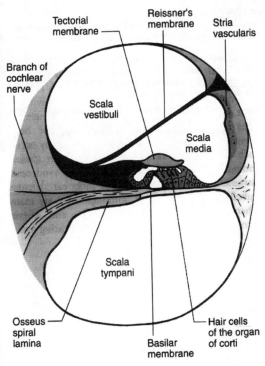

Fig. 14.2. Cross section of the cochlea

Vestibular system

The vestibular system functions to provide information about angular and linear acceleration for the brain. It is also encased in the petrous temporal bone.

5 separate neuroepithelial elements work in combination to provide this information: 3 semicircular canals, the utricle and the saccule.

The semicircular canals are paired to provide complimentary information about the direction of travel (Fig. 14.3.).

The inferior and superior vestibular nerves pass the information to the brain.

The ultrastructure of these neuroepithelial elements is shown in Fig. 14.4.

Fig. 14.3. Paired motion of the semicircular canals

Fig. 14.4. Ultrastructure of semicircular canals/utricle

Sensorineural hearing loss

The aetiology of such a hearing loss can usually be determined by careful consideration of the patient's history, a clinical examination and the findings of special investigations.

The age of onset of the patient's hearing loss is important, as is any family history of hearing loss. Careful consideration of a patient's pregnancy and perinatal history are also important.

Examination

This examination will aim to discover any congenital abnormality or inherited syndrome in which hearing loss may play a part.

Ears   Pre-auricular pits present?
                shape and location of the pinnae
                size of the EAC
                appearance of the TM
Eyes   Eyebrows
                Interpupillary distance
                Colour of iris
                External ocular movements
                Appearance of fundus
                Retinal pigment
Face   Shape
                Symmetry
Skin   Texture
                Pigmentation
Extremities   Shape of fingers and toes
                Carrying angle

Investigations

These investigations aim to confirm and assess the extent of the patient's hearing loss and to look for any evidence of an inherited condition.

Audiological assessment
Radiology including CT/MRI
Blood tests U+Es
Glucose
TFTs
ECG
Cytogenetics

Specialist opinions

You may need to consult an Opthalmologist and/or a Clinical Geneticist.

Table 14.1 Classification of patients presenting with inner ear hearing loss

Non hereditary	Hereditary
Presbyacusis	Syndromic
Noise Induced Hearing Loss	Non Syndromic
Idiopathic Sudden Hearing Loss	
Autoimmune Hearing Loss	
Vascular causes	
Ototoxicity	
Non Organic Hearing Loss	

Presbyacusis

This term describes a decreased peripheral auditory sensitivity. It is usually age related, and affects men more than women.

Signs and symptoms

This condition shows itself as bilateral, progressive, symmetrical sensorineural hearing loss, with no history of noise exposure. The patient may have worse speech discrimination than expected when reviewing the audiogram. Decreasing central auditory discrimination leads to phonemic regression.

Investigations

Otoscopy.
Pure tone audiogram. (See Fig. 14.5.).

Types of Presbyacusis

Based on the shape of the audiogram and the site of loss, presbyacusis can be subdivided into the following subtypes:

- *Sensory presbyacusis:* steep sloping audiogram above speech frequency. It starts in mid life so speech discrimination is preserved. Degeneration in Organ of Corti.
- *Neural presbyacusis:* down sloping high frequency loss. Flatter than sensory presbyacusis. Thought to be 1st order neurone loss. Disproportionate discrimination score.
- *Strial presbyacusis:* flat audiogram. Good discrimination.
- *Cochlear conductive/indeterminate presbyacusis:* Down sloping audiogram. Increasing stiffness of basilar membrane.
- *Central presbyacusis:* Loss of GABA in Inferior Colliculus
- *Middle ear aging:* Loosening of ligaments or ossicular articulation problem.

Management

The patient may be given counselling and advice about hearing loss, and Given a hearing aid where the symptoms are troublesome.

Fig. 14.5. Investigation of presbyacusis: pure tone audiogram for (a) right ear; (b) left ear

Noise induced hearing loss

This is defined as damage to the inner ear caused by exposure to loud noise. There is a relationship between the volume of sound and its duration which causes damage. Eight hours of exposure to a sound level of 85 dB usually causes damage. Louder sounds will cause damage at shorter exposure times.

Acoustic trauma is caused by sounds greater than 180 dB. Rupture of the tympanic membrane and ossicular fracture may occur.

Signs and symptoms

The patient will usually present with bilateral and symmetrical hearing loss. There may be a noise induced temporary threshold shift (TTS)—for example, hearing may improve over the weekend if the problem is noise at work. The patient may have difficulty hearing in background noise or they may have tinnitus.

Investigations

Use audiometry. For a typical pattern see Fig. 14.6.

Pathology

Hearing loss is greatest in 3–6kHz region of cochlea. Below 2kHz the acoustic reflex is protective. EAC resonant frequency is 1–4kHz so energy delivered at these frequencies is greater. The actual loss of cochlea cells occurs where noise damage is greatest. Outer hair cells lose rigidity and the stereocilia fuse.

Management

Consider the following to prevent further noise damage:
• Health and safety at work
• Provision of ear defenders
• Routine hearing screening for occupations at risk
For established damage consider:
• Hearing aids
• Counselling for tinnitus

▶ Rifle Shooting

This will sometimes result in an asymmetric SNHL with the noise damaged pattern. When firing a rifle, one ear is nearer to the gun barrel. If the patient shoots right handed, their LEFT ear is most affected as it is nearer to the barrel of the gun.

Fig. 14.6. Audiogram of NIHL

Idiopathic sudden hearing loss

See emergencies section, p.420.

Tinnitus

This is a sensation of a noise in the ear. It can exist with a hearing loss of any cause and can even occur in patients with normal hearing. However it is most commonly associated with sensorineural hearing loss. Most people will experience tinnitus at some time in their lives and for most it is no more than a transient nuisance, however in some it is a troublesome symptom, which can trigger depression or even suicide. Tinnitus is usually intrinsic, i.e. only heard by the patient.

Causes of intrinsic tinnitus
- Drugs
- Labyrinthitis
- Trauma
- Vascular
- Presbycusis
- Meniere's disease
- Noise induced hearing loss
- Otosclerosis
- Acoustic neuroma

Cause of extrinsic tinnitus
- Insects in the ear canal
- Vascular malformations
- Palatal myoclonus

The tinnitus model (see Fig. 14.7.)

Experiments have shown that 95% of normal people will experience a degree of tinnitus when put into a sound proofed room. This means that the ear/auditory pathways are producing 'noise' or electrical activity that even normally hearing people can recognize, however our central auditory pathways filter out this useless information and we do not normally perceive it. In fact our CNS is constantly monitoring our surroundings but little of this is brought to our attention, e.g. up to this point YOU were not aware of your shoes on your feet, or the noise of passers-by and traffic, but now they have been brought to your attention, you become aware of them.

This screening system is essential in order to avoid sensation overload! It is believed that tinnitus becomes problematic when this screening or filtering process breaks down, and the 'noise' that the ear generates is not discarded as useless information, but is perceived as a threat, which in itself triggers an emotional reaction via the limbic system.

Tinnitus retraining therapy seeks to reverse this process by counselling and removing the perception of noise as a threat.

NB: When meeting patients with tinnitus it is very important to avoid negative counselling, e.g. '*Tinnitus–oh that's awful I would hate to have that*' or '*Tinnitus–well there is nothing that can be done about that you will just have to put up with it*'. Sentiments such as these will only serve to reinforce the negative feelings patients have about their condition and turn their feelings of 'threat' to feelings of hoplessness.

Fig. 14.7. Tinnitus retraining—diagram of model

Autoimmune ear disease

Autoimmune ear disease is classified as either organ specific, or as a systemic disease.

Organ specific
Vestibuloauditory autoimmunity or evidence of cell mediated immunity against inner ear antigens.

Systemic disease
Part of a recognised systemic autoimmune disease. Common diseases which have auditoryvestibular involvement are shown opposite.
Patients with autoimmune ear disease are usually middle-aged and are more likely to be female than male.

Signs and symptoms
- Bilateral unexplained SNHL
- May be fluctuant dizziness or Meniere's like syndrome with aural fullness
- Rapidly progressive hearing loss over days or weeks
- Associated VIIth nerve palsy
- Normal otoscopic examination
- Coexistent systemic immune disease.

Investigations
Take a full history and give a full oto-neurological examination, including a pure tone audiogram. Do a MRI scan to exclude acoustic neuroma with unilateral presentation.

Carry out the following blood tests
- Antigen specific antibodies
- Antigen non specific antibodies
- Acute phase reactants
- Lyme titres

Treatment
Treatment should be given under the guidance of neurotolgist and/or a rheumatologist.
Give steroids such as Prednisolone 1mg/kg per day PO
Or give steroid sparing alternatives:
- Cyclophosphamide
- Methotrexate
- Plasmaphoresis

The following conditions are thought to have an auto-immune basis and can cause hearing loss:

Polyarteritis nodosa

This condition affects the small and medium arteries. There is a rare association with an inner ear hearing loss.

Cogan's syndrome

This is a non syphilitic interstitial keratitis with vestibuloauditory dysfunction. It presents with photophobia and lacrimation one to six months before vestibuloauditory symptoms develop.

Atypical cogan's

This interstitial keratitis develops one to two years before auditory vestibular problems.

Wegener's granulomatosis

This is a necrotising granulomatous vasculitis of the lower and upper respiratory tract which also affects the kidneys causing focal necrotising glomerulonephritis. 90 per cent of patients have a sensorineural hearing loss and 20 per cent have a conductive hearing loss with effusion. cANCA positive 90 per cent.

Relapsing polychondritis

In this condition, giant cell arteritis and systemic vasculitis cause recurrent episodes of inflammatory necrosis. There is a raised ESR and a false positive VDRL.

Rheumatoid arthritis

Very common condition with characteristic arthropathy.

Ototoxicity

Drugs can damage the cochlea and vestibular system. It is worth taking a careful drug history, as a wide range of drugs can cause symptoms. Cross check with the BNF for side effects.

Aminoglycoside antibiotics

These antibiotics have a narrow therapeutic index and can cause damage to the inner ear. Common side effects are drug induced vestibular symptoms and hearing loss.

Patients requiring parenteral aminoglycoside antibiotics should have the plasma levels of the drug monitored during therapy. Local policy varies; often trough levels of antibiotic are used to determine future dose levels.

Topical antibiotics

Most topical antibiotics available contain an aminoglycoside antibiotic. These drugs are experimentally ototoxic in guinea pigs and other animals. They are believed to enter the inner ear through the round window membrane causing direct ototoxic effects. Drug data sheets also warn of the risks of using these preparations when there are grommets in situ or where there is a perforation of the TM.

▶ Short courses of these topical antibiotics—less than 10 days—are safe with perforations or grommets in the presence of infection. Oedema of the middle ear mucosa with a thickened round window membrane, limits the entry of antibiotic into the inner ear. *Untreated infection is a greater risk to hearing than the antibiotic.*

Therapeutic uses

Aminoglycosides can be used to treat patients with Menieres disease by causing a vestibulopathy when instilled into the middle ear. Much higher doses are used compared with the standard drops.

Other drugs

Chemotherapy, especially cisplatin, induces SNHL. Aspirin and Erythromycin can cause a reversible SNHL. Patients present with tinnitus.

Hereditary hearing loss

Heredited hearing loss may be divided into syndromic and non syndromic types. Non syndromic or non organic hearing loss is most common, representing about two thirds of cases.

As the loci of genes associated with hearing loss are identified, it becomes more obvious that the classifying of these conditions on syndromic basis may be misleading. Many patients with apparently non syndromic hereditary hearing loss have the same gene alterations as their syndromic counterparts but are not phenotypically syndromic.

Other classifications of hereditary hearing loss are:

Genetics	See Table 14.2
Age of onset	Early (Birth to age 2) Known congenital Suspected congenital Delayed (3 to 20) Adult (>21 years)
Hearing loss	Sensorineural Conductive Mixed hearing loss
Laterality	Unilateral/bilateral
Stability	Stable Fluctuating Progressive
Frequencies	Low (250–1kHz) Medium (>1kHz–4kHz) High (>4kHz)
Associations	Radiological abnormalities Vestibular dysfunction

Table 14.2 Genetic inheritance of hearing loss

Inheritance	Percentage	Condition
Autosomal recessive	60–70%	Non syndromic SNHL
		Pendreds
		Ushers
		Jervell-Lange-Nielsen
Autosomal dominant	20–25%	Waardenburg's
		BOR
		Alports
X-linked recessive	2–3%	X-linked mixed hearing loss with stapes gusher
X-linked dominant	Uncertain	Alports
Chromosomal	<1%	
Mitochondrial	<1%	
Multifactorial	Uncertain	

Syndromic hearing loss

Goldenhaars syndrome (Oculoauricularvertebral OAV syndrome)

This is the most common syndrome occurring in approximately 1 in 10,000 live births. It is sporadic, not caused by genetic inheritance.

Features of Goldenhaars syndrome

Face	25% Marked asymmetry
	Maxilla and temporal bones reduced and flattened
	Hypolpasia/aplasia of mandible.
Ear	Flattened helical rim
	Pre-auricular tags
	EAC atretic/small
Hearing loss	CHL
	SNHL 15%
Associations	Skeletal abnormalities c-spine/skull base
	Cleft lip/palate
	Velopharyngeal insufficiency
	Mental retardation 15%

Treacher collins

Patients have a mandibulofacial dysostosis due to 1st/2nd branchial arch, groove and pouch abnormalities. This is the commonest syndrome of hearing loss. 60% of cases are sporadic rather than genetic. This abnormality has been found to occur on gene 5q 31–4.

Features of Treacher Collins syndrome

Face	Depressed cheeks
	Narrow midface
	Malformed pinnae cup shaped
	Hypertelorism
Ear	Narrow EAC
	Malformed ossicles, cochlea and labyrinth
Associations	Cleft palate
	Palatopharyngeal incompetence 30–40%
	Normal intelligence

Fig. 14.8. Features of Goldenhaars syndrome

Fig. 14.9. Features of Treachers Collins syndrome

Syndromic hearing loss II

Waardenburg's Syndrome

2–5% of congenitally deaf children have Waardenburg's syndrome

Features of Waardenburg's Syndrome

Appearance	Dystopia canthorum in type 1
	Synophrys—confluent eyebrows 85% type 1
	Heterochromia iridis (Different colour irides)
	Broad nasal root
	Sapphire eyes
	White forelock 30–40%
	Vitiligo
	Premature grey hair
Hearing loss	Congenital SNHL
	20% of those with type 1 WS and 50% of those with type 2 have a hearing loss
	50% of people with WS have normal hearing

Branchial-oto-renal syndrome(BOR)

In this rare condition there is an association of branchial fistulas/cysts with hearing problems and renal abnormalities.

Alport's syndrome

This is a rare hereditary progressive glomerulonephritis with SNHL. It presents as hearing loss and renal problems. There are six subtypes of Alport's syndrome classified by type of inheritance, age of onset of renal failure, presence of hearing loss and ocular abnormalities. The diagnosis of Alport's syndrome depends on three out of four of the following being found:

• Positive family history of haematuria and renal failure
• Electronmicroscopic evidence of glomerulonephritis on renal biopsy
• Characteristic ophthalmic signs
• Progressive high frequency SNHL starting in childhood

Pendred's syndrome

This is a rare autosomal recessive inherited condition where a non-toxic goitre is found in association with profound congenital SNHL. It is associated with the mondini deformity of the cochlea.

Jervell-Lange-Nielsen syndrome

This condition is believed to be autosomal recessive. The abnormality is located on chromosome 11. There is a prolonged QT interval on ECG. Multiple syncopal episodes may occur from the age of 3–5 years onwards.

Usher's syndrome

This is an autosomal recessive condition consisting of retinitis pigmentosa and hearing impairment.

Non-organic hearing loss (NOHL)

This describes a situation where a patient claims to have a hearing loss where none exists, or where a patient exaggerates a hearing loss which does exist.

A typical example may be a child who is having difficulties at school or at home, and who presents with a very poor hearing test result. Often the hearing loss documented on the audiogram will seem out of keeping with the child's participation in the consultation. Another example is a patient who is pursuing a claim for damages as a result of a hearing loss.

The clues to look for when diagnosing this condition are: concerns raised by the audiologist about inconsistent results, if there is litigation involved or if the parent-child interaction is unusual.

Investigations

- Pure tone audiometry
- Tuning fork tests—Stenger test
- Speech audiogram—more difficult to fabricate abnormal response
- Stapedial reflex testing
- Delayed speech feedback—the patient reads aloud and their speech is played into the affected ear. The playback is slightly delayed which will cause the patient to hesitate or stutter if they can hear.
- Brain stem evoked auditory response—this is the gold standard in litigation cases.

Management

Careful handling of non-organic hearing loss is required. It may be wise to suggest to affected children that you know their hearing is better, but don't be too confrontational. Bring them back for another audiogram and suggest that they try to be a little more accurate.

Litigation claims needs more tact and multiple investigations before any confrontation.

Stenger test

Use two 512Hz tuning forks.

Step 1

The patient closes their eyes and the examiner stands behind.
The tuning fork is activated and placed at 5cm from each ear in turn
The patient will hear the note in their good ear but deny hearing it in the non hearing ear.

Step 2

Both tuning forks are used without the patient realizing it.
One is held 5cm from the ear with the alleged poor hearing. The other is held, at the same time, 15cm away from the good ear.
The patient with NOHL will deny hearing any sound. The tuning fork held near the bad ear will mask the sound of the tuning fork near the good ear. The genuine patient will only hear the tuning fork near the good ear.

Labyrinthitis (vestibular neuronitis)

This presents as a sudden episode of vertigo in a previously well person. It is equally common in men and women, with the usual age of onset being thirty to forty years. Attacks are usually single, but people may occasionally experience multiple attacks, and it can be recurrent. It normally lasts 1–2 days and improves over weeks. Vertigo is usually unilateral, or rarely, bilateral. Epidemics can occur in the spring or summer. There may be an associated URTI two weeks prior to the vertigo. It occasionally leaves a BPPV symptom complex.

Pathology
- Axonal loss—endoneurial fibrosis and atrophy of the nerve
- Suspected viral aetiology e.g. Rubeola, HSV, Reovirus, CMV, influenza and mumps.

Investigations
- Pure tone audiograms
- Nystagmus away from affected side
- Quix Test +ve (Seated Rombergs Test)
- ENG if there is clinical doubt about the diagnosis
- MRI if there is asymmetry or recurrent episodes

Treatment
- Vestibular suppressant for acute attack—Stemetil 5mg sub-buccal/12.5mg IM
- Steroids if SNHL—Prednisolone 1mg/kg for 1 week
- Patients usually compensate well for this condition.
- Vestibular rehabilitation—for patients who do not compensate.

Benign paroxysmal positional vertigo

This is the most common cause of peripheral vertigo. It usually starts around the age of 50 years. The patient experiences brief episodes of vertigo caused by changes in position, in particular looking up and rolling over in bed. It is worse in the morning and the evening. This condition is believed to occur as a result of stimulation of the semi-circular canals by otoliths which have become mis-placed.

There are three typical patterns in benign paroxysmal positional vertigo:
• Acute form—resolves in three months
• Intermittent form—active and inactive periods over years
• Chronic form—has continuous symptoms over longer duration.

Investigations
• Full otoneurological examination
• Dix-Hallpike test
• Pure tone audiogram
• ENG—if there is diagnostic uncertainty
• MRI scan—if symptoms persistent for more than 3 months

Dix-Hallpike test

Place the patient on the examining couch, positioned in such a way that when they lie back their head will be over the end of the bed. While the patient is sitting turn their head 30° towards the examiner. This leads to maximal stimulation of the PSCC on lying down. Then ask the patient to lie down, looking at the examiner's nose. The examiner supports the head and allows the head to extend over the edge of the bed. A positive test results in rotatory nystagmus after a delay of 1–5 seconds. This lasts between 10 to 30 seconds. Reversal to the upright position changes the direction of the nystagmus. This process is fatiguable and sensitivity of the test can be improved with Frenzel glasses which do not allow optic fixation.

Treatment

Fatiguing exercises: if the patient has significant symptom free episodes (see Fig. 14.10.)
Epleys manoeuvre: can bring 90% relief if the patient has had symptoms by repositioning the displaced otoliths (see Fig. 14.11.).
Surgery: this is rare. A singular neurectomy may lead to SNHL in 10–20% of patients. A retrosigmoid vestibular nerve section may result in 1% mortality as the proceure involves craniotomy. A posterior canal occlusion via a mastoid operation will control the symptoms, but a SNHL may complicate 5% of cases.

Fig. 14.10. Brandt Doroff exercises

Fig. 14.11. Epley manoeuvre

Meniere's disease/syndrome

Meniere's disease presents itself as increasing fullness in the ear and roaring tinnitus, with a sensation of blocked hearing, and episodic vertigo. Alternatively there may be a sudden onset of vertigo with no warning (see Signs and symptoms, p.314). 30–50% of people with Meniere's disease have bilateral symptoms within 3 years of presentation.

Meniere's disease occurs in between 50–150 people per 100,000 of the population. It is more common in females than in males and usually occurs between the ages of 35–40.

Causes
- Idiopathic Meniere's disease
- Post traumatic head injury or ear surgery
- Post infectious delayed e.g. in mumps and measles
- Late-stage syphilis
- Classical Cogan's
- Atypical Cogan's

Signs and symptoms
Of people with Meniere's disease:
- 42% have hearing loss alone
- 11% have vertigo alone
- 44% have vertigo and hearing loss
- 3% have tinnitus

Vertigo lasts more than 20 minutes and is associated with nausea, vomiting and autonomic effects. Most episodes last 2–4 hours (although some last for more than 6 hours).
Horizontal or horizonto-rotatory nystagmus is always present.
The patient may experience disequilibrium after an attack for several days.
A fluctuating SNHL is found in the early stages of the disease. Later, the hearing loss becomes permanent. The hearing may not change for some days after an attack.

Types of hearing loss
- Low frequency SNHL
- Flat moderately severe SNHL
- Bilateral SNHL with >25dB asymmetry

Poorly controlled patients have progressive hearing loss, stabilizing at 50-60dB

Variant Presentations of Meniere's disease include
- Lemoyez variant—hearing improves with vertigo attacks
- Otolithic crisis of Tumarkin—patient has drop attacks with vertigo (decompression of saccule)
- Cochlear Meniere's—auditory symptoms only
- Vestibular Meniere's—vestibular symptoms only

Investigations

There is no single diagnostic test.
- Otoneurological examination
- Pure tone audiogram
- MRI scan if there is asymmetry
- Autoantibodies—ESR, ANA, RhF, IgGs
- Echocochleography (ECoG)—this test involves placing a recording electrode either in the EAC or through the tympanic membrane to rest against the promontory of the cochlea. Sound is then applied to the test ear and the electrical activity in the ear is documented. Several components can be identified and measured. An increased ratio of the summating potential compared to the action potential >0.4 suggests hydrops (Fig 14.12.).

Pathology

On sectioning the inner ear in affected patients, the scala media is found to be expanded, as if there has been too much pressure in the endolymph. This is known as Endolymphatic hydrops.

Fig. 14.12. Diagram of ECoG waveform

Treatment of Meniere's disease

Medical management

- **Prophylaxis**—no added salt in diet, Serc 16mg tds PO
- **For acute attacks of vertigo**—stemetil, 5 mg sub-buccal
- Six monthly review with symptom diary recording vertigo (spinning) episodes and the length of each episode.

Surgical intervention

Patients whose symptoms are not improved by maximum medical therapy will require active intervention.

▶ Principles of intervention

All treatments balance the control of vertiginous episodes with the risk of hearing loss and the associated morbidity of the procedure. Treatment should not be undertaken for non-vertiginous symptoms. Care should be undertaken when dealing with the better hearing ear.

Factors affecting the choice of intervention

- Patient choice
- Surgeon's preference
- Cost of treatment
- Hearing level in affected ear
- Patient fitness

Measuring success

Guidelines from the American Academy of Otorhinolaryngologists and Head and Neck Surgeons (AAOHNS) measure success as comparing number of vertiginous episodes in 6 months prior to treatment with the number of episodes 6 months after treatment and followed up for 2 years.

Table 14.3 Interventional treatments for Menieres disease

Procedure	Indications	Control of Vertigo	Hearing Loss	Cost	Risk
Transtympanic gentamicin injection	Hearing loss <50dB	85%	5%	Low	Low
Endolymphatic sac decompression	Fluctuating SNHL	65%	<5%	Medium	Low
Total labyrinthectomy	Hearing loss >60dB	95%	Total Loss	Medium	Low–Med
Vestibular Nerve Section	Longstanding disease. Hearing loss <50dB	90%	<5%	High	Medium

Vascular causes of inner ear dysfunction

Vascular occlusion of the labyrinthine artery can cause the sudden onset of vertigo and hearing loss. This occlusion leads to widespread necrosis of membranous structures and labyrinthitis ossificans. The patient may have a prior history of transient ischaemic attacks (TIA's)—62% of TIA patients have episodic vertigo. Compensation usually occurs in 4–6 months.

Occlusion of anterior vestibular artery

Produces hearing loss and vertigo.
As the posterior circulation remains intact, the patient may simply present with a BPPV like symptom complex.

Recurrent vestibulopathy/vascular loop syndrome

Seven per cent of vertigo patients experience this syndrome. It is believed to occur as a result of an abnormally placed blood vessel impacting upon the vestibular nerve in the internal auditory meatus.

Females with this syndrome outnumber males by a 2:1 ratio. The usual age is 35–55 years old. The patient has usually had symptoms of episodic vertigo for 3 years at presentation. 80% have had episodic vertigo within the previous year and 10 per cent have BPPV. PTA high-frequency loss is found in 50% of patients and a middle frequency loss in 20%. The resulting histological abnormality is axonal loss and endoneurial fibrosis.

Investigations

- Full neurotological examination
- Spontaneous nystagmus
- Non Classical Dix Hall Pike test—no fatigue
- Pure tone audiograms
- MRI/MRA

Treatment

Vestibular suppressants—Stemetil 5mg sub-buccal tds for vertigo.
Consider microvascular nerve decompression.

Temporal bone fractures

These can occur as the result of serious head injury. Patients with this injury often present late to the ENT surgeon. Other injuries usually take precedence.

Types of fracture

These fractures are described according to their orientation to the axis of the temporal bone. Most fractures are complex and do not fit with the standard patterns:
- 80% are longitudinal
- 20% are transverse

Management

Treat head injury and other trauma according to the ATLS protocol.
As part of a secondary survey:
- Examine behind ear for bruise (Battle's sign)
- Examine EAC for blood/CSF/step
- Examine TM for disruption of annulus
- Test facial nerve function.

Investigations

CT scan—often a head injury scan will not show a fracture.
Doing a CT scan of the temporal bone with fine cut bony windows gives the best diagnostic information and prognosis for hearing loss.

Classical pattern of temporal bone fractures

Longitudinal fracture
- Blood in EAC
- Haemotymapnum
- Disruption of annulus
- SNHL only temporary
- Facial nerve injury rare—it can occur if not exactly longitudinal
  Statistically this type of fracture causes more facial nerve palsies

Transverse fracture
- EAC normal
- Haemotympanum
- SNHL permanent
- Facial nerve injury in 50%
- Vertigo and nystagmus

Chapter 15

The skull base

Overview

The skull base is a specialized area of clinical work. The ENT surgeon is actively involved in this area, often as part of a team including a neurosurgeon or plastic/craniofacial surgeon.

Access to these difficult areas has increased with the development of image guidance systems and the ability to extend endoscopic sinus surgery approaches via the sphenoid to the skull base.

Acoustic neuroma

An acoustic neuroma is a benign, slow growing tumour. It is more correctly called the vestibular schwannoma, because of its origin on the vestibular nerve. Post mortem data shows that this tumour is under-diagnosed. An acoustic neuroma may be an incidental finding on MRI.

Acoustic neuromas account for 6% of all intracranial neoplasms, the majority of which are sporadic (95%). 5% are genetic—part of the inherited condition of NF2 (neurofibromatosis Type 2) on chromosome 22.

Presentation

The patient may experience some of the following:
- Sudden SNHL or progressive high frequency SNHL.
- Vertiginous episodes—but these are rare as the patient unknowingly compensates.
- Symptoms of raised intracranial pressure such as headache or visual disturbance.
- Brainstem compression—ataxia is a late symptom of this.

Investigations

- PTA.
- MRI scan with gadolinium contrast.
- Full otoneurological exam.
- Hitselbergers sign—postauricular numbness due to facial nerve compression.
- Reduced corneal reflex.
- Unterberger's test positive—patient marches on the spot with the eyes closed. A positive test is a rotation to one side or the other.

Management

Management options balance the risk of hearing loss, facial nerve palsy and surgical morbidity. There are several possibilities:
- Watchful waiting—with serial MRI scans for slow growing tumours.
- Retrosigmoid approach—preserves the hearing
- Translabyrinthine approach—destroys the hearing but is an easier approach. It is useful if there is little hearing to preserve.
- Middle fossa approach—is technically challenging as it involves opening the middle fossa. No driving for one year due to the risk of fitting.
- Intracapsular removal—useful to decompress large tumours in elderly patients with brainstem compression.
- Stereotactic radiosurgery—this multiplanar radiotherapy is useful in small tumours as it avoids surgery.

Complications

- Any intracranial procedure e.g. craniotomy—carries a 1% risk of mortality.
- Facial nerve palsy.
- Total hearing loss

Box 15.1 Differential diagnosis of cerebello-pontine angle (CPA) tumour

Acoustic neuroma 80%
Meningioma
Epidermoid cyst
Cholesterol granuloma
Arachnoid cyst
Posterior cerebellar artery (PCA) aneurysm

Nasopharyngeal carcinoma (NPC)

There are two distinct types of this cancer of the back of the nose:
- Undifferentiated non-keratinizing squamous cell carcinoma (SCC)—this is more common in people from southern China and Chinese people from Hong Kong. It is associated with EBV.
- Differentiated keratinizing SCC—this has similar at risk groups to the majority of head and neck cancers.

Presentation
- Epistaxis
- Nasal obstruction
- Lymph node metastasis
- Middle ear effusion
- Extensive tumours can involve the skull base and cause cranial nerve palsies.

Investigations
Patients will be given a CT and/or an MRI scan.

▶ Important
Every patient presenting with a unilateral middle ear effusion must have their postnasal space visualized to exclude an NPC.

Treatment
Radiotherapy is given for all stages. Neck dissection may be necessary if there are extensive lymph node metastases.

Juvenile angiofibroma

This is a rare tumour almost exclusively seen in males. (If the patient is female consider chromosomal analysis.) It originates from the spheno-palatine foramen and is locally invasive but not malignant. It is a combination of fibrous tissue with endothelial spaces in vascular tissue.

Presentation

- Recurrent epistaxis in young male (average age 14)
- Large posterior nasal mass
- Pulsatile mass palpated prior to adenoidectomy
- Nasal obstruction.

Investigations

- Clinical examination with endoscope
- CT scan and MRI
- Angiography
- *Do not* do a biopsy for fear of life threatening haemorrhage

Management

The treatment is surgical removal, with pre-operative embolisation to reduce the blood loss during the operation. There are several ways to gain access to the area, but the most common is via the midface in an operation called midfacial degloving.

Sinonasal malignancy

This term describes a diverse group of malignant tumours affecting the nose and sinus system. SCC account for 70% of sinonasal malignancy, adenocarcinoma 10%, and adenoid cystic carcinoma 10%.

Nickel workers are at risk of developing SCC, woodworkers are at risk of adenocarcinoma. This is often delayed up to 20 years after exposure. The prognosis is poor with less than 50% of patients surviving for 5 years.

Common sites for sinonasal malignancy are:
• Maxillary sinus
• Nasal cavity
• Ethmoid sinus.

Presentation

Some or all of the following features may be seen:
• Nasal obstruction
• Epistaxis
• Sinusitis
• Maxillary symptoms
  • Loose teeth
  • Ulcer on palate
  • Cheek swelling
• Ethmoid symptoms
  • Unilateral obstruction
  • Diplopia
  • Headache.

Investigations
• CT and/or MRI
• Endoscopy and biopsy
• FNA if cervical metastases.

Treatment

Surgical resection and/or radiotherapy may be required. Treatment decisions should be made by an MDT in a specialist head and neck clinic taking into account the type of tumour and the staging.

TNM Staging of sinonasal malignancy

Maxillary sinus
- T1—Tumour limited to antral mucosa.
- T2—Tumour causing erosion or destruction into hard plate/lateral nasal wall.
- T3—Tumour eroding posterior wall/subcutaneous/cheek/medial orbit.
- T4—Intracranial extension/orbital apex/skin of nose.

Ethmoid sinus
- T1—confined to ethmoid.
- T2—Extends to nasal cavity.
- T3—Extemds to anterior orbit/maxillary sinus.
- T4—Intracranial extension.

Common operations

The consent process

General principles

The GMC has issued clear guidelines to assist the consent process. Its recommendations are summarized below:

- Patients must be given sufficient information—in a way that they can understand—to enable them to exercise their right to make informed decisions about their care.
- Patients' rights are protected by law.
- Effective communication is the key to informed consent.

Consent to investigation and treatment

A doctor who is undertaking a procedure or investigation will need to obtain consent from the patient. If this is not possible, then consent can be obtained by a nominated person who is suitably trained and qualified, who understands the risks involved, and who has sufficient knowledge of the proposed investigation or treatment.

It is important that patients make their own decisions about treatment. Ensuring voluntary decision making involves giving the patient a balanced view of the options and explaining the need for informed consent.

Forms of consent

Consent can be either express or implied consent.

Implied consent—is when the patient's actions may be, but are not necessarily an agreement to treatment.

Express consent—is written consent. It must be obtained and documented in the notes when:

- the treatment or procedure is complex, or involves significant risks and/or side effects.
- providing clinical care is not the primary purpose of the investigation or examination.
- there may be significant consequences for the patient's employment, social or personal life.
- the treatment is part of a research programme.

In an emergency, when no consent can be obtained, life-saving treatment can be given without consent.

Reviewing consent

Previously obtained consent must be reviewed prior to investigation or treatment, and especially where:

- significant time has elapsed between obtaining consent and the start of treatment.
- there have been material changes in the patient's condition, or in any aspects of the proposed treatment plan, which might invalidate the patient's existing consent.
- new, potentially relevant information has become available, about the risks of the treatment, for example, or about other treatment options.

Consent to research

See Research section, p.14.

Giving patients sufficient information

- Answer questions honestly, accurately, and objectively.
- Give details of the diagnosis and prognosis, including the likely prognosis if the condition is left untreated.
- Say if there are any uncertainties about the diagnosis, including options for further investigation prior to treatment.
- Give options for treatment or management of the condition, including the option not to treat.
- State the purpose of a proposed investigation or treatment, give details of the procedures or therapies involved, including subsidiary treatment such as methods of pain relief.
- Tell the patient how they should prepare for each procedure and give details of what they might experience during or afterwards, including common and serious side effects.
- Explain the likely benefits and the probabilities of success for each option, discuss any serious or frequently occurring risks, including any lifestyle changes which may be necessary as a result of the treatment.
- Say if a proposed treatment is experimental.
- State how and when the patient's condition and any side effects will be monitored or re-assessed.
- Give the name of the doctor who will have overall responsibility for the treatment and, where appropriate, give the names of the senior members of his or her team.
- State whether doctors in training will be involved, and the extent to which students may be involved in an investigation or treatment.
- Remind patients that they can change their minds about a decision at any time and that they have a right to seek a second opinion.
- Give details of any costs or charges which the patient may have to meet.
- Only withhold information that could cause a patient harm. Any information withheld from the patient shall be recorded in the notes.

Presenting information to patients

- Where possible, use up-to-date written material, visual and other aids to explain complex aspects of investigation, diagnosis or treatment.
- Make arrangements to meet particular language and communication needs wherever possible. This could involve translations, independent interpreters, signers, or the patient's representative.
- Where appropriate, discuss with patients the possibility of bringing a relative or friend, or of making a tape recording of the consultation.
- Use accurate data to explain the probabilities of success, the risk of failure of, or any harm associated with their treatment options.
- Be considerate when giving distressing information. Give patients information about counselling services and patient support groups.
- Allow patients sufficient time to reflect, before and after making a decision, especially where the information is complex or the risks are serious.
- Where patients have difficulty understanding information, or where there is a lot of information to absorb, provide it in manageable amounts over a period of time, alongside written or other back-up material. You may need to repeat it.
- Involve nursing staff or other members of the health care team who may have valuable knowledge of the patient's background or particular concerns. They could help in identifying what risks the patient should be told about.
- If treatment is not to start until some time after consent has been obtained, the patient should be given a clear route for reviewing their decision with the person providing the treatment.

Establishing capacity to make decisions

Fluctuating capacity

Patients who have difficulty retaining information, or are only intermittently competent to make a decision, should be given assistance to reach an informed decision. Record any decision made while the patient is competent, including the key elements of the consultation. Review these decisions at appropriate intervals before treatment starts, to establish that this decision can be relied on.

Mentally incapacitated patients

If patients lack the capacity to make an informed decision, you may carry out an investigation or a treatment that is judged to be in their best interests—including treatment for any mental disorder—provided that they comply with it.

Advance statements

Living Wills or Advance Directives must be respected if they are relevant to the current circumstances.

Children and consent

At 16 years old a young person can be treated as an adult and can be presumed to have the capacity to make an informed decision. A child under 16 may have the capacity to make an informed decision, depending on their ability to understand what is involved.

Where a competent child refuses treatment, a person with parental responsibility or the court, may authorize an investigation or treatment which is in the child's best interests. The position is different in Scotland, where those with parental responsibility cannot authorize procedures a competent child has refused. Legal advice may be helpful on how to deal with such cases.

Box 16.1 'Best interests' principle

This involves looking at the following questions;
- Are there any alternative options for treatment or investigation which are clinically indicated?
- Is there any evidence of the patient's previously expressed preferences, including an advance statement?
- What is your own and the health care team's knowledge of the patient's background, such as cultural, religious, or employment issues?
- What are the views about the patient's preferences given by a third party who may have knowledge of the patient, for example the patient's partner, family, carer, tutor-dative (Scotland), or a person with parental responsibility?
- Which option least restricts the patient's future choices, where more than one option (including non-treatment) seems reasonable in the patient's best interest?

Applying to the court

Application to the court may be needed if a patient's capacity to consent is in doubt or if there are differences of opinion over the patient's best interest. This can occur for non-therapeutic or controversial treatments such as organ donation, sterilisation or turning off life support.

Complications of ear surgery

There are risks with all surgical procedures. The degree of risk is related to both the specific procedure and to the underlying pathology. The patient should be given an indication of the likely risk in a sensitive way, so that they are not frightened into abandoning surgery.

A full explanation of the underlying condition will highlight the risks of leaving an ear disease untreated. Risks should be documented in the case notes and on the consent form.

The list of complications for CSOM is similar to that of the operation—the untreated disease carries similar risks as the operation. These are:

- Hearing loss—temporary and permanent. Always obtain an audiogram at least within 3 months of surgery, but preferably nearer to surgery and perform pre-op tuning fork tests and document your findings
- Tinnitus—temporary and permanent
- Vertigo or unsteadiness—temporary and permanent
- Facial nerve palsy—temporary and permanent
- Wound infection
- Need for further surgery
- Formation of mastoid cavity
- Need for ongoing care e.g. aural toilet for mastoid cavities.

Inter-operative considerations

These can be avoided by taking precautions, e.g. always setting up and checking items such as facial nerve monitors yourself. The precautions undertaken in theatre, such as the use of a facial nerve monitor, should be recorded on the operation note. Any inter-operative unusual findings or complications should be witnessed and recorded by a senior colleague if available.

Immediate post-operative period

Check for facial nerve palsy in recovery.

Post-operative ward review

Facial nerve function should be checked, along with the eye movements for nystagmus. Webber's tuning fork test should be done. The patient should localise to the operated ear.

Complications of nasal surgery

Nasal surgery includes a large range of procedures on both the external and the internal nose. Procedures on the sinuses are also included.

Complications of external nose surgery

- Imperfect cosmetic result
- Poor healing of incisions/granuloma and keloid formation
- Bruising
- Ecchymosis
- Need to wear a nasal splint for a week
- Swelling
- Need for packing.

Complications of internal nose surgery

- Bleeding and need for packing
- Infection
- Change in nasal shape e.g. supratip depression with sub-mucous resection (SMR)
- Persistence of nasal blockage for 3 months
- Need for adjunctive medication.

Complications of sinus surgery

- Bleeding
- Infection
- Orbital damage
- Optic nerve damage
- CSF leak
- Orbital haematoma.

Prevention of complications

Intra-operative considerations

- Good vasoconstriction to maximize vision in operative field and prevent blood loss
- Head up position to improve venous drainage
- Using preoperative CT scans displayed during surgery to avoid unexpected anatomical variations
- Use of steroids to reduce oedema in rhinoplasty
- Swab samples for infected sinus problems.

Post-operative problems

- Observation for bleeding—repack if necessary
- Check for orbital haemorrhage
- Check for visual disturbance.

Complications of head and neck surgery

These procedures are often prolonged. They can have high morbidity rates and sometimes an associated mortality. The patient group is older and the co-morbidities associated with heavy smoking and alcohol abuse make the risks even higher.

Major risks
- Death
- Cardiovascular complications
- MI
- DVT
- Chest infections
- PE
- Flap failure.

Pre-operative considerations
- Prophylactic antibiotics
- Thromboembolic prophylaxis
- Chest physiotherapy
- Pre-operative nutrition—involve dietician
- Stop smoking
- Admit early for assessment and alcohol detox if necessary.

Post-operative considerations
- Continued thromboembolic prophylaxis and early mobilisation
- Antibiotics
- Chest physiotherapy
- Balance between analgesia and respiratory depression
- Early removal of central and peripheral lines
- Removal of urinary catheter
- Tracheostomy care
- Avoidance of pressure sores
- Early action if suspected complication
- Postoperative care on ITU for selected patients
- Nursing protocols and flap observations (see p.368).

Tonsillectomy

Indications

- Recurrent acute tonsillitis
- Chronic tonsillitis
- Obstructive sleep apnoea syndrome
- Oropharyngeal obstruction
- Following 2 quinsies
- Suspected malignancy
- Diagnosis of variant CJD.

Pre-operative checks

Confirm that the operation is still needed and examine the ENT system for associated features. Discuss the surgery, complications, and the need for time off work or school.

Procedure

Give the patient a GA and keep them supine with a bolster under shoulder and their head in a head ring. This position extends head on body. The postnasal space is lower than the oropharynx, so blood collects there (Fig. 16.1). Insert a Boyle–Davis gag with Doughty modification for anaesthetic tube. Place the Draffin bipod to suspend gag. Incise the mucosa over the anterior pillar.

The tonsil is removed by dissection in the peritonsillar space. Ensure that there is adequate tonsil bed haemostasis.

Post-operative care

Give appropriate pain relief and encourage the patient to move around. Give food as and when it is tolerated. Monitor the patient for blood loss. Major blood loss is obvious, but minor loss in a young child manifests itself as a rising pulse without increasing pain.

Complications

- Primary haemorrhage <1% (see p.430)
- Secondary haemorrhage 5–10% (see p.430)
- Infection
- Poor pain control.

Length of stay

Depends on the unit, the patient may stay in for the day, or overnight.

Discharge advice

Regular analgesia should be taken as the pain often increases around five to seven days after the operation. Give the patient contact details and advice in case of haemorrhage. They should stay off work or school for two weeks and avoid boisterous activity for two weeks.

Fig. 16.1. Diagram showing tonsillectomy position

Adenoidectomy

Indications

The patient may have adenoid problems as a result of, or alongside glue ear treatment. Removal of the adenoids aids the resolution of glue ear. Patients may experience recurrent adenoiditis or obstructive sleep apnoea syndrome.

Pre-operative checks

- Confirm the diagnosis and the presence of glue with tympanometry.
- Discuss the surgery, complications, and need for time off work or school.
- Examine the ENT system for associated features and check the palate for bifid uvula.

Procedure

- Administer the patient a general anaesthetic.
- Position them supine with the cervical spine straight. If the spine is extended as in a tonsillectomy position, the vertebral body of C2 is very prominent and can lead to excess bleeding from PNS after curettage if inadvertently damaged.
- Check for bifid uvula or submucous cleft.
- Insert an adenoid curette through the mouth into the PNS—curette the adenoidal pad.
- Alternatively, the adenoid can be removed under direct vision with suction monopolar diathermy.
- Haemostasis with pressure from swab placed in PNS.

Post-operative care

Give the patient analgesia and observe them for primary haemorrhage.

Complications

Primary haemorrhage is rare at less than 1%. If it is uncontrolled it needs a PNS pack, sedation and an ITU stay for very young children.

A hyper nasal voice (called rhinolalia aperta) may occur if there is a defect in the soft palate. Subtle malformations such as submucous cleft can be easy to miss and should be looked for before performing an adenoidectomy.

Length of stay

An adenoidectomy is usually a daycase, with the patient discharged after 4 hours, unless it is with a tonsillectomy.

Discharge advice

Advise the patient to take regular analgesia and stay off school for 1 week.

Grommet insertion

Indications

The patient may present with glue ear, recurrent acute otitis media and/or persistent middle ear effusion. They may have Eustachian tube dysfunction. Rarely, the patient may be undergoing hyperbaric oxygen therapy and cannot equalize pressure.

Pre-operative checks

Check that the operation is still required and check tympanometry ± audiogram. Examine the patient's EAC to check access if the operation is being done under local anaesthetic.

Procedure

- Use a local or a general anaesthetic.
- If a local anaesthetic is used, EMLA cream should be instilled under microscope control. Wait for 60 minutes (send the patient for a cup of tea). Remove the cream by microsuction.
- Using a microscope, insert an ear speculum and identify the antero-inferior segment. Perform a radial myringotomy using a myringotome. Enough fluid is aspirated to allow the grommet to be inserted. The grommet is placed in the myringotomy hole with crocodile forceps, and then adjusted with a needle as required.
- If bleeding occurs, use steroid drops to help prevent the grommet blocking.

Post-operative care

Use minimal analgesia and give a course of steroid ear drops if there is bleeding at the time of insertion.

Complications

This procedure has very few complications. Occasionally, there may be an infective discharge. Treat this with antibiotic and steroid drops for 1 week.

Length of stay

This procedure is done as a daycase.

Discharge advice

Avoid swimming for 2 weeks. Many children will swim with grommets in place and have no problem, however precautions should be taken if discharge follows swimming. Use vaseline and cotton wool earplugs with a swimming hat when bathing. Use similar ear plugs for hair washing. Request a grommet check—community audiogram after 6 weeks—to see if there has been any improvement in hearing.

Septoplasty

Indications
The patient may present with nasal obstruction or may be having treatment for epistaxis. A bent septum can limit surgical access to the sinuses—a septoplasty may be needed to correct this before sinus surgery.

Pre-operative checks
Discuss the surgery, complications and the need for time off work with the patient. Examine their ENT system for associated features of rhinitis. Discuss their need for possible continuing treatment for associated rhinitis.

Procedure
Give a general anaesthetic, or a local anaesthetic if the patient is very infirm. Lay the patient supine with their head flexed on head ring. The patient's head should be tilted up.

The local anaesthetic and adrenaline mixture should be infiltrated into the septum. Approach the septum via a hemitransfixion incision. The mucoperichondrial flaps should be elevated and the cartilage repositioned. Resect gross deviations. The 1cm dorsal and anterior struts should be preserved to keep support. The incision should be sutured and the nose packed if necessary.

Post-operative care
Advise the patient to keep their head up and to avoid blowing their nose for 1 week. They should undertake minimal activity for 2 weeks.

Complications
There may be some bleeding.

Length of stay
Daycase or overnight stay.

Discharge advice
Avoid strenuous activity for 2 weeks. Nasal toilet with saline sniffs should be performed 4 times a day for 2 weeks.

Chapter 17

Ward care

Pre-operative care

Pre-assessment

The process of pre-assessment has become established. In many units nurse-led pre-assessment clinics can identify problems ahead of the planned surgery date, thus avoiding costly delays in the operating schedule. These clinics can only run efficiently if there is good communication between the doctor, nurse, and the anaesthetist.

Protocols have been developed to ensure that only appropriate investigations are ordered, to avoid unnecessary expense.

Clerking

- Effective documentation is important for improved care and to fulfill medico-legal requirements.
- The minimum standard is a confirmation of the need for the surgery or investigation, an ENT examination, a list of medications with known allergies and a list of the results from any investigations ordered.
- Documentation of the consent process is usually provided by the consent form, which is kept in the patient's notes.

Investigations

- Any investigations ordered should be based on the protocol, and discussed with the anaesthetist
- The first step is ordering investigations; but most important is finding and documenting the results of the investigations.

Special considerations

Deep vein thrombosis (DVT) prophylaxis

The risk of DVT for all surgical patients should be classified as low/medium/high. This is determined by the length of surgery, the patient's underlying condition and their past thromboembolic history.

Low	Compression stockings
Medium	Compression stockings + LMW heparin + intraoperative compression boots
High	Stockings + LMW heparin and intraoperative pneumatic compression boots

---

Box 17.1 Low molecular weight heparin e.g. dalteparin sodium

Medium risk	2500U 1–2 hrs pre-op
	2500U every 24hrs until ambulatory
High risk	2500U 1–2 hrs pre-op
	5000U every 24hrs

Antibiotic prophylaxis

Antibiotics may be given to patients with pre-existing cardiac problems such as valve problems, or for patients who have had major head and neck surgery, to reduce the risk of post-operative infection and fistula formation.

- Cefuroxime 1.5g 8hrly for 5 days
- Metronidazole 500mg PR 8hrly 5 days

Diabetic patients

Diabetic patients should be placed first on the operating list. Take regular BM-stix to monitor sugar level. Use a sliding scale insulin regime until eating if insulin dependent.

Post-operative care

Documentation

It is important to document the patient's daily progress and ward round instructions. Any important changes during the day should also be documented. Use a system approach for major head and neck patients e.g. CVS/RS/nutrition etc.

Drain care

Monitor drainage for a 24 hour period. Remove when it has drained less than 30ml in a 24 hour period. If the drain loses its vacuum or becomes 'devacced', examine drain position, change the drain bottle for a new one, and consider pressure to the wound or connect the drain to continuous low pressure wall suction.

Nutrition/fluid balance

Involve dietician for long term feeding requirements.

Fluid and electrolytes

Calculate 24 hour maintenance fluid requirements by the patient's weight:
- 0–10kg   100ml/kg per 24hrs
- 11–20kg   1000ml + 50ml/kg/24hrs
- 20kg+   1500ml + 20ml/kg/24hrs

This volume of fluid requires a composition of 1–2 mEq of Na^+ and 0.5 mEq K^+ per kg/24hrs.

- 1 litre N/saline contains 154mEq of Na^+
- 1 litre D/saline contains 77mEq of Na^+

Maintenance is best undertaken with dextrose/saline to avoid sodium overload plus addition of 20mmol/L of K^+.

- **Properly kept fluid balance charts are essential in order to monitor the patient's fluid input and output.**

Calories

Post-operative patients require between 40 and 70 Kcal per kg per day. Most ENT patients will be able to be fed either via the mouth or via a nasogastric tube—enteral feeding.

Monitoring intake of calories and other vital substances
- Check weight daily
- Keep a food record chart
- Do regular urinalysis for glucose
- Check levels of FBC, calcium, magnesium, phosphate, zinc, LFTs, U+Es as required
- Vitamins and trace elements screen.

Box 17.2 How to unblock a blocked nasogastric tube

- Flush with water
- Flush with soda water
- Flush with a 5% sodium bicarbonate solution
- Aspirate tube with empty syringe
- Flush tube with smaller syringe
- Use Creon powder with sodium bicarbonate to flush the tube.

Care of myocutaneous flaps

It is very important to monitor the viability of these flaps accurately. Often patients are nursed on wards with limited plastic surgery expertise.

- Ask your local plastic surgeon about the post-operative protocol for the care of free flaps.

General principles

- Maintain intravascular volume
- Maintain oxygen carrying haematocrit but not polycythaemia
- Monitor flap appearance by using a flap chart
- Monitor flap blood supply e.g. Doppler flow.

Protocol example

- Keep pulse <100
- Maintain systolic BP >100mmHg
- Keep urine output >35ml/hr
- Aim for haemoglobin level of 8.5–10.5g/dl
- If haematocrit <25 give blood
- If haematocrit >35 give colloid

Flap observations

- Doppler and colour observations
- Every 30 min for the first 4 hours, then
- Every hour for the next 48 hours, then
- Every 2 hours for the next 48 hours

Tracheostomy care

The formation of a tracheostomy causes some physiological problems; mainly because it bypasses the nose. The initial requirements of inspired air are humidification, warming and filtering. After 48 hours the mucous glands in the trachea hypertrophy and help in this process.

Irritation caused by the tube

- The presence of the tube can cause coughing and excess secretion from the bronchopulmonary tree.
- Regular suction and inner tube cleaning may be needed as often as every 30 minutes in the initial stages.

Securing the tube

The first tube is usually sutured to the skin to prevent dislodgement. Tapes are then applied, unless there is a free flap where the feeding vessels may be occluded.

In the first week after a tracheostomy the tube should be treated very carefully to prevent dislodgement. The tract between the skin and the trachea is poorly developed and tube displacement during this time could be catastrophic.

▶ Important

Always keep a spare tracheostomy tube and tracheal dilators by the bedside of tracheostomy patients.

Communication with patients and relatives

This is a very important area and one that can cause difficulties. Always treat patients and relatives as you would expect to be treated in a similar situation.

Communication is not just about sitting down and talking with a patient. It can be as informal as saying good morning in the corridor, or smiling at a patient in a bed near the nurses' station.

Basic principles
- Read the patient's notes thoroughly and be prepared before any formal talk with a patient or their relatives.
- Speak to the nurse looking after the patient for any relevant information.
- Take the nurse with you as a witness or mediator.
- Always speak plainly and try to be honest.

▶ If you are kind and courteous you will have few problems.

Discharge planning

- There is always pressure to discharge patients from the ward with the greatest of haste. Prior planning, often before surgery, can help with this process.
- Nursing staff have good protocols—so liaise with them and seek their advice.

General points

Consideration of the following questions will help in planning effective discharge:

- Is the patient fit to leave—are they orientated, mobile and pain free?
- Is the patient's nutritional support catered for?
- Is their wound satisfactory?
- Does the patient need transport?
- Do they have enough medication—both that prescribed in hospital and their regular medication?
- Do any medications need monitoring—such as warfarin?
- Does the patient's GP need to know that the patient is leaving hospital before the discharge letter arrives?
- Is a district nurse required?
- Is outpatient follow up organised?

Allied health professionals

Who are allied health professionals?

This term covers a number of different professional groups including:
• Audiologists
• Hearing therapists
• Speech and Language Therapists (SALT)
• Head and Neck Specialist Nurses
• Dietician
• Aural Care Nurse.

They all have different roles and these are explained in the following pages.

Modern ENT practice has become multidisciplinary and the involvement of these professionals, alongside members of the medical team, has enhanced patient care significantly.

There are many other personnel who are equally important to patient care such as physiotherapists and occupational therapists. These are not discussed in this handbook.

▶ It is important to use these professional services properly. Get to know the names of the staff in your department, and find out their particular skills and interests. Try to sit in on their clinics to obtain first hand knowledge of their areas of expertise.

Communicate with these other professionals and give them the respect that their expertise deserves.

The audiologist

The majority of an audiologist's work is with older people and young children. These age groups comprise the majority of hearing problems. The audiologist has a wide-ranging role, encompassing many aspects of patient care.

The main duties of an audiologist are:
• To assess hearing problems
• To rehabilitate hearing loss with aids
• To assess balance disorders
• To rehabilitate balance disorders
• To give counselling for hearing problems.

Many audiologists specialise within the field of audiology. Particular specialities include:
• Paediatric audiology
• Cochlear implant rehabilitation.

The role of the audiologist is extended to allow for liaison with peripatetic services in the community. A child of school age will require support in school if their hearing loss has an educational impact. The audiologist can provide an effective route of communication between the school and the ENT department.

▶ You will need to understand audiological tests and investigations, as they are an important aspect of ENT care. Audiologists are able to offer advice on appropriate tests and their interpretation.

Every practicing otolaryngologist should be able to perform an audiogram and a tympanogram. This is important for clinical practice, in particular, for out of hours assessment when no audiological staff are available. Watching an experienced audiologist perform an audiogram is a good way to become familiar with the technique.

The hearing therapist

This profession has evolved from duties previously undertaken in the audiology department. Many hearing therapists are fully trained audiologists.

The duties of a hearing therapist can include:
- Tinnitus counselling
- Auditory training
- Counselling for people with hearing impairment
- Supportive counselling for families
- Providing lipreading advice.

The hearing therapist can spend a considerable amount of time with each patient. This allows for an in-depth discussion of a person's difficulties. This can help to improve the quality of life of affected individuals.

Vestibular rehabilitation

Many patients have vestibular dysfunction arising from the causes discussed in Chapter 13. Central compensation for these problems is often complete and unaided. However, a large number of patients have problems in fully compensating for this type of problem. Their symptoms are often compounded by psychological problems caused by the fear of experiencing a vertigo attack. Targeted exercise programmes combined with counselling by a hearing therapist can overcome these difficulties.

Fig. 18.1. Tinnitus retraining–diagram of model

Speech and language therapists (SALT)

Speech and language therapists have an important role to play in some ENT conditions. Many patients who are under the care of the ENT department will need specialist input from the SALT team. A major component of their work is dealing with swallowing disorders.

The main duties of a speech and language therapist are:
- Managing communication disorders. This includes:
  - Assessing the communication capacity of a patient
  - Helping to determine the prognosis for regaining speech
  - Determining the patient's need for communication and the aids required
  - Providing appropriate advice.
- Managing dysphagia. This includes:
  - Assessing the type of swallowing problem
  - Assessing the risk of aspiration
  - Assessing possible interventions.

As well as their general duties, the SALT team form part of the multidisciplinary team managing patients with head and neck cancer and voice disorders.

Voice rehabilitation after laryngectomy

Patients undergoing laryngectomy often fear that they will be unable to communicate after surgery. SALTs may help by introducing patients who have already undergone surgery to demonstrate the range of options for rehabilitation. The options for communication after surgery can include:
- Pen and paper
- Magnetic writing tablets such as Etch-a-sketch
- Oesophageal speech
- Electric larynx
- Tracheo-oesophageal valves.

The head and neck specialist nurse

This nurse specialist is often the glue which holds the head and neck cancer multidisciplinary team together. The role of the head and neck specialist nurse spans the whole of patient care from diagnosis to pre-operative planning to follow up.

These nurses are uniquely placed to manage patient care; their job flexibility allows them to be active in the community and to extend their care into the home environment. Patients will often view the head and neck nurse as their first point of contact. They are involved early on at the diagnosis stage, up to the patient's final discharge from the clinic.

The main duties of the head and neck specialist nurse are :
• Counselling the patient and their family
• Explaining and giving information on every aspect of care
• Liaising with other members of the multidisciplinary team
• Assessing the suitability of care options—for example, how the patient might cope with radical surgery
• Mobilising support from the family and community services.

Background of head and neck specialist nurses

These are usually very experienced senior grade nurses from head and neck specialties. They will have had previous responsibility, usually at ward sister/charge nurse level. They will have have a degree level qualification and experience in head and neck or oncological care.

They will also have good counselling skills and the personality to cope with this demanding job.

Extended roles

A head and neck specialist nurse may also have additional roles:
• Nurse trainer
• Research co-ordinator
• Protocol design
• Independent follow-up clinics.

Dietician

From a nutritional point of view, head and neck cancer patients present a wide variety of challenges. The dietician is an extremely important member of the multidisciplinary team.

The main duties of a dietician are:
- To assess the nutritional status of patients
- To identify specific nutritional concerns
- To plan dietary interventions
- To monitor the patient's response to an intervention.

On-going research is often an important part of a dietician's role. For example, the role of salicylates in patients with ASA triad and nasal polyps.

Specific problems and areas of work dealt with by a dietician:

- Pre-operative malnutrition
  - Due to dysphagia from primary tumour
  - Cachexia of malignancy
  - Associated alcohol abuse
- Planning pre-operative feeding regime
- Planning pre-operative route of nutrition such as PEG/NG tube
- Post-operative nutrition
  - Avoiding re-feeding syndrome
  - Managing nutrition in the absence of swallowing
  - Non functioning alimentary tract
  - Intolerance to enteral nutrition
  - Electrolyte disturbance
- Discharge planning
- On-going care including liaising with community nurses and the patient's family
- Dietary review in outpatients.

Box 18.1 Houseman's tip

Dieticians often have essential knowledge of electrolyte replacement and supplementation. This expert knowledge can help in planning nutritional requirements for the optimum care of patients. They will also give advice about the frequency and type of investigations needed to monitor these parameters.

Aural care nurse

Aural care nurses provide an important service in the management of ear disorders and have taken on many aspects of otological care. They are trained to recognise problems in the ear canal and the tympanic membrane. They are also skilled in using the operating microscope. Shared care of patients is important and these nurses should be supervised by, or in close contact with, an otologist.

Areas of expertise of an aural care nurse include:
- Wax removal
- Pre and post-operative care of patients undergoing ear surgery
- Continued aural care for chronic ear disorders
- Diagnosis and management of otitis externa
- Treatment of mastoid cavity problems.

The aural care nurse's efficient management of these conditions—which represent a large amount of clinical otological practice—has led to increased capacity in the outpatient department.

Aural care nurses are graded 1–3 depending on their level of experience. Grade 3 aural care nurses are able to undertake the full range of aural care from a simple de-wax to the maintenance and cleaning of complex ears with distorted anatomy.

Areas of potential for extending the role of aural care nurses are:
- Direct referral from GP or A&E
- Nurse prescribing
- Research and development
- Guideline and protocol development.

▶ Time spent working and learning from an aural care nurse can help you develop the skills necessary to perform ear surgery. Experience in using instruments with the operating microscope significantly enhances hand and eye co-ordination.

Chapter 19

Practical procedures

How to cauterize the nose

Always ensure that you have performed adequate first aid steps before attempting to pack or cauterize the nose (see Chapter 20, p.418).

Procedure

- Apply one or two cotton buds or a dental roll soaked in 1:200,000 adrenaline or 5% cocaine solution to the area, and apply pressure for at least two minutes.
- Silver nitrate sticks may be applied to the bleeding point for one or two seconds at a time. Avoid using this form of cautery if the nose is actively bleeding since the blood will simply wash the chemical away. In addition to being ineffective, this will cause unwanted burns to the lip, nose or throat. Instead, wait for the vasoconstrictive effects of the cocaine to work, then apply pressure to the bleeding point. This will nearly always stop the bleeding temporarily before cautery.
- Apply the silver nitrate in a circle starting a few mm from the bleeding point. This will allow any feeding blood vessels to be dealt with prior to cauterizing the main bleeding vessel.
- It may be necessary to reapply the adrenaline or cocaine soaked cotton wool to reduce the bleeding between attempts at cautery.
- If the nose is still bleeding reapply pressure, and consider packing the nose.
- Electro or hot wire cautery may be used to good effect in experienced hands.

How to pack the nose

N.B. always ensure that you have performed adequate first aid steps before attempting to pack or cauterise the nose (see Chapter 20, p.418).

When packing the nose, the aim is to put pressure on the bleeding vessel and prevent an active haemorrhage, so that the normal thrombotic mechanisms can act. Nasal packs are usually left in place for 24–48 hours. They must be secured anteriorly to prevent them falling back into the airway. Prophylactic antibiotics are often used. Patients should be admitted and are often lightly sedated. Different methods and materials are used to pack the nose.

Anterior nasal packing
Nasal tampons

Nasal tampons are the simplest way to pack the nose (see Fig. 19.1.). They consist of a dry sponge, which is placed into the nasal cavity and then hydrated with water or saline. The sponge then dramatically increases in size, putting pressure on the bleeding area. The nasal tampon should be lubricated with a little antibiotic cream (Naseptin). Then simply lift the tip of the nose and slide the tampon into the nasal cavity ensuring that it is passed parallel to the floor of the nose and not towards the top of the head. A little water or saline is then dripped onto the tampon, which is secured by taping the attached string to the face.

BIPP packing

In this procedure, bismuth iodine and paraffin paste is used to impregnate a length of ribbon gauze. This mixture is antiseptic. Some skill and a good light is needed to place this form of nasal pack effectively. Topical analgesia such as cocaine spray is essential prior to packing.

Posterior nasal packing
Epistaxis balloon or urinary catheter

A variety of special nasal balloons are available (see Fig. 19.2.). They are easy to insert and are particularly helpful when the bleeding point is posterior. A Foley urinary catheter is also effective. This is passed into the nasopharynx, inflated and then pulled anteriorly so that it occludes the posterior choana. It is prevented from slipping back into the nasopharynx or mouth by means of a clamp, which is placed at the nasal vestibule. It is important to put some padding between the skin and a clamp to ensure no pressure damage is caused. Additional anterior nasal packs may be inserted as above where needed.

Fig. 19.1. Nasal tampons

Fig. 19.2. Epistaxis balloons

How to remove foreign bodies

You will need
- A good light
- A cooperative patient
- Good equipment.

The first attempt will usually be the best tolerated. If you are not confident that you will be able to remove the foreign body, refer to ENT for more experienced help.

Foreign bodies in the ear

Signs and symptoms
- Pain
- Deafness
- Unilateral discharge
- Bleeding
- May be symptomless.

Management
- Children will usually require a general anaesthetic unless they are remarkably cooperative.
- Insects may be drowned with olive oil.
- Syringing may be used if you can be certain there is no trauma to the ear canal or drum.
- Use a head lamp or mirror, an operating auroscope or an operating microscope.
- Soft foreign bodies such as cotton wool may be grasped with a pair of crocodile or Tilley's forceps.
- Solid foreign bodies such as a bead, are best removed by passing a wax hook or Jobson–Horne probe beyond the foreign body and gently pulling towards you.

Refer to senior staff ± GA if:
- Failed attempt
- Uncooperative child
- Suspected trauma to the drum.

Foreign bodies in the nose

Signs and symptoms
- Unilateral foul smelling discharge
- Unilateral nasal obstruction
- Unilateral vestibulitis
- Epistaxis.

Management
- An auroscope can easily be used to examine a child's nose.
- Ask the child to blow their nose if they are able.
- Solid foreign bodies such as beads are best removed by passing a wax hook or Jobson–Horne probe beyond the foreign body and gently pulling it towards you. Avoid grasping the object with a pair of forceps, since this may simply push it further back into the nose or airway.
- Soft foreign bodies may be grasped and removed with crocodile or Tilley's forceps.

Refer to senior staff if:
- Failed removal
- Uncooperative child.

Foreign bodies in the throat
See also Oesophageal foreign bodies, Chapter 20, p.428. The cause is often fish, chicken or lamb bones.

Signs and symptoms
- Acute onset of symptoms (not days later)
- Constant pricking sensation on every swallow
- Drooling
- Dysphagia
- Localised tenderness in the neck, if above the thyroid cartilage then look carefully in the tongue base and tonsil regions
- Pain on rocking the larynx from side to side
- Soft tissue swelling.

Management
- Use a good light to examine the patient.
- Anaesthetise the throat using Xylocaine spray.
- Try feeling for a foreign body (FB) even if you cannot see one in the tonsil or tongue base.
- Perform an AP & lateral soft tissue X-ray of the neck looking for foreign bodies at the common sites (see Fig. 19.3.). Pay particular attention to the:
- Flecks of calcification around the thyroid cartilage are common on X-ray.
  - Tonsil
  - Tongue base/vallecula
  - Posterior pharyngeal wall.
- Tilley's forceps are best for removing foreign bodies in the mouth.
- McGill's intubating forceps may be useful for removing foreign bodies in the tongue base or pharynx.

Refer for endoscopy under GA in case of:
- Airway compromise—**URGENT**
- Failed removal
- Good history but no FB seen
- X-ray evidence of a FB.

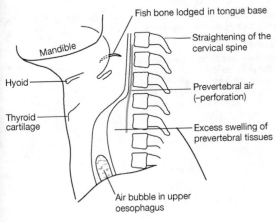

Fig. 19.3. Lateral soft tissues X-ray of the neck

How to syringe an ear

See Fig. 19.4. Check that the patient has no previous history of TM perforation, grommet insertion, middle ear or mastoid surgery.

Procedure
- Warm the water to body temperature
- Pull the pinna up and back
- Use a dedicated ear syringe
- Aim the jet of water towards the roof of the ear canal
- STOP if the patient complains of pain.

Water jet aimed along roof of ear canal

Reciver to collect water, placed under the ear.
Held in position by the patient

Fig. 19.4. How to syringe an ear

How to dry mop an ear

A dry mop should be performed in any ear which is discharging, before topical antibiotics and steroid ear drops are instilled.

Procedure
- Tease out a clean piece of cotton wool into a flat sheet
- Twist this onto a suitable carrier such as an orange stick, a Jobson–Horne probe, or even a clean matchstick see Fig. 19.5
- Gently rotate the soft end of the mop in the outer ear canal
- Discard the cotton wool and make a new mop—continue until the wool is returned clean

Fig. 19.5. Diagram of an ear mop

How to instill ear drops

See Fig. 19.6.

Procedure

- Lie the patient down with the affected ear uppermost
- Straighten the ear canal by pulling the pinna up and back
- Squeeze in the appropriate number of drops
- Use a gentle pumping motion of your finger in the outer ear canal. This will encourage the drops to penetrate into the deep ear canal.

Consider using an 'otowick'. This is like a preformed sponge and it acts as a reservoir, helping to prevent the drops leaking out of the ear canal. An otowick is particularly useful in otitis externa.

HOW TO INSTILL EAR DROPS

Lie the patient down
with the ear uppermost

Pull the pinna
'upward and
backwards'

Apply digital pumping

(a)

(b)

Fig. 19.6. How to instill ear drops

How to drain a haematoma of the pinna

This usually occurs after direct trauma to the pinna. It is often caused by a sports injury such as boxing or rugby. If left untreated it may leave a permanent deformity such as a 'cauliflower' ear.

Do not neglect the associated head injury which may take priority over the ear injury.

Procedure

- Aspiration may be satisfying, but the collection nearly always reforms, so it is probably best avoided.
- Refer for drainage in sterile conditions.
- Incise the skin of the pinna under local anaesthesia in the helical sulcus (see Fig. 19.7.).
- Milk out the haematoma.
- Do not close the wound.
- Apply pressure to the ear to prevent recollection, either by packing the contours of the ear with proflavine or saline soaked cotton wool, and apply a head bandage. Alternatively use a through and through mattress suture tied over a bolster or dental roll.
- Give antibiotics.
- Review in 4–5 days.

Fig. 19.7. Haematoma pinna incision

How to drain a quinsy

Signs and symptoms

- Sore throat—worse on one side
- Pyrexia
- Trismus
- Drooling
- Fetor
- Peritonsillar swelling
- Displacement of the uvula away from the affected side (see Fig. 19.8.).

Procedure

- This procedure usually requires admission.
- Re-hydrate with IV fluids.
- IV antibiotics.
- Spray the throat with xylocaine or inject lignocaine into the mucosa as shown.
- Lie the patient down.
- Get a good light and a sucker.
- Use a 5ml syringe and a large bore needle or IV cannula to perform 3 point aspiration (see Fig. 19.8.).
- Send any pus obtained to microbiology.
- Reserve incision for those cases which recur or fail to resolve within 24 hrs.

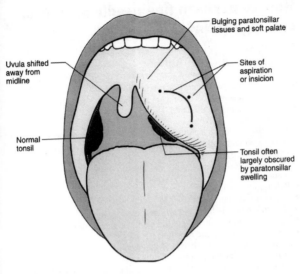

Fig. 19.8. Quinsy/incision/aspiration

How to perform fine needle aspiration cytology (FNAC)

Procedure

- Lie the patient down
- Clean the skin with alcohol
- Fix the lump between finger and thumb
- Use a fine needle (blue or orange) attached to a 10ml syringe
- Pass the needle into the lump
- Apply suction
- Move the needle back and forth through the lump using small vibration type movements—this can prevent contamination by sampling other tissues
- Make some rotary movements in order to remove a small core of tissue
- Release the suction
- Then remove the needle
- Detach the needle from the syringe and fill it with air
- Replace the needle and expel the contents onto a microscope slide
- Remove the needle and repeat as necessary
- Check the inside of the barrel of the needle for any tissue which may have become lodged there
- Take a second slide and place it on top of the first, sandwiching the sample between the two
- Briskly slide the two apart, spreading the sample thinly and evenly
- Fix and label the slides.

Emergency airway procedures

(See Chapter 8, p.184)

Chapter 20

ENT emergencies

Epistaxis

Epistaxis, or a nosebleed, is a common problem, which will affect most of us at sometime in our lives. It is usually mild and self-limiting.

Causes of epistaxis

Local causes
- Nose picking
- Idiopathic
- Trauma
- Infection
- Tumours.

Systemic causes
- Hypertension
- Anticoagulant drugs
- NSAIDs
- Coagulopathy (haemophilia, leukaemia, DIC, Von Willebrand's disease)
- Hereditary haemorrhagic telangiectasia (an inherited condition with a weakness of the capillary walls leading to haemangioma formation).

The anterior part of the nasal septum is the most frequent site for bleeding. It has a rich blood supply and a propensity for digital trauma. This part of the nose is known as Little's area (see Fig. 20.1.).

Firstaid for epistaxis

See Fig. 20.2. The patient should be advised to:
- Lean forward
- Pinch the fleshy part of the nose (not the bridge) for 10 minutes
- Avoid swallowing the blood
- Put an icepack on the nasal bridge
- Suck an ice cube.

Resuscitation

- Assess blood loss
- Take the pulse
- Measure the blood pressure
- Gain intravenous access
- Set up intravenous infusion
- Full blood count
- Group and save.

See How to cauterize/pack the nose, pp.394–6.

Fig. 20.1. Little's area

Fig. 20.2. Epistaxis first aid

Sudden onset hearing loss

Acute sensorineural hearing loss (SNHL) is an ENT emergency. It usually has an acute onset and is sometimes associated with balance disturbance.

Investigations

- Take a full drug history
- Exclude head or acoustic trauma
- Check the ear canal to exclude wax
- Check the ear drum to exclude glue ear
- Tuning fork tests:
  - Weber goes to other ear
  - Rinne AC>BC in affected ear
- Audiogram confirms hearing loss and no air/bone gap
- ESR and auto-antibodies—may be abnormal if there is an auto immune cause for the hearing loss
- MRI to exclude acoustic neuroma—request this as a routine priority unless there is associated neurology.

Management

If the patient presents within 24–48 hours of onset try empirical treatment as below, but there is little evidence base to support it:

- Admission for bed rest
- Oral steroids (prednisolone 60mg)
- Oral betahistine
- Acyclovir
- Carbogen gas (a mixture of CO_2 and O_2 given for 5min inhalation per waking hour)
- Daily audiograms.

If there is any improvement in the hearing at 48 hours, continue with the treatment. If not, discharge on a reducing course of prednisolone and acyclovir.

- Give a two week outpatient assessment and re-test the hearing.
- Chase blood and/or MRI results. Consider a hearing aid referral.

Facial palsy or VII nerve palsy

Examination of the patient will reveal if the palsy is upper or lower motor neurone type. The House–Brackmann scoring system is frequently used to record the degree of facial weakness (see Box 20.1).

Upper motor neurone palsy
- Usually as part of a stroke (CVA)
- Forehead spared
- Look for other neurological signs.

Lower motor neurone palsy
- The entire face is affected, including the forehead
- Taste disturbance may be present as taste fibres run with the chorda tympani branch of the facial nerve.

Management
- General neurological and cranial nerve exam—to exclude other neurology
- Exclude serious head injury—fracture of the temporal bone may lead to disruption of the facial nerve in its intra-temporal section.
- Examine the ear—looking for cholesteatoma, haemotympanum or disruption of the drum or canal.
- Test the hearing.
- Check the parotid for lumps.

Causes of LMN facial palsy
- Bell's palsy
- Ramsay Hunt syndrome
- Acute otitis media
- Cholesteatoma
- CPA tumours such as acoustic neuroma
- Trauma
- Parotid gland malignancies

Bell's palsy: probably viral in origin, but the diagnosis is made by excluding the other causes shown above. Starting prednisolone (40–60mg) within 48 hours improves recovery rates. Prognosis is good, 80% of patients fully recover, although returning to full function may take months. As with other causes of facial palsy, the failure of complete eye closure can lead to corneal ulceration so eye drops or lubricating gel and an eye pad at night may be required. Refer the patient to ophthalmology.

Ramsay Hunt syndrome: due to herpes zoster infection of the facial nerve. The features are similar to Bell's palsy with the addition of vesicles on the drum/ear canal/pinna/palate. The prognosis is less good.

Box 20.1 House–Brackmann grading of facial palsy

1 Complete eye closure, normal movement
2 Complete eye closure, mild weakness, barely perceptible
3 Complete eye closure, obvious weakness
4 Incomplete eye closure, obvious weakness
5 Incomplete eye closure, flicker of movement
6 Incomplete eye closure, no movement.

Periorbital cellulitis

This is a serious and sight-threatening complication of ethmoidal sinusitis. Treatment should be aimed at the underlying sinus infection, although a combined approach should be followed with input from ENT and Ophthalmology.

Presentation
- Preceding URTI
- Swelling of the upper lid and periorbital tissues
- Difficulty opening the eye
- Pain around the eye
- ± nasal discharge.

Investigations
Look for:
- Proptosis
- Pain on eye movement
- Reduced range of eye movement
- Diplopia
- Change in colour vision (red goes first)
- Change in visual acuity.

Management
- Have a high index of suspicion. If you are concerned, get a CT scan
- Get an Ophthalmic opinion
- Take a nasal swab
- Start IV broad spectrum antibiotics (e.g. Augmentin)
- Order a CT sinuses coronal (and axial views through the orbits)
- Any compromise in visual acuity/colour vision or suggestion of an intra-orbital abscess requires urgent surgical intervention.

If you are treating conservatively, ensure that regular eye observations are performed, as these patients can progress quickly towards blindness.

Fractured nose

Any patient with a fractured nose must have sustained a blow or an injury to the head. Direct trauma to the nose or face is usually from a punch, a clash of heads or a fall. Brisk but short lived epistaxis is common afterwards.

In patients with a nasal fracture always consider a head injury and/or cervical spine injury.

Investigations

The diagnosis is made on finding a new deformity to the nose, often with associated epistaxis, facial swelling and black eyes. Ask the patient if their nose has changed shape as a result of their injury. In the first few days after a nasal injury it can be difficult to assess if there is a bony injury due to the degree of associated soft tissue swelling.

- Try examining the patient from above and behind and looking along the nose from bridge to tip. See Fig. 20.3.
- X-rays are not required to make the diagnosis, but may be helpful in excluding other bony facial fractures.
- Exclude a septal haematoma by looking for a boggy swelling of the septum, which will cause total or near total nasal obstruction. This will require urgent treatment by incision and drainage in theatre.

Treatment

- Treat the head injury appropriately
- Administer first aid for epistaxis (see p.418)
- Consider nasal packing if the bleeding continues (see p.396)
- Clean and close any overlying skin injuries
- Make an ENT outpatient appointment for 5–7 days time. By then, much of the soft tissue swelling will have resolved, allowing assessment of the bony injury. If manipulation under anaesthetic (MUA) is required it can be arranged for 10–14 days after the original injury.

Fig. 20.3. Fractured nose examination (Nasal deformity is best appreciated by examining the patient from above + behind.)

Oesophageal foreign bodies

Foreign bodies often impact in the oesophagus. Most pass harmlessly, but hazardous and potentially life-threatening complications may arise. These include: para-oesophageal abscess, mediastinitis, airway obstruction, stricture formation and tracheo-oesophageal fistula.

Sharp foreign bodies carry a much higher risk of perforation. Take a good history to establish if the patient could have ingested a bone or something similar.

Signs and symptoms
- Immediate onset of symptoms
- Early presentation—hours not days
- Pain—retrosternal or back pain
- A feeling of an obstruction in the throat
- Drooling or spitting out of saliva
- Point tenderness in the neck
- Pain on rocking the laryngeal skeleton from side to side
- Hoarseness—rare
- Stridor—rare but serious.

X-ray findings (see Fig. 19.3, p.400)
- Order a plain soft tissue X-ray of the neck—lateral and AP.
- Not all bones will show on X-ray—so look for soft tissue swelling in addition to a radio-opaque object.
- Look for an air bubble in the upper oesophagus.
- Look for soft tissue swelling of the posterior pharyngeal wall—more than half a vertebral body is abnormal above C4 and more than a whole vertebral body below C4.
- If there is prevertebral air—the oesophagus has been perforated.
- Surgical emphysema is a sign of perforation.
- Loss of the normal cervical spine lordosis suggests inflammation of the pre-vertebral muscles due to an impacted foreign body or an abscess.

Treatment

Endoscopic removal under GA is often required, and is mandatory if there is any suggestion of a sharp foreign body. If the obstruction is a soft bolus, a short period of observation is appropriate with a trial of a fizzy drink (e.g. Coca-Cola) and IV smooth muscle relaxants (Buscopan).

Secondary tonsillar haemorrhage

Bleeding which occurs 5–10 days after a tonsillectomy operation is known as a secondary tonsillar haemorrhage. (A primary haemorrhage is bleeding in the first 24 hours after surgery.) A secondary haemorrhage occurs in less than 10% of cases and may result from an infection of the tonsillar fossa. This condition should not be underestimated.

- Admit the patient
- Gain intravenous access
- Give antibiotics and IV fluids.

Occasionally surgical intervention may be needed to achieve haemostasis.

Glossary of ENT terms and eponyms

Acoustic neuroma (vestibular schwannoma): A benign tumour of the eighth cranial nerve

ANCA: Anti nuclear cytoplasmic antibody: +ve in Wegeners granulomatosis

Anosmia: Loss of the sense of smell

Antrostomy: An artificially created opening between the maxillary sinus and the nasal cavity

A's: Adenoids/adenoidectomy

BAWO: Bilateral antral washouts

BINA: Bilateral intranasal antrostomy

BINP: Bilateral intranasal polypectomy

BNF: British National Formulary

BOR: Branchial-oto-renal

BPPV: Benign paroxysmal positional vertigo

BSER: Brainstem evoked response—an objective test of hearing

Cachosmia: The sensation of an unpleasant odour

Caloric tests: Tests of labyrinthine function

CAT: Combined approach tympanoplasty. A type of mastoid surgery, usually performed for cholesteatoma in which the posterior canal wall is left intact, unlike a modified radical mastoidectomy.

CHL: Conductive hearing loss

CJD: Creutzfeldt–Jakob disease

CSOM: Chronic suppurative otitis media

CT: Computerized tomography

CXR: Chest X-ray

Dohlman's operation: an endoscopic operation on a pharyngeal pouch

DL: Direct laryngoscopy

DO: Direct oesophagoscopy

DP: Direct pharyngoscopy

EAC: External auditory canal

EAM: External auditory meatus

ENG: Electronystagmography

ENT: Ear, nose, and throat

ESR: Erythrocyte sedimentation rate

EUA: Examination under (general) anaesthesia

EUM: Examination under the microscope—usually of the ears

FBC: Full blood count

FESS: Functional endoscopic sinus surgery

FNAC: Fine needle aspiration cytology

FOSIT: Medical shorthand for a feeling of something in the throat

Free flap: The movement of a piece of tissue (skin ± muscle ± bone) with a supplying artery and vein from one site in the body to another. The blood supply is connected to local blood vessels via a micro vascular anastomsis. This is most frequently performed in reconstructing surgical defects following resection of head and neck malignancies.

Freys syndrome: Gustatory sweating, a complication of parotidectomy.

GA: General anaesthetic

GORD: Gastro-oesophageal reflux disease

Globus: A sensation of a lump in the throat, when on examination no lump can be found. (see also FOSIT)

Glottis: Another name for the vocal cords

Glue ear: A common cause of conductive hearing loss, due to Eustachian tube dysfunction. The middle ear fills with thick sticky fluid, hence its name. Also known as otitis media with effusion (OME) and secretory otitis media (SOM)

Grommet: A ventilation tube placed in the eardrum in the treatment of glue ear also known as 'G's', 'tympanostomy tubes' or 'vent tubes'

HHT: Hereditary haemorrhagic telangiectasia

HIB: Haemophyllus influenza type B

HME: Heat & moisture exchanger

HPV: Human papilloma virus

IJV: Internal jugular vein

IV: Intravenous

Ludwig's angina: Infection of the submandibular space

MDT: Multi disciplinary team

MLB: A diagnostic endoscopy. Microlaryngoscopy and bronchoscopy

ML/Microlaryngoscopy: Microscopic surgical examination of the larynx using a suspended rigid laryngoscopy and a microscope

MMA: Middle meatal antrostomy. A surgical enlargement of the natural maxillary sinus ostium. See FESS

MOFIT: Multiple out fracture of the inferior turbinate. See also SMD and TITs

MRI: Magnetic resonance imaging

MRM: Modified radical mastoidectomy. Mastoid surgery performed for cholesteatoma.

MRND: Modifed radical neck dissection

MUA: Manipulation under anaesthetic

NARES: Non-allergic rhinitis with eosinophilia

NIHL: Noise induced hearing loss

od: Once daily

OME: See glue ear

OSA: Obstructive sleep apnoea

Osteomeatal complex (OMC): The area between the middle turbinate and the lateral nasal wall. The maxillary, frontal and anterior ethmoid sinuses drain into this area—the final common pathway.

Otorrhea: Ear discharge

Panendoscopy (Pan): Full ENT examination performed under general anaesthetic in order to evaluate/exclude a malignancy of the upper aerodigestive tract.

Pec. major: Pectoralis major myocutaneous flap. Frequently used to reconstruct surgical defects in the head and neck region.

PEG: Percutaneous endoscopic gastrostomy

PND: Post nasal drip

po: Per oral

post-op: Post-operative

PPI: Proton pump inhibitor

pre-op: Pre-operative

Presbycusis: The common hearing loss of old age, high frequency, bilateral and sensorineural in type.

PSCC: Posterior semi circular canal

Quinsy: Paratonsillar abscess

Ramsay Hunt Syndrome: Herpes zoster infection of the facial nerve.

Reinkes oedema: Benign oedema of the vocal cords caused by smoking.

Rhinorrhoea: Nasal discharge

SALT: Speech and language therapist

SCC: Squamous cell carcinoma

Second look: A planned staged operation to ensure that cholesteatoma has not recurred in the mastoid after CAT.

Secretory otitis media (SOM): Glue ear

Serous otitis media (SOM): Glue ear

SHO: Senior House Officer

SMR: Sub-mucous resection (of the nasal septum)

SMD: Sub-mucous diathermy to the inferior turbinates, performed to reduce the nasal obstruction associated with inferior turbinate hypertrophy.

SNHL: Sensorineural hearing loss

SOHND: Supra omohyoid neck dissection. A type of selective neck dissection

SPR: Specialist Registrar

STIR: Short tau inversion recovery

T's: Tonsils/tonsillectomy

tds: Three times daily

TITs: Trimming of the inferior turbinates. A surgical procedure performed to reduce the nasal obstruction associated with inferior turbinate hypertrophy, sometimes associated with spectacular heamorrhage!

TM: Tympanic membrane

TMJ: Temporo mandibular joint

TSH: Thyroid stimulating hormone

T-tube: Long term grommet

TTS: Temporary threshold shift

Tympanometry: The indirect measurement of the middle ear pressure or compliance of the ear drum.

Tympanostomy tube: A grommet

URT: Upper respiratory tract

URTI: Upper respiratory tract infection

VOR: Vestibulo-ocular reflux

WS: Waardenburg's syndrome

Index

CONTENTS

SECTION B

BIOCHEMICAL PRESENTATIONS

SECTION C

HAEMATOLOGICAL PRESENTATIONS

CHURCHILL'S P

Differential Diagnosis

Commissioning Editor: Laurence Hunter
Development Editor: Clive Hewat
Project Manager: Anne Dickie and Nayagi Athmanathan
Designer: Kirsteen Wright

CHURCHILL'S POCKETBOOK OF

Differential Diagnosis

Andrew T. Raftery BSc MD FRCS(Eng) FRCS(Ed)
Formerly Consultant Surgeon, Sheffield Kidney Institute, Sheffield Teaching Hospitals NHS Foundation Trust, Northern General Hospital, Sheffield; Member (formerly Chairman), Court of Examiners, Royal College of Surgeons of England; Formerly Member of Panel of Examiners, Intercollegiate Speciality Board in General Surgery; Formerly Member of Council, Royal College of Surgeons of England; Formerly Honorary Clinical Senior Lecturer in Surgery, University of Sheffield, UK

Eric Lim MB ChB MD MSc FRCS(C-Th)
Consultant Thoracic Surgeon, Royal Brompton Hospital, London; Senior Lecturer, National Heart and Lung Institute, Imperial College, London, UK

Andrew J. K. Östör MB BS FRACP
Consultant Rheumatologist and Associate Lecturer, Addenbrooke's Hospital; Director, Rheumatology Clinical Research Unit, School of Clinical Medicine, Addenbrooke's Hospital, University of Cambridge, Cambridge, UK

THIRD EDITION

CHURCHILL
LIVINGSTONE

ELSEVIER

EDINBURGH LONDON NEW YORK OXFORD
PHILADELPHIA ST LOUIS SYDNEY TORONTO 2010

CHURCHILL
LIVINGSTONE
ELSEVIER

First Edition © Harcourt Publishers Limited 2001
Second Edition © Elsevier Limited 2005
Third edition © Elsevier Limited 2010. All rights reserved.

ISBN 978-0-7020-3222-6
Reprinted 2010
International ISBN 978-0-7020-3223-3

British Library Cataloguing in Publication Data
A catalogue record for this book is available from the British Library

Library of Congress Cataloging in Publication Data
A catalog record for this book is available from the Library of Congress

Notice

Knowledge and best practice in this field are constantly changing. As new research and experience broaden our knowledge, changes in practice, treatment and drug therapy may become necessary or appropriate. Readers are advised to check the most current information provided (i) on procedures featured or (ii) by the manufacturer of each product to be administered, to verify the recommended dose or formula, the method and duration of administration, and contraindications. It is the responsibility of the practitioner, relying on their own experience and knowledge of the patient, to make diagnoses, to determine dosages and the best treatment for each individual patient, and to take all appropriate safety precautions. To the fullest extent of the law, neither the Publisher nor the Authors assumes any liability for any injury and/or damage to persons or property arising out of or related to any use of the material contained in this book.

The Publisher

We are grateful to the publishers, Elsevier, for the invitation to produce a third edition of the *Pocketbook of Differential Diagnosis*. Being in the twilight of his career, the senior author (A.T.R) felt that a further, younger co-author would be helpful in bringing the book up to date. We are pleased that Andrew Ostor, Consultant Rheumatologist at Addenbrooke's Hospital, Cambridge, has agreed to fill this role. It is now eight years since the first edition and four years since the second and in that time Eric Lim has progressed from Senior House Officer on the first edition, to Registrar on the second and is now a Consultant Thoracic Surgeon. Much has changed in that time and most of the chapters have been updated. New chapters on halitosis, hallucinations, nail abnormalities, rashes, thirst, tiredness and vaginal discharge have been added. We have also attempted to indicate the relative frequency of the various conditions by colour coding them according to whether they are considered common (green), occasional (orange) or rare (red).

We have also added new sections on biochemistry (Section B) and haematology (Section C). These list the causes of such things as hypokalaemia, hypercalcaemia, leucocytosis and anaemia and have been written in a slightly different style from the main clinical section. They provide a ready check for assessing abnormal biochemical and haematological results.

We have welcomed comments from teachers and students who have suggested additions and corrections and these have been taken into account when writing this third edition. We are pleased with the way that the first and second editions have sold and that, in these days of self-directed problem-based learning, medical students still see the need for a book offering a didactic approach.

When we originally wrote the first edition of this book, we hoped it would fit into the 'white coat pocket' and be useful on the wards. Now with the 'bare below the elbow' edict, we hope that you will have large enough pockets in the new dress code-compliant uniforms to accommodate it! We hope it will continue to help you on the wards and in the clinics – and in examinations.

A.T.R.   Sheffield
E.L.   London
A.J.K.O.   Cambridge

ACKNOWLEDGEMENTS

We wish to thank all those who have contributed to the successive editions of this book. We would particularly like to express our thanks to our junior staff and medical students who have suggested corrections, amendments and improvements to the book. Any errors that may have occurred however remain our responsibility. We would also like to thank our wives for their patience and encouragement shown throughout the production of this third edition. Mr Raftery would like to thank his secretary, Mrs Denise Smith, for the hard work and long hours she has put in to typing and re-typing the manuscript into its final form for publication (Mr Raftery cannot use a word processor!).

This book has been written in three sections: Clinical Presentations, Biochemical Presentations and Haematological Presentations.

In the Clinical Presentations section (Section A), we have attempted to indicate the relative frequency of the conditions causing the various symptoms and signs by colour coding them in green, orange and red, according to whether they are considered common, occasional or rare, respectively.

●   A common cause of the symptom or sign

●   Might occasionally give rise to the symptom or sign

●   Will only rarely cause the symptom or sign

This has been no easy task (and indeed in the Biochemical Presentations and Haematological Presentations sections we found it so difficult that we abandoned it) but we hope that it will indicate to readers whether they are dealing with a common, occasional or rare disorder. It is appreciated that some conditions may be common in the UK and rare in other parts of the world (and *vice versa*). Where this is the case, the appropriate colour coding is indicated in brackets, e.g. *Campylobacter* is a common cause of diarrhoea in the UK and therefore coded green but rare in tropical Africa and therefore coded red and in brackets. We have tried to indicate the importance of the condition, not only in causing a particular symptom or sign, but also in its overall incidence, e.g. diverticular disease is a common condition and is a common cause of pain in the left iliac fossa and is therefore coded green. It is only an occasional cause of large bowel obstruction and in this context is coded orange.

At the end of each chapter the reader will find a box containing either what we consider to be important learning points, or indicating symptoms and signs suggestive of significant pathology which require urgent action.

ABC	airway, breathing and circulation
ABGs	arterial blood gases
AC	air conduction
ACE	angiotensin-converting enzyme
ACTH	adrenocorticotrophic hormone
ADH	antidiuretic hormone
AF	atrial fibrillation
AFP	alpha fetoprotein
AIDS	acquired immunodeficiency syndrome
ANA	antinuclear antibody
ANCA	antineutrophil cytoplasmic antibody
ANF	antinuclear factor
anti-CCP	anti-cyclic citrullinated peptide
AP	anteroposterior
APTT	activated partial thromboplastin time
ARF	acute renal failure
AXR	abdominal X-ray
BC	bone conduction
BCG	bacille Calmette–Guérin
BPPV	benign paroxysmal positional vertigo
BUN	blood urea nitrogen
c-ANCA	cytoplasmic-staining antineutrophil cytoplasmic antibody
CAPD	continuous ambulatory peritoneal dialysis
CCF	congestive cardiac failure
CK-MB	creatine kinase–myocardial type
CMV	cytomegalovirus
CNS	central nervous system
COPD	chronic obstructive pulmonary disease
CRF	chronic renal failure
CREST	calcinosis cutis–Raynaud phenomenon–oesophageal hypomobility–sclerodactyly–telangiectasia
CRP	C-reactive protein
C&S	culture and sensitivity
CSF	cerebrospinal fluid
CT	computerised tomography
CVA	cerebrovascular accident
CVP	central venous pressure
CXR	chest X-ray
DDAVP	1-deamino-8-D-arginine vasopressin
DDH	developmental dysplasia of the hip
DHEA	dehydroepiandrosterone
DIC	disseminated intravascular coagulation
DIP	distal interphalangeal
DMSA	dimercaptosuccinic acid
DVT	deep venous thrombosis
EBV	Epstein–Barr virus
ECG	electrocardiogram

EEG	electroencephalogram
ELISA	enzyme-linked immunosorbent assay
EM	electron microscope
EMG	electromyography
EMSU	early morning specimen of urine
ERCP	endoscopic retrograde cholangiopancreatography
ESR	erythrocyte sedimentation rate
FBC	full blood count
FEV1	forced expiratory volume (1 second)
FNAC	fine-needle aspiration cytology
FSH	follicle-stimulating hormone
FVC	forced vital capacity
GBM	glomerular basement membrane
GCS	Glasgow Coma Scale
GI	gastrointestinal
GORD	gastro-oesophageal reflux disease
G6PD	glucose-6-phosphate dehydrogenase
GTN	glyceryl trinitrate
GUM	genito-urinary medicine
Hb	haemoglobin
βHCG	β-human chorionic gonadotrophin
5HIAA	5-hydroxyindoleacetic acid
HIV	human immunodeficiency virus
IGF-1	insulin growth factor-1
Ig	immunoglobulin
IP	interphalangeal
ITP	idopathic thrombocytopenic purpura
IVC	inferior vena cava
IVU	intravenous urography
JVP	jugular venous pressure
KUB	kidney ureter bladder (plain X-ray)
LDH	lactate dehydrogenase
LFTs	liver function tests
LH	luteinising hormone
LIF	left iliac fossa
LVF	left ventricular failure
MAG3	mercapto acetyl triglycine
MCH	mean corpuscular haemoglobin
MCHC	mean corpuscular haemoglobin concentration
MCP	metacarpophalangeal
MCV	mean corpuscular volume
ME	myalgic encephalomyelitis
MEN	multiple endocrine neoplasia
MRA	magnetic resonance angiography
MRCP	magnetic resonance cholangiopancreatography
MRI	magnetic resonance imaging
MSU	midstream specimen of urine
MTP	metatarsophalangeal

NSAID	non-steroidal anti-inflammatory drug
NSTEMI	non-ST elevation myocardial infarction
OGD	oesophagogastroduodenoscopy
PAS	periodic acid–Schiff
PCR	polymerase chain reaction
PCV	packed cell volume
PIP	proximal interphalangeal
PR	per rectum
PSA	prostate specific antigen
PT	prothrombin time
PTC	percutaneous transhepatic cholangiography
PTH	parathyroid hormone
PV	per vaginam
RAST	radio allergen sorbent test
RBC	red blood cell
RDW	red cell distribution width
RF	rheumatoid factor
RTA	road traffic accident
SIADH	syndrome of inappropriate ADH secretion
SLE	systemic lupus erythematosus
STD	sexually transmitted disease
STEMI	ST segment elevation infarction
T_4	thyroxine
TATTS	'tired all the time' syndrome
TB	tuberculosis
TFT	thyroid function test
TIA	transient ischaemic attack
TIBC	total iron-binding capacity
TPN	total parenteral nutrition
TSH	thyroid-stimulating hormone
TT	thrombin time
U&Es	urea and electrolytes
US	ultrasonography
UTI	urinary tract infection
VDRL	Venereal Disease Research Laboratory
V/Q	ventilation/perfusion ratio
WCC	white cell count

CONTENTS

SECTION A

CLINICAL PRESENTATIONS

SECTION B

BIOCHEMICAL PRESENTATIONS

SECTION C

HAEMATOLOGICAL PRESENTATIONS

SECTION A

CLINICAL PRESENTATIONS

ABDOMINAL PAIN

Abdominal pain is an extremely common presenting symptom. The pain may be acute (sudden onset) or chronic (lasting for more than a few days or presenting intermittently). It is important to be able to distinguish causes of abdominal pain which need urgent surgery, e.g. ruptured aortic aneurysm, perforated diverticular disease, from those that do not, e.g. biliary colic, ureteric colic, acute pancreatitis. The causes of abdominal pain are legion and the list below contains some of the more common causes but is not intended to be comprehensive.

CAUSES

GASTROINTESTINAL

GUT
Gastroduodenal
- Peptic ulcer
- Gastritis
- Malignancy
- Gastric volvulus

Intestinal
- Appendicitis
- Obstruction
- Diverticulitis
- Gastroenteritis
- Mesenteric adenitis
- Strangulated hernia
- Inflammatory bowel disease
- Intussusception
- Volvulus
- TB
  - (common in parts of the world where TB is endemic)

HEPATOBILIARY
- Acute cholecystitis
- Chronic cholecystitis
- Cholangitis
- Hepatitis

PANCREATIC
- Acute pancreatitis
- Chronic pancreatitis
- Malignancy

SPLENIC
- Infarction
- Spontaneous rupture

URINARY TRACT
- Cystitis
- Acute retention of urine
- Acute pyelonephritis
- Ureteric colic
- Hydronephrosis
- Tumour
- Pyonephrosis
- Polycystic kidney

GYNAECOLOGICAL
- Ruptured ectopic pregnancy
- Torsion of ovarian cyst
- Ruptured ovarian cyst
- Salpingitis
- Severe dysmenorrhoea
- Mittelschmerz
- Endometriosis
- Red degeneration of a fibroid

VASCULAR
- Aortic aneurysm
- Mesenteric embolus
- Mesenteric angina (claudication)
- Mesenteric venous thrombosis
- Ischaemic colitis
- Acute aortic dissection

PERITONEUM
- Secondary peritonitis
- Primary peritonitis

ABDOMINAL WALL
- Strangulated hernia
- Rectus sheath haematoma
- Cellulitis

RETROPERITONEUM
- Retroperitoneal haemorrhage, e.g. anticoagulants

REFERRED PAIN

- Myocardial infarction
- Pericarditis
- Testicular torsion
- Pleurisy
- Herpes zoster
- Lobar pneumonia
- Thoracic spine disease, e.g. disc, tumour

'MEDICAL' CAUSES

- Hypercalcaemia
- Uraemia
- Diabetic ketoacidosis
- Sickle cell disease
- Addison's disease
- Acute intermittent porphyria
- Henoch–Schönlein purpura
- Tabes dorsalis

HISTORY

Age

Certain conditions are more likely to occur in certain age groups, e.g. mesenteric adenitis in children, diverticular disease in the elderly.

Pain

- Time and mode of onset, e.g. sudden, gradual.
- Character, e.g. dull, vague, cramping, sharp, burning.
- Severity.
- Constancy, e.g. continuous (peritonitis); intermittent (pain of intestinal colic).
- Location: where did it start? Has it moved?
- Radiation, e.g. loin to groin in ureteric colic.
- Effect of respiration, movement, food, defecation, micturition and menstruation.
- Vomiting.
- Did vomiting precede the pain?
- Frequency.
- Character, e.g. bile, faeculent, blood, coffee grounds.

Defecation

- Constipation: absolute constipation with colicky abdominal pain, distension and vomiting suggests intestinal obstruction.
- Diarrhoea: frequency, consistency of stools, blood, mucus, pus.

Fever

- Any rigors.

Past history

- Previous surgery, e.g. adhesions may cause intestinal obstruction.
- Recent trauma, e.g. delayed rupture of spleen.
- Menstrual history, e.g. ectopic pregnancy.

EXAMINATION

General

Is the patient lying comfortably? Is the patient lying still but in pain, e.g. peritonitis? Is the patient writhing in agony, e.g. ureteric or biliary colic? Is the patient flushed, suggesting pyrexia?

Pulse, temperature, respiration

Pulse and temperature are raised in inflammatory conditions. They may also be raised with impending infarction of bowel. An increased respiratory rate might suggest chest infection referring pain to the abdomen.

Cervical lymphadenopathy

Associated with mesenteric adenitis.

Chest

Referred pain from lobar pneumonia.

Abdomen

- Inspection. Does the abdomen move on respiration? Look for scars, distension, visible peristalsis (usually due to chronic obstruction in patient with very thin abdominal wall). Check the hernial orifices. Are there any obvious masses, e.g. visible, pulsatile mass to suggest aortic aneurysm?
- Palpation. The patient should be relaxed, lying flat, with arms by side. Be gentle and start as far from the painful site as possible. Check for guarding and rigidity. Check for masses, e.g. appendix mass, pulsatile expansile mass to suggest aortic aneurysm. Carefully examine the hernial orifices. Examine the testes to exclude torsion.
- Percussion, e.g. tympanitic note with distension with intestinal obstruction; dullness over bladder due to acute retention.
- Auscultation. Take your time (30–60 s); e.g. silent abdomen of peritonitis; high-pitched tinkling bowel sounds of intestinal obstruction.

Rectal examination

Always carry out a rectal examination.

Vaginal examination

There may be discharge or tenderness associated with pelvic inflammatory disease. Examine the uterus and adnexa, e.g. pregnancy, fibroids, ectopic pregnancy.

GENERAL INVESTIGATIONS

- **FBC, ESR**
  Hb ↓ peptic ulcer disease, malignancy. WCC ↑ infective/ inflammatory disease, e.g. appendicitis, diverticulitis. ESR ↑ Crohn's disease, TB.

- **U&Es**
  Urea and creatinine ↑ uraemia. Electrolyte disturbances in vomiting and diarrhoea.

- **LFTs**
  Abnormal in cholangitis and hepatitis. Often abnormal in acute cholecystitis.

- **Serum amylase**
  Markedly raised in acute pancreatitis. Often moderately raised with perforated peptic ulcer or infarcted bowel.

- **MSU**
  Blood, protein, culture positive in pyelonephritis. Red cells in ureteric colic.

- **CXR**
  Gas under diaphragm (perforated viscus). Lower lobar pneumonia (referred pain).

- **AXR**
  Obstruction – dilated loops of bowel. Site of obstruction. Local ileus (sentinel loop) – pancreatitis, acute appendicitis. Toxic dilatation – dilated, featureless, oedematous colon in ulcerative colitis or Crohn's disease. Renal calculi. Calcified aortic aneurysm. Air in biliary tree (gallstone ileus). Gallstones (10% radio-opaque).

- **US**
  Localised abscesses, e.g. appendix abscess, paracolic abscess in diverticular disease. Free fluid – peritonitis, ascites. Aortic aneurysm. Ectopic pregnancy. Ovarian cyst. Gallstones. Empyema, mucocele of gall bladder. Kidney – cysts, tumour.

SPECIFIC INVESTIGATIONS

- **Blood glucose**
  Raised in diabetic ketoacidosis.

- **Serum calcium**
  Hypercalcaemia.

- **CRP**
  Crohn's disease.

- **VDRL**
  Syphilis (tabes dorsalis).

- **Sickling test**
  Sickle cell disease.

SECTION A

- **Urinary porphobilinogens**
  Acute intermittent porphyria.
- **ABGs**
  Metabolic acidosis, e.g. uraemia, infarcted bowel, sepsis, diabetic ketoacidosis.
- **βHCG**
  Pregnancy. Ectopic pregnancy.
- **ECG**
  Myocardial infarction (referred pain).
- **OGD**
  Peptic ulcer. Malignancy.
- **IVU**
  Stones. Obstruction.
- **Barium enema**
  Carcinoma. Volvulus. Intussusception.
- **Small bowel enema**
  Small bowel Crohn's disease. Lymphoma of small bowel. Carcinoma of small bowel.
- **Duplex Doppler**
  Superior mesenteric artery stenosis (mesenteric angina). Superior mesenteric artery thrombosis. Mesenteric venous thrombosis.
- **Angiography**
  Superior mesenteric embolus or thrombosis.
- **CT**
  Aneurysm. Pancreatitis. Tumour.
- **MRCP**
  Biliary tract disease.

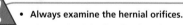

- Always examine the hernial orifices.
- Always check for localised tenderness if colicky abdominal pain becomes constant. Tachycardia, fever and a raised white cell count suggests infarction.

ABDOMINAL SWELLINGS

Abdominal swellings may be divided into generalised and localised swellings. Abdominal swellings are a common surgical problem. They are also frequently the subject of examination questions! Generalised swellings are classically described as the 'five Fs', namely fat, faeces, flatus, fluid or fetus. For the purpose of description of localised swellings, the abdomen has been divided into seven areas, i.e. right upper quadrant, left upper quadrant, epigastrium, umbilical, right lower abdomen, left lower abdomen and suprapubic area. Hepatomegaly, splenomegaly and renal masses, although referred to in this section, are dealt with under the relevant heading in the appropriate section of the book.

RIGHT UPPER QUADRANT

CAUSES

LIVER

See hepatomegaly, p. 215.

GALL BLADDER

- Secondary to carcinoma of the head of the pancreas
- Mucocele
- Empyema
- Carcinoma

RIGHT COLON

- Carcinoma
- Faeces
- Diverticular mass
- Caecal volvulus
- Intussusception

RIGHT KIDNEY

- Carcinoma
- Polycystic kidney
- Hydronephrosis
- Pyonephrosis
- Perinephric abscess
- TB
- Solitary cyst
- Wilms' tumour (nephroblastoma)

HISTORY

Liver

See hepatomegaly, p. 215.

Gall bladder

Known history of gallstones. History of flatulent dyspepsia. Jaundice. Dark urine. Pale stools. Pruritus. Recent weight loss may suggest carcinoma of the head of the pancreas or carcinoma of the gall bladder.

Right colon

Lassitude, weakness, lethargy suggesting anaemia from chronic blood loss. Central abdominal colicky pain, vomiting and constipation and change in bowel habit will suggest colonic carcinoma. There may be a history of gross constipation to suggest faecal loading. Known history of diverticular disease. History of attacks of crying, abdominal pain and blood and mucus in the stool ('redcurrant jelly' stool) will suggest intussusception in infants.

Right kidney

See kidney swellings, p. 282.

EXAMINATION

Liver

See p. 215.

Gall bladder

A mucocele is either non-tender or only mildly tender. It is large and smooth and moves with respiration, projecting from under the ninth costal cartilage at the lateral border of rectus abdominis. Empyema presents with an acutely tender gall bladder, which is difficult to define due to pain and tenderness. The patient may be jaundiced due to Mirizzi syndrome (external pressure from a stone impacted in Hartmann's pouch on the adjacent bile duct). Carcinoma of the gall bladder may present as a hard, irregular mass in the right hypochondrium, but normally presents as obstructive jaundice due to secondary deposits in the nodes at the porta hepatis causing external compression of the hepatic ducts. A smooth enlarged gall bladder in the presence of jaundice may be due to carcinoma of the head of the pancreas (Courvoisier's law: 'in the presence of obstructive jaundice, if the gall bladder is palpable the cause is unlikely to be due to gallstones').

Right colon

Faeces are usually soft and putty-like and can be indented but may also feel like a mass of rocks. Carcinoma is usually a firm to hard irregular mass, which may be mobile or fixed. A diverticular mass is usually tender and ill-defined, unless there is a large paracolic abscess. With caecal volvulus, there is a tympanitic mass which may be tender with impending infarction. With intussusception, there will be a smooth, mobile tender sausage-shaped mass in the right hypochondrium. The mass may move as the intussusception progresses.

Right kidney

See kidney swellings, p. 282.

GENERAL INVESTIGATIONS

■ **FBC, ESR**
   Hb ↓ anaemia, e.g. carcinoma of the colon, haematuria with renal lesions. Hb ↑, e.g. hypernephroma (polycythaemia associated with hypernephroma). WCC ↑, e.g. empyema, diverticular mass. ESR ↑, malignancy.

■ **U&Es**
   Vomiting and dehydration, e.g. gall bladder and bowel lesions. Ureteric obstruction with renal lesions leading to uraemia.

■ **LFTs**
   Liver lesions. Secondary deposits in liver.

■ **MSU**
   Renal lesions – red blood cells, pus cells, malignant cells. C&S.

■ **AXR**
   Intestinal obstruction due to carcinoma of the large bowel. Gallstones (10% are radio-opaque). Caecal volvulus. Constipation. Calcification in renal lesions.

■ **US**
   Liver lesions. Gallstones. Mucocele. Empyema. Bile duct dilatation.

SPECIFIC INVESTIGATIONS

■ **Barium enema**
   Carcinoma of the colon. Diverticular disease. Intussusception.

■ **Colonoscopy**
   Carcinoma of the colon. Diverticular disease.

■ **CT**
   Liver lesions. Gall bladder lesions. Renal lesions.

LEFT UPPER QUADRANT

CAUSES

SPLEEN

See splenomegaly, p. 410.

STOMACH
- Carcinoma
- Gastric distension (acute dilatation, pyloric stenosis)

PANCREAS
- Pseudocyst
- Carcinoma

KIDNEY
See right upper quadrant, p. 9.

COLON
- Carcinoma of the splenic flexure
- Faeces
- Diverticular mass

HISTORY

Spleen
See splenomegaly, p. 410.

Stomach
Vomiting will suggest pyloric stenosis, acute dilatation of the stomach and carcinoma. Vomiting food ingested several days previously suggests pyloric stenosis. Lethargy, loss of appetite and weight loss are seen in carcinoma of the stomach.

Pancreas
There may be a history of acute pancreatitis, which would suggest the development of a pseudocyst. Weight loss, backache and jaundice will suggest carcinoma of the pancreas. Recent onset of diabetes may occur with carcinoma of the pancreas.

Kidney
See kidney swellings, p. 282.

Colon
Lower abdominal colicky pain and change in bowel habit may suggest carcinoma or diverticular disease. A long history of constipation may suggest faecal masses.

EXAMINATION

Stomach
Gastric distension may present with a vague fullness and a succussion splash. Carcinoma will present with a hard, craggy, immobile mass.

Pancreatic tumours may be impalpable or present as a fixed mass, which does not move with respiration. Pancreatic pseudocysts are often large, smooth and may be tender.

Colon

See right upper quadrant, p. 9.

GENERAL INVESTIGATIONS

- **FBC, ESR**
  Hb ↓ carcinoma. Hb ↑ hypernephroma (polycythaemia is associated with hypernephroma). WCC ↑ diverticular disease, renal infections.

- **U&Es**
  Vomiting, dehydration (with gastric and colonic lesions). Renal lesions.

- **LFTs**
  Liver lesions. Secondary deposits in liver.

- **Serum amylase**
  Acute pancreatitis.

- **US**
  Splenomegaly. Renal lesions. Paracolic abscess.

SPECIFIC INVESTIGATIONS

- **Blood glucose**
  May be raised in pancreatic carcinoma.

- **Barium enema**
  Carcinoma. Diverticular disease.

- **Colonoscopy**
  Carcinoma. Diverticular disease.

- **Gastroscopy**
  Carcinoma of the stomach. Pyloric stenosis.

- **CT**
  Carcinoma of the pancreas. Pancreatic pseudocyst. Liver secondaries. Splenomegaly. Paracolic abscess.

EPIGASTRIUM

Many of the swellings that occur here will have been described under swellings in other regions of the abdomen. Although a full list of epigastric swellings is given below, only those not referred to in other sections will be discussed in the history and examination sections.

CAUSES

ABDOMINAL WALL

- Lipoma
- Epigastric hernia
- Xiphisternum
- Metastatic deposits

STOMACH

- Congenital hypertrophic pyloric stenosis
- Carcinoma
- Acute gastric volvulus

PANCREAS

See left upper quadrant, p. 11.

TRANSVERSE COLON

- Carcinoma
- Faeces
- Diverticular mass

LIVER

See hepatomegaly, p. 215.

RETROPERITONEUM

- Aortic aneurysm
- Lymphadenopathy (lymphoma, secondaries from testicular carcinoma)

OMENTUM

- Omental secondaries, e.g. stomach and ovary

HISTORY

Abdominal wall

The patient may indicate a soft, subcutaneous swelling, which may be a lipoma or an epigastric hernia containing extraperitoneal fat. The latter always occurs in the midline through a defect in the linea alba. They may become strangulated, in which case they are tender, and occasionally the skin is red. Occasionally a patient may indicate a firm bony lump in the upper epigastrium, which is in fact a normal xiphisternum. This may have become apparent due to either a deliberate attempt to lose weight or sudden weight loss as a result of underlying disease. Metastatic deposits may present as single or multiple fixed lumps in the skin or subcutaneous tissue, e.g. from breast or bronchus.

Stomach

A baby may present with projectile vomiting. The infant thrives for the first 3–4 weeks of life and then develops projectile vomiting after feeds. The first-born male child in a family is most commonly affected. There may be a history of a familial tendency, especially on the maternal side.

Retroperitoneum

A history of backache may suggest an aortic aneurysm or the patient may complain of a pulsatile epigastric swelling. Backache may also be a presenting symptom of retroperitoneal lymphadenopathy.

EXAMINATION

Abdominal wall

A soft, lobulated mass suggests a lipoma. It will be mobile over the tensed abdominal musculature. A fatty, occasionally tender, non-mobile swelling in the midline will suggest an epigastric hernia. The majority of epigastric hernias are composed of extraperitoneal fat, although there may be a sac with bowel contents. A cough impulse will be palpable. The swelling may be reducible. Hard, irregular, fixed lumps in the abdominal wall suggest metastatic deposits, especially if there is a history of carcinoma of the breast or bronchus.

Retroperitoneum

An aneurysm presents as a pulsatile expansile mass. Check the distal circulation (emboli, associated peripheral ischaemia). Retroperitoneal lymph node metastases from testicular cancer may present as a large retroperitoneal mass. Check the testes for swellings. Check all other sites for lymphadenopathy (especially the left supraclavicular node). Lymphadenopathy may also result from lymphoma. Check for lymphadenopathy elsewhere and for splenomegaly. A hard, craggy, mobile mass, especially in the presence of ascites, suggests omental secondaries (ovary, stomach – check for Virchow's node, i.e. left supraclavicular node).

GENERAL INVESTIGATIONS

- **FBC, ESR**
  Hb ↓ carcinoma of the stomach, carcinoma of the colon, carcinomatosis. WCC ↑ diverticulitis.
- **U&Es**
  Vomiting and dehydration with gastric and colonic lesions.

- **LFTs**
  Liver lesions.
- **US**
  Aortic aneurysm. Lymphadenopathy. Pancreatic pseudocyst.

SPECIFIC INVESTIGATIONS

- **Blood glucose**
  May be abnormal with pancreatic carcinoma or previous pancreatitis.
- **CT**
  Pancreatic tumours. Pancreatic pseudocyst. Lymphadenopathy. Aortic aneurysm. Omental deposits. Guided biopsy/FNAC.
- **Barium enema**
  Carcinoma of the colon. Diverticular disease.
- **Colonoscopy**
  Carcinoma of the colon. Diverticular disease.
- **Gastroscopy**
  Carcinoma of the stomach.
- **Laparoscopy**
  Carcinoma of the ovaries. Omental secondaries. Carcinomatosis peritonei.
- **Biopsy.**

UMBILICAL

Many of the swellings here will already have been described under swellings in other regions of the abdomen. Only those not referred to in those sections will be discussed in the history and examination sections.

CAUSES

SUPERFICIAL

- Sister Joseph's nodule (malignant)

HERNIA

- Paraumbilical
- Umbilical (children)

STOMACH

- Carcinoma

TRANSVERSE COLON

- Carcinoma
- Faeces
- Diverticular mass

SMALL BOWEL

- Crohn's disease
- Carcinoma
- Mesenteric cysts

OMENTUM

- Secondary deposits, e.g. stomach, ovary

RETROPERITONEUM

- Aortic aneurysm
- Lymph nodes, e.g. lymphoma, secondaries from testicular carcinoma

HISTORY

Superficial

Sister Joseph's nodule presents as a hard lump at the umbilicus. It is due to secondary deposits of carcinoma of the stomach, colon, ovary or breast.

Hernia

An umbilical hernia presents in infancy as an umbilical swelling which is reducible, and will usually have been noted at birth. Paraumbilical hernias usually occur in obese adults, often female. The patient may have had a lump for a long time. It may present with incarceration or with a tender painful swelling, suggesting strangulation.

Small bowel

The patient may present with central abdominal colicky pain, vomiting and diarrhoea, suggestive of Crohn's disease or more rarely a carcinoma of the small bowel.

EXAMINATION

Superficial

Sister Joseph's nodule presents as a hard lump or lumps at the umbilicus. Check for carcinoma of the stomach, colon, ovary or breast.

SECTION A

Hernia

In infants there may be an obvious large umbilical defect. The swelling is usually wide-necked and reducible. In adults there may be a reducible paraumbilical hernia. Occasionally it is soft, containing extraperitoneal fat. Frequently there is a sac containing omentum. Incarceration may occur. A tender red swelling suggests strangulation. A Richter's-type hernia may occur at this site.

Small bowel

Small bowel masses are usually very mobile, may be sausage-shaped, and may be tender.

GENERAL INVESTIGATIONS

■ FBC, ESR
Hb ↓ carcinoma. WCC ↑ diverticular disease.

■ U&Es
Vomiting. Dehydration, e.g. carcinoma of the stomach, carcinoma of the bowel, Crohn's disease.

■ LFTs
Alkaline phosphatase raised with liver secondaries.

■ US
Aortic aneurysm. Retroperitoneal lymphadenopathy.

SPECIFIC INVESTIGATIONS

■ CT
Aortic aneurysm. Retroperitoneal lymphadenopathy. Omental deposits. Guided biopsy/FNAC.

■ Barium enema
Carcinoma of the colon. Diverticular disease.

■ Colonoscopy
Carcinoma of the colon. Diverticular disease.

■ Gastroscopy
Carcinoma of the stomach.

■ Small bowel enema
Crohn's disease. Lymphoma. Carcinoma.

■ Laparoscopy
Carcinoma of the ovaries. Omental secondaries. Carcinomatosis peritonei.

■ Biopsy
Benign versus malignant.

RIGHT AND LEFT LOWER QUADRANTS

CAUSES

ABDOMINAL WALL

- Lipoma
- Spigelian hernia

LARGE BOWEL

RIGHT LOWER QUADRANT

- Appendix mass/abscess
- Carcinoma of the caecum
- Carcinoma of the ascending colon
- Faeces
- Crohn's disease
- Caecal volvulus
- Intussusception

LEFT LOWER QUADRANT

- Carcinoma of the sigmoid colon
- Diverticular mass
- Faeces
- Sigmoid volvulus
- Crohn's disease

SMALL BOWEL

- Crohn's disease
- Carcinoma
- Lymphoma
- Ileo-caecal TB

OVARY/UTERUS/FALLOPIAN TUBE

- Ovarian cyst
- Ovarian neoplasm
- Ectopic pregnancy
- Tubo-ovarian abscess
- Uterine fibroid

KIDNEY

See kidney swellings, p. 282.

SPLEEN (MASSIVE SPLENOMEGALY)

See splenomegaly, p. 410.

RETROPERITONEUM

- Iliac artery aneurysm
- Lymphadenopathy
- Neoplasm of iliac bone, e.g. osteogenic sarcoma, Ewing's tumour

HISTORY

Anterior abdominal wall

The patient may have the development of a soft mass that is slow growing, suggestive of a lipoma. A spigelian hernia occurs just lateral to the rectus muscle, halfway between the umbilicus and symphysis pubis. It is usually reducible.

Large bowel

A short history of central abdominal, colicky pain followed by a sharply localised pain in the right iliac fossa will suggest the diagnosis of acute appendicitis. After 48 hours, if there is not generalised peritonitis, an appendix mass will have formed and an abscess may subsequently form in the right iliac fossa. With carcinoma of the caecum the patient will either have noticed a mass or will present with alteration in bowel habit and the symptoms of anaemia, e.g. tiredness, lethargy. The same applies to carcinoma of the ascending colon. Faeces will be indentable and hard, rock-like masses will be felt around the colon. Caecal volvulus will present with central abdominal colicky pain and abdominal distension. Intussusception is more common in infants and usually presents with colicky abdominal pain and the classic 'redcurrant jelly' stool. Crohn's disease will present with malaise and diarrhoea with central abdominal colicky pain.

Carcinoma of the sigmoid colon will present with lower abdominal colicky pain, a change in bowel habit and bleeding PR. Diverticular disease may present with similar symptoms. Sigmoid volvulus will present with lower abdominal colicky pain and a tense, palpable mass in the left abdomen, which is tympanitic on percussion. Large bowel Crohn's disease will present with a sausage-like, palpable mass, which may be tender and is associated with diarrhoea.

Small bowel

If there is a mass palpable in the right iliac fossa the site of pathology is likely to be in the terminal ileum. This usually involves central abdominal colicky pain and a change in bowel habit. Ileo-caecal TB causes abdominal pain, diarrhoea which is associated with malaise and weight loss.

Spleen

With massive splenomegaly, the spleen may be palpable extending into the right lower quadrant.

Ovary/fallopian tube/uterus

The patient herself may feel a lump in the abdomen (ovarian cyst, fibroid) or notice generalised abdominal swelling, which may be associated with a massive ovarian cyst or ascites associated with ovarian cancer. Ectopic pregnancy will present with a missed period and abdominal pain, bleeding PV, and collapse with hypovolaemic shock if it ruptures. Salpingo-oophoritis will present with lower abdominal pain and tenderness and associated fever, and often a purulent vaginal discharge. Menorrhagia, lower abdominal pain and dyspareunia may suggest fibroids.

Retroperitoneum

The patient may present having noticed a pulsatile swelling in the iliac fossa. Pelvic lymphadenopathy may be suspected by history of removal of a malignant lesion from the lower limb, especially malignant melanoma. There may be an existing lesion present on the limb. A dull, boring pain may be suggestive of an iliac bone lesion. A palpable bony lesion suggests an osteogenic sarcoma or Ewing's tumour of bone.

EXAMINATION

The features of most of the lesions described above have been described in the other sections on abdominal swellings. Only those findings relevant to the ovary, uterus and fallopian tube will be described here. Examination may reveal a greatly distended abdomen, which may be due to a huge ovarian cyst or ascites associated with an ovarian neoplasm. Huge ovarian cysts are often smooth and loculated. It is impossible to get below them as they arise out of the pelvis. Signs of ascites include shifting dullness and a fluid thrill. With ectopic pregnancy, there may be a palpable mass in either iliac fossa. This may be associated with shock if rupture of the ectopic pregnancy has occurred. Shoulder-tip pain may occur from irritation of the undersurface of the diaphragm with blood. With tubo-ovarian abscess there may be a palpable mass arising out of the pelvis, or merely lower abdominal tenderness. Vaginal examination will reveal tenderness in the pouch of Douglas. Uterine fibroids may be extremely large and palpable as nodules on the underlying uterus.

GENERAL INVESTIGATIONS

■ FBC, ESR
   Hb ↓ Crohn's disease, carcinoma. ESR ↑ carcinoma, Crohn's disease, ileo-caecal TB. WCC ↑ appendicitis, diverticulitis.

■ U&Es
   Vomiting. Dehydration. Obstruction from carcinoma or Crohn's disease.

- **LFTs**
  Alkaline phosphatase ↑ with liver secondaries.
- **US**
  Ovarian lesions. Uterine lesions. Tubo-ovarian abscesses.
  Pregnancy. Ectopic pregnancy. Iliac artery aneurysms.
  Lymphadenopathy. Appendix mass. Crohn's mass.
- **AXR**
  Obstruction. Dilated loops of bowel. Ovarian teratoma (teeth,
  etc.). Erosion of iliac bone – bone tumours.

SPECIFIC INVESTIGATIONS

- **βHCG**
  Raised in pregnancy.
- **Mantoux test**
  Ileo-caecal TB.
- **CT**
  Ovarian lesions. Uterine lesions. Abscess. Ectopic pregnancy.
  Iliac artery aneurysm. Lymphadenopathy. Appendix mass. Bone
  tumours.
- **Barium enema**
  Carcinoma. Diverticular disease.
- **Small bowel enema**
  Crohn's disease. Carcinoma. Lymphoma.
- **Colonoscopy**
  Carcinoma (biopsy). Diverticular disease.
- **Laparoscopy**
  Carcinoma, Crohn's disease, ileo-caecal TB.
- **Bone scan**
  Bone tumour.

SUPRAPUBIC

CAUSES

BLADDER

- Acute retention
- Chronic retention
- Carcinoma

UTERUS

- Pregnancy
- Fibroids
- Carcinoma

BOWEL

- Diverticular mass
- Crohn's disease
- Carcinoma

OTHER

- Urachal cyst.

HISTORY

Bladder

Sudden onset of suprapubic pain with inability to pass urine suggests acute retention. There will usually be a past history of difficulty in starting and a poor stream. A history of dribbling may suggest acute renal failure associated with upper tract problems from chronic outflow obstruction. Haematuria, frequency, dysuria may suggest bladder carcinoma.

Uterus

Missed periods and early morning vomiting will suggest pregnancy. Menorrhagia and dyspareunia will suggest fibroids. Intermenstrual bleeding suggests carcinoma.

Urachus

Umbilical discharge may suggest a urachal cyst or abscess.

EXAMINATION

In acute retention there will be a smooth, tender swelling extending towards (but not above) the umbilicus. It is dull to percussion and it is impossible to get below it. Digital rectal examination will usually reveal benign prostatic hypertrophy or occasionally a hard, irregular prostate associated with carcinoma. With carcinoma of the bladder, a hard, irregular craggy mass may be felt arising out of the pelvis.

Uterus

A smooth, regular swelling arising out of the pelvis suggests a pregnant uterus. Later, as the uterus enlarges, fetal heart sounds may be heard. Fibroids are usually smooth and firm and may become very large. Uterine carcinoma is hard and craggy. Bimanual examination may confirm the diagnosis.

GENERAL INVESTIGATIONS

- FBC, ESR
  Hb ↓ tumour. WCC ↑ infection.

- **MSU**
  Red cells. White cells. Organisms, (infection precipitating) retention. Malignant cells with carcinoma.
- **US**
  Pregnancy. Fibroids. Bladder tumour. Urachal cyst.

SPECIFIC INVESTIGATIONS

- **βHCG**
  Pregnancy.
- **PSA**
  Carcinoma of the prostate.
- **Cystoscopy**
  Bladder tumour. Biopsy.
- **Barium enema**
  Colonic carcinoma. Diverticular disease. Crohn's disease.
- **Colonoscopy**
  Carcinoma. Diverticular disease.
- **CT**
  Ovarian lesions. Uterine lesions. Bladder lesions. Urachal cyst.

- Abdominal mass in conjunction with weight loss is suggestive of malignancy and requires urgent investigation.
- An abdominal mass in association with pyrexia, tachycardia and localised tenderness suggests an acute inflammatory cause.
- Always check the βHCG in women of childbearing age.
- A hard, craggy, mobile mass, especially in the presence of ascites, suggests omental secondaries, e.g. ovary, stomach. Check for Virchow's node, i.e. in the left supraclavicular fossa.

ANORECTAL PAIN

Anorectal pain is a common problem. The majority of patients have an obvious cause, e.g. fissure-in-ano, perianal abscess or thrombosed haemorrhoids.

CAUSES

ACUTE

- Fissure-in-ano
- Perianal haematoma
- Thrombosed haemorrhoids
- Perianal abscess
- Intersphincteric abscess
- Ischiorectal abscess
- Trauma
- Anorectal gonorrhoea
- Herpes

CHRONIC

- Fistula-in-ano
- Anorectal malignancy
- Chronic perianal sepsis, e.g. Crohn's disease, TB
- Proctalgia fugax
- Solitary rectal ulcer
- Cauda equina lesions

HISTORY

Constipation with pain on defecation and blood (usually on the paper) will suggest fissure-in-ano. A sudden onset of pain with a tender lump in the perianal region will suggest perianal haematoma. A past history of prolapsing piles, with failure to reduce them, associated with pain and tenderness suggests thrombosed haemorrhoids. Gradual onset of pain and tenderness with swelling is suggestive of abscess formation. A careful history must be taken of trauma. A history of anal sexual exposure will suggest gonorrhoea or herpes. With gonorrhoea there may be irritation, itching, discharge and pain. With herpes there will be pain and irritation. Proctalgia fugax is diagnosed on the history of perineal pain, which is spasmodic, the spasms lasting up to 30 min. The pain often feels deep inside the rectum. The cause is unknown but may be related to paroxysmal contraction of levator ani. Anorectal malignancies will be suggested in alteration of bowel habit and bleeding on defecation. Pain will only be apparent if the tumour involves the anal canal below the dentate line, where sensation is of the somatic type. Solitary rectal ulcer may present with pain but more usually presents with bleeding PR, passage of mucus, and difficulty with defecation. Chronic perianal sepsis may be the presenting symptom of Crohn's disease or TB. These diseases may already be manifest at other sites of the body. Rarely lesions of the cauda equina may cause anal pain.

EXAMINATION

Inspection may reveal a chronic fissure-in-ano, perianal haematoma, thrombosed piles, or a tumour growing out of the anal canal. A tense, red, tender area may be present, representing a perianal abscess. A fullness in the buttock with redness may indicate a large ischiorectal abscess. A digital rectal examination should be carried out unless the diagnosis is obvious. With gonococcal proctitis, proctoscopy may reveal pus and blood in the rectal ampulla with oedematous and friable mucosa. The presence of vesicles in the anal area will suggest herpes. Solitary rectal ulcer is usually diagnosed on sigmoidoscopy when redness and oedema of the mucosa is seen, usually, but not always, in association with frank ulceration. If a cauda equina lesion is suspected a full neurological examination should be carried out. No abnormality is usually found with proctalgia fugax.

GENERAL INVESTIGATIONS

- ■ FBC, ESR
  WCC ↑ infections, e.g. abscess. ESR ↑ Crohn's disease, TB and malignancy.
- ■ Blood glucose
  Sepsis may be a presentation of diabetes mellitus.
- ■ Proctoscopy
  Haemorrhoids. Anorectal malignancy. Anorectal gonorrhoea. Swab ↑ Gram-negative intracellular diplococci.
- ■ Sigmoidoscopy
  Anorectal malignancy.

SPECIFIC INVESTIGATIONS

- ■ Endo-anal ultrasound
  This may demonstrate intersphincteric abscesses or fistulae-in-ano.
- ■ MRI
  This will delineate complex fistula problems or may indicate a cauda equina lesion.
- ■ Antigen detection tests
  Herpes.

- **Electron microscopy**
  Identification of virus in vesicle fluid.

- **PCR**
  For fast diagnosis of herpes.

- Recurrent perianal abscesses may be the first presentation of diabetes. Ask about thirst and urinary frequency.
- Recurrent perianal problems, especially fissures in unusual places, may be a presentation of Crohn's disease.
- Do not treat perianal abscesses with antibiotics. Perianal abscesses should be incised and drained. Failure to do so may result in development of a fistula-in-ano.

ARM PAIN

This section deals with pain in the upper limb unrelated to joint pains. The majority of causes of arm pain are related to either neurological or vascular lesions.

CAUSES

CERVICAL LESIONS

- Disc lesion
- Cervical spondylosis
- Syringomyelia
- Infection, e.g. osteitis, TB
- Tumours
  - Spinal cord
  - Meninges
  - Nerves
  - Vertebral bodies

BRACHIAL PLEXUS

- Cervical rib
- Malignant infiltration, e.g. Pancoast's tumour
- Thoracic inlet syndrome

VASCULAR LESIONS

- Myocardial ischaemia (left arm)
- Embolism
- Axillary venous thrombosis
- Subclavian artery stenosis
- Arterial thrombosis

OTHERS

- Repetitive strain injury
- Carpal tunnel syndrome
- Peripheral neuropathy
- Bone tumours
- Compartment syndrome
  - Acute, e.g. crush injuries
  - Chronic, e.g. exertional

HISTORY

Symptoms of cervical lesions include: pain and stiffness in the neck; pain radiating down the arm. Cervical cord compression may occur.

Cervical spondylosis represents 'wear and tear' of the cervical spine. It is common over the age of 60 years. Acute disc lesions usually occur in the younger patient. A careful history is needed to exclude trauma.

Brachial plexus lesions refer pain down the arm and may result from localised lesions, e.g. a cervical rib causing extrinsic compression will affect T1 and cause wasting of the small muscles of the hands and paraesthesia in the dermatomal distribution, i.e. the inner aspect of the upper arm.

Subclavian artery stenosis will result in 'claudication' in the arm, i.e. pain brought on by exercise, relieved by rest, due to inadequate blood flow. A history of cardiac problems, e.g. AF or widespread arterial disease, will suggest embolism or thrombosis. A sudden onset of a painful, swollen, cyanotic limb will suggest axillary vein thrombosis. Pain radiating into the left arm brought on by exercise and related to central chest pain and pain radiating into the neck suggests myocardial ischaemia. Pain associated with occupation, e.g. writing, word-processing (keyboard occupations), will suggest repetitive strain injury. A history of diabetes mellitus, renal failure, liver failure, alcohol abuse, vitamin B_{12} deficiency, drugs, e.g. phenytoin, vincristine, suggests peripheral neuropathy.

Pain, paraesthesia in the thumb, index and middle finger, which is worse in bed at night and relieved by hanging the arm out of bed, would suggest carpal tunnel syndrome. The latter may be associated with pregnancy, rheumatoid arthritis, myxoedema, anterior dislocation of the lunate, gout, acromegaly, amyloidosis and arteriovenous fistula at the wrist created for haemodialysis.

Localised bone pain may be due to primary or secondary tumours. The latter are most common and may result from a primary in the breast, bronchus, thyroid, prostate or kidney. Pathological fractures may occur. With compartment syndrome there may be a history of crush injury, vascular injury or vascular surgery. Chronic compartment syndrome may result from unusual exertion, e.g. weight-lifting.

EXAMINATION

A full neurological examination should be carried out, looking for cervical lesions, brachial plexus lesions or carpal tunnel syndrome. There may be limitation in movements of the cervical spine. The limbs should be examined for swelling, e.g. axillary vein thrombosis, when there will be cyanosis and dilated veins. Examine for signs of ischaemia and feel for pulses. The classical signs of an ischaemic limb, i.e. pain, pallor, pulselessness, paraesthesia, 'perishing cold' and paralysis, may be present. Occupation will suggest repetitive strain injury and there will usually be little to find on examination. Horner's syndrome (ptosis, miosis, enophthalmos and anhidrosis) suggests Pancoast's tumour. With bone tumours there will be localised swelling and tenderness. With compartment syndrome there will be a swollen tender compartment in the forearm, paraesthesia and paralysis. Pulses may be normal initially; later they are reduced or absent.

GENERAL INVESTIGATIONS

- **FBC, ESR**
  WCC ↑ infection, e.g. osteomyelitis or cervical spine TB. ESR ↑ infection and malignancy.

- **CRP**
  ↑ Infection/inflammatory cause.

- **Cervical spine X-ray**
  Cervical spondylosis, bony metastases, cervical spine fractures.

- **CXR**
  Malignancy resulting in bone secondary. Pancoast's tumour (apical lung tumour spreading to involve brachial plexus). Cervical rib (13 ribs).

- **ECG**
  Cardiac ischaemia.

- **Cardiac enzymes**
  Cardiac ischaemia

SPECIFIC INVESTIGATIONS

- **CT**
  Cervical disc lesions, tumours.

- **MRI**
  Cervical disc lesions, tumours.

- **Nerve conduction studies**
  Brachial plexus lesions, peripheral neuropathy, carpal tunnel syndrome.

- **Duplex Doppler**
  Arterial or venous lesions.

- **Arteriography**
  Arterial lesions.

- **Venography**
  Venous lesions, e.g. axillary vein thrombosis.

- **Angina may present only with pain in the left arm. Take a careful history**

- **Paraesthesia and weakness in association with arm pain suggests nerve compression.**

ARM SWELLINGS

Swelling may be localised or generalised. Localised swellings may be related to joints or fractures. Localised swellings around joints are covered in the section on joint disorders (p. 250). This section includes only those conditions that may cause generalised swelling of the arm.

CAUSES

- Trauma
- Infection
  - e.g. cellulitis, lymphangitis
- Axillary vein thrombosis
- Lymphoedema
  - Congenital
  - Acquired
    - Axillary node lesions
      - Carcinoma
      - Infection, e.g. filariasis
      - Excision
      - Radiotherapy
- Other
  - Reflex sympathetic dystrophy (Sudek's atrophy)

HISTORY

A history of trauma will be obvious in many cases, although pathological fractures may occur with little trauma. Reflex sympathetic dystrophy may follow trauma, e.g. Colles' fracture. Congenital lymphoedema of the arm is rare; however, secondary lymphoedema is not and a history of carcinoma of the breast, operations on the axilla or radiotherapy to the axilla should be sought. There may be a history of a puncture wound or flea bite, suggesting cellulitis or lymphangitis. Streptococcal cellulitis is common following puncture wounds in patients who already have lymphoedema of a limb. Axillary vein thrombosis may come on after excessive or unusual exercise and has been nicknamed 'effort thrombosis'. An example is a patient who has been painting a ceiling who is not used to doing that sort of thing. It may occur in patients with cervical ribs or thoracic inlet obstruction. Thrombosis may also occur following insertion of a central line.

EXAMINATION

There may be localised swelling and tenderness together with crepitus associated with a fracture. There may be generalised non-pitting oedema suggestive of lymphoedema. Examination of the axilla may reveal a mass of lymph nodes, a scar suggestive of previous surgery or the skin changes of previous radiotherapy. Examination of the breast may reveal the site of a primary tumour that has resulted in secondary axillary lymphadenopathy. With axillary vein thrombosis there will be swelling, cyanosis and prominent dilated veins on the arm. With cellulitis there may be redness and heat in the arm, and in lymphangitis there may be red, inflamed streaks along the line of lymphatic vessels. With reflex sympathetic dystrophy the limb becomes painful, swollen and stiff with a reddened, smooth, shiny appearance to the skin.

GENERAL INVESTIGATIONS

■ **FBC, ESR**
   Hb ↓ tumour. WCC ↑ infection. ESR ↑ tumour or infection.

■ **Swab**
   C&S of any lesion that may have resulted in cellulitis or lymphangitis.

■ **CXR**
   Cervical rib (associated with axillary vein thrombosis).

■ **Arm X-ray**
   Patchy porosis of bone with reflex sympathetic dystrophy. Possible foreign body associated with cellulitis.

SPECIFIC INVESTIGATIONS

■ **US or CT**
   Axillary mass.

■ **Mammography**
   Breast carcinoma – axillary lymphadenopathy.

■ **Duplex Doppler**
   Axillary vein thrombosis.

■ **Venography**
   Axillary vein thrombosis.

- **Always take a careful and detailed history. Trauma may have been minimal and forgotten, e.g. an insect bite.**
- **Always examine the breast and axillary nodes.**

ASCITES

Ascites is the accumulation of excess free fluid in the peritoneal cavity.

CAUSES

HEPATIC

- Cirrhosis
- Hepatic tumours

MALIGNANT DISEASE

- Carcinomatosis
- Abdominal/pelvic tumour (primary or secondary)
- Pseudomyxoma peritonei
- Primary mesothelioma

CARDIAC

- Cardiac failure
- Constrictive pericarditis
- Tricuspid incompetence

RENAL

- Nephrotic syndrome

PERITONITIS

- TB
- Spontaneous bacterial

VENOUS OBSTRUCTION

- Budd–Chiari syndrome
- Veno-occlusive disease
- Hepatic portal vein obstruction
- Inferior vena cava obstruction

GASTROINTESTINAL

- Pancreatitis
- Malabsorption
- Bile ascites

HISTORY

Symptoms

Patients with ascites can present with abdominal discomfort, increasing abdominal girth, weight gain and ankle or sacral swelling.

Onset

The development of ascites is usually gradual, but sudden onset can result from acute decompensation of liver cirrhosis, malignancy, portal or splenic vein thrombosis and Budd–Chiari syndrome.

Past medical history

Any history of malignancy in the abdomen or pelvis is relevant; however, abdominal metastasis can also result in ascites, especially from breast, ovarian, prostatic, testicular and haematological malignancies. Cirrhosis of the liver may result from alcoholism, previous hepatitis, Wilson's disease, primary and secondary biliary cirrhosis and haemochromatosis. A previous history of TB should raise suspicion of secondary disease.

Associated symptoms

Shortness of breath can result from splinting of the diaphragm due to tense ascites itself, or secondarily as part of the syndrome of cardiac failure when it is the underlying cause.

EXAMINATION

Classical findings are shifting dullness and a fluid thrill. As liver disease and carcinomatosis account for 90% of the cases presenting with ascites, a detailed examination of all systems is required. The next commonest causes are cardiac failure and nephrotic syndrome.

Inspection

Evidence of liver disease would be suggested by the presence of jaundice, spider naevi, loss of body hair, gynaecomastia, palmar erythema and caput medusae. The jugular venous pressure (JVP) is elevated in the presence of cardiac failure, and a prominent *v* wave is seen with tricuspid regurgitation. Further elevation of the JVP on inspiration (Kussmaul's sign) may be observed with a pericardial effusion.

Palpation

Careful abdominal examination should be performed to look for possible abdominal or pelvic tumours. 'Dipping' may be required to feel masses in the presence of gross ascites. Hepatomegaly and splenomegaly can occur with portal hypertension and hepatic and haematological malignancies. Displacement of the apex beat with cardiomegaly may result from cardiac failure. Pedal oedema occurs with cirrhosis, cardiac failure, malabsorption, obstruction of lymphatic flow due to intra-abdominal or pelvic tumours, and nephrotic syndrome.

Auscultation

A third heart sound, systolic murmurs (functional tricuspid and mitral regurgitation) and crepitations (pulmonary oedema) may be audible with cardiac failure. Heart sounds are muffled with pericardial effusions. A pericardial friction rub or knock is occasionally audible in pericarditis.

Percussion

Dullness of the lung bases occurs with pulmonary oedema and pleural effusions (which may occur secondary to ascites).

Internal examination

A rectal examination may reveal ulceration or a fixed mass suggestive of a carcinoma. In women, an adnexal mass PV may be the first indication of a pelvic tumour.

GENERAL INVESTIGATIONS

History and examination findings may reveal the underlying cause. General investigations can be used to confirm or indicate the possible aetiology.

- **Urine dipstick**
  Will be strongly positive for protein in nephrotic syndrome. If so, a 24-hour urine collection for protein should be undertaken: more than 3.5 g/24 h is indicative of nephrotic syndrome.

- **FBC**
  A raised white count may indicate an infective aetiology but a differential white count is more specific.

- **U&Es**
  Elevated urea and creatinine implies severe renal impairment, and may occur as a component of hepatorenal syndrome, which is renal impairment secondary to liver failure.

- **LFTs**
  May be deranged in the presence of liver disease. The serum albumin will be able to indicate hypoalbuminaemia but the underlying cause must still be sought.

- **CXR**
  Findings suggestive of cardiac failure are cardiomegaly, upper venous diversion of blood, the presence of Kerley B lines,

pulmonary oedema and pleural effusions. Occasionally the presence of carcinoma may be suggested by a lesion in the lung fields.

■ **US abdomen/pelvis**
In addition to confirming the presence of ascites, US will detect any intra-abdominal masses that are not palpable on clinical examination, and visualise fatty deposits in the liver in the presence of cirrhosis. Dilated collateral veins may be seen in conditions that result in obstruction of the venous outflow of the liver, including cirrhosis and Budd–Chiari syndrome.

■ **Abdominal paracentesis**
Aspiration of the ascitic fluid is very useful to help determine the underlying cause. A sample should be sent to microbiology, clinical chemistry and pathology.

Ascitic fluid

Appearance

Chylous   The milky white appearance of chylous ascites is due to obstruction of the lymphatic ducts.

Bile-stained   Is suggestive of bile peritonitis.

Haemorrhagic   Can occur in malignancy, trauma and TB.

Straw-coloured   The usual appearance with most other causes.

Biochemistry

Protein   The ascitic protein levels are often used to classify the ascites as a transudate or an exudate; however this may not always be reliable. A transudate would be ascitic fluid with the protein concentration of less than 25 g/L in the sample or 11 g/L lower than the serum protein level, while an exudate is the opposite.

Amylase   Usually elevated in pancreatic ascites.

Glucose   Low in bacterial infections.

Triglyceride   Elevated in chylous ascites; may indicate obstruction of drainage of the thoracic duct.

Bilirubin   Elevated in bile ascites.

Microbiology

Gram and Ziehl–Neelsen staining with cultures may be positive with a bacterial aetiology.

Cytology

WCC   Neutrophilia is suggestive of a bacterial peritonitis, while tuberculous peritonitis usually results in a lymphocytosis. Malignant cells may be identified and a primary source may possibly be located.

SPECIFIC INVESTIGATIONS

■ Echocardiography
   Cardiac failure will manifest as a dilated and poorly contracting
   ventricle with a reduced ejection fraction. A pericardial effusion
   is visible as an echo-free space between the left ventricle and
   the pericardium. Tricuspid regurgitation can be visualised with
   colour-flow Doppler imaging.

■ Liver biopsy
   Will be able to confirm and may be able to ascertain the
   underlying cause of liver cirrhosis.

■ Renal biopsy
   Reveals the underlying cause of nephrotic syndrome.

■ Portal venography
   Is indicated if obstruction to the venous outflow of the liver is
   suspected and can confirm Budd–Chiari syndrome and veno-
   occlusive disease.

   • Ascites can result from abnormalities in a number
      of different systems and a detailed examination of
      all systems is required to avoid missing potentially
      treatable conditions, such as cardiac failure and TB.

AXILLARY SWELLINGS

The great majority of axillary swellings are enlarged lymph nodes. Axillary nodes are often enlarged due to secondary deposits from carcinoma of the breast. Most axillary swellings are easily diagnosed on clinical examination alone.

CAUSES

SUPERFICIAL

- Acute abscess
- Sebaceous cyst
- Lipoma
- Hidradenitis suppurativa

DEEP

- Lymphadenopathy
- Breast lump (in the axillary tail)
- Lipoma
- Chronic abscess, e.g. TB
- Axillary artery aneurysm

HISTORY

Superficial

Acute abscess

This presents as a tender swelling in the skin. There may be a purulent discharge. Common in diabetics.

Sebaceous cyst

A sebaceous cyst will present as a firm swelling in the skin, often with a punctum. It may be tender if it becomes inflamed and there may be discharge from it.

Lipoma

This presents as a soft, lobulated swelling in the subcutaneous tissue.

Hidradenitis suppurativa

The patient presents with multiple tender swellings in the superficial tissue of the axilla, the infection occurring in the apocrine sweat glands. A purulent discharge usually occurs. There may be a history of diabetes.

Deep

Lymphadenopathy (p. 304)

The patient may have noticed a lump in the axilla, which may be tender or non-tender. Check for a site of infection or malignancy in the region of drainage of the nodes, i.e. the arm, the chest wall and the abdominal wall as far down as, and including, the umbilicus, the skin of the back as far down as the iliac crest and the breast. Has the patient noticed any lumps elsewhere? Check for malaise, pyrexia, night sweats, cough. There may be a history of bruising or epistaxis to suggest a blood dyscrasia. Is there any evidence of scratches on the arm to suggest cat scratch disease?

Breast lumps

Occasionally a lump in the medial wall of the axilla may be a swelling in the axillary tail of the breast, e.g. fibroadenoma or carcinoma.

Lipoma

Occasionally the patient may notice a firm swelling which appears intermittently, slipping out from under cover of the muscles.

Chronic abscess

Check for a history of TB. There may be night sweats.

Axillary artery aneurysm

This is rare. The patient may notice a pulsatile swelling under the arm. When the swelling becomes large, the patient may notice the arm moving away from the side of the body with each heart beat. Occasionally there may be symptoms in the hand due to distal embolisation.

EXAMINATION

Superficial

Acute abscess

There may be a tender, red, fluctuant swelling with purulent discharge.

Lipoma

There will be a soft, lobulated swelling in the subcutaneous tissue.

Sebaceous cyst

A small, well-defined swelling in the skin. A punctum may be visible. If it is infected, the surrounding skin will be red and the lesion tender. Discharge may be present.

Hidradenitis suppurativa

Multiple tender swellings with surrounding erythema and discharge of pus are present.

Deep

Chronic abscess

A fluctuant swelling presents in the axilla. With TB there may be little or no signs of inflammation.

Lymphadenopathy

Single discrete node, e.g. lymphoma. Numerous hard nodes or matting of nodes (carcinoma). Tender fluctuant nodes (abscess). Check for infection or tumour in the area of drainage of the lymphatics. Examine the breast. Check all other sites of nodes, e.g. cervical, inguinal; check for hepatosplenomegaly.

Lipoma

Deep lipomas are usually intermuscular and may be felt only in certain positions. They may slip in and out between the pectoral muscles. They may be firmer and not have the lobulated feel of a more superficial lipoma.

Axillary artery aneurysm

A pulsatile mass will be palpable within the axilla. Check the distal circulation. If an axillary artery aneurysm is large, when the patient stands with the arms by the sides, the arm moves away from the side of the body as the lump pulsates.

Breast lumps

A lump on the medial wall of the axilla may be a lump in the axillary tail of the breast.

GENERAL INVESTIGATIONS

- **FBC, ESR**
  Hb ↓ malignant disease. WCC ↑ infection or leukaemia. ESR ↑ infection and malignancy. Platelets ↓ leukaemia.

- **Swab**
  C&S, microscopy of any discharge.

SPECIAL INVESTIGATIONS

- **CXR**
  TB.

- **US**
  Lymphadenopathy, lipoma, aneurysm.

- **Mantoux test**
  TB.

- **FNAC**
  Benign versus malignant.
- **Mammography**
  Carcinoma of the breast.
- **Arteriography**
  Assess distal circulation with axillary artery aneurysm.

- **Always examine the breast – in both male and female patients.**
- **Always examine all other potential sites for lymphadenopathy.**

BACKACHE

Backache is one of the most common complaints seen in general practice and orthopaedic clinics. It accounts for about 20% of referrals to orthopaedic clinics. Most causes are either traumatic or degenerative but other causes are numerous and may occur as a result of pathology in almost any system of the body.

CAUSES

CONGENITAL

- Kyphoscoliosis
- Spina bifida
- Spondylolisthesis

ACQUIRED

TRAUMATIC
- Vertebral fractures
- Ligamentous injury
- Joint strain
- Muscle tears

INFECTIVE
- Osteomyelitis – acute and chronic
- TB
- Discitis

INFLAMMATORY
- Ankylosing spondylitis
- Rheumatology disorders

NEOPLASTIC
- Metastases
- Primary tumours

DEGENERATIVE
- Osteoarthritis
- Intervertebral disc lesions

METABOLIC
- Osteoporosis
- Osteomalacia

ENDOCRINE
- Cushing's disease (osteoporosis)

IDIOPATHIC
- Paget's disease
- Scheuermann's disease

PSYCHOGENIC
- Psychosomatic backache

VISCERAL
- Penetrating peptic ulcer
- Carcinoma of the pancreas
- Carcinoma of the rectum

VASCULAR
- Aortic aneurysm
- Acute aortic dissection

RENAL
- Renal calculus
- Carcinoma of the kidney
- Inflammatory disease

GYNAECOLOGICAL
- Pelvic inflammatory disease
- Endometriosis
- Uterine tumours

HISTORY

Congenital

The diagnosis is usually apparent from the history, although with spondylolisthesis the symptoms, i.e. low lumbar backache, worse on standing, may not present until late childhood or early adult life.

Acquired
General

The speed of onset is important. Sudden onset back pain may be due to trauma or disc lesions, whereas gradual onset of pain may be due to conditions such as degenerative disease. Mechanical lesions impinging on the cord can result in neurological symptoms such as bladder dysfunction (urinary retention). Symptoms worse on movement and relieved by rest suggest a mechanical cause, whereas pain that is severe and unrelenting can occur with malignant causes. In addition there may be symptoms (other than musculoskeletal) related to the underlying cause such as abdominal pain, dysuria or menorrhagia.

Traumatic

There will usually be a clear history of trauma. Care must be taken in moving the patient. Neurological sequelae may be obvious.

Infective

There may be a history of TB; the patient may have had night sweats or cough. Osteomyelitis of the spine may also occur in diabetes and the immunocompromised, in which case the organism is more commonly *Staphylococcus aureus*. With spinal TB the patient is usually young and complains of malaise, fever, pain, tenderness and limitation of movement of the spine. Discitis usually presents with mild backache accompanied by leg pain.

Inflammatory

Ankylosing spondylitis usually affects young adult males. The sacroiliac joints are affected initially, then the whole spine. The patient usually presents with lumbar stiffness, especially when rising in the morning. Iritis and plantar fasciitis may also occur. Rheumatology disorders may present with symptoms in other joints.

Neoplastic

The patient is usually unwell with severe unrelenting pain, often localised to a particular area of the spine. There may be a past history of a primary tumour (e.g. bronchus, breast, thyroid, prostate or kidney), or the primary may not be apparent. The pain may have been of sudden onset with a pathological fracture resulting in a collapsed vertebra. Rarely paraplegia may be a presenting symptom. Myeloma may present with backache.

Degenerative

Osteoarthritis usually presents in the older patient, with pain made worse on movement and relieved by rest. With intervertebral disc lesions there is usually sudden onset of pain radiating down the back of the leg (sciatica). The pain is worse on movement, coughing and straining. Neurological symptoms may be present, e.g. weakness of a limb, bladder symptoms.

Metabolic

Osteoporosis is commonest in post-menopausal women. Bone pain and pathological fractures occur. Osteomalacia may occur in adults with a history of gastrectomy, steatorrhoea, renal failure or anticonvulsant therapy.

Endocrine

There may be a history of Cushing's disease or long-term steroid therapy.

Idiopathic

Paget's disease of bone may cause backache. This usually occurs over the age of 40 years. The patient may have noted other changes, e.g. enlargement of the face or bowing of the leg. Scheuermann's disease is osteochondritis of the spine. It causes backache in adolescence. The patient may present because the parents have noticed round shoulders.

Psychogenic

This is very common. Check for malingering, anxiety, depression and compensation neurosis.

Visceral

With penetrating peptic ulcer the patient complains of epigastric pain radiating straight through to the back. The pain may be relieved by food and antacids. With carcinoma of the pancreas the patient will describe a boring pain in the back, which is unrelenting. There will be a history of anorexia and weight loss. The patient may be jaundiced. With carcinoma of the rectum invasion of the sacrum and the sacral plexus may occur, causing low back pain with sciatica.

Vascular

Aortic aneurysm may cause back pain by eroding into the vertebral bodies. Alternatively it may cause severe back pain due to rupture. The patient may have noticed a pulsation in the abdomen. Acute aortic dissection usually gives a severe tearing back pain associated with chest pain. The patient is usually shocked.

Renal

There is usually a dull, boring ache with carcinoma of the kidney. The patient may also complain of haematuria. With ureteric colic the pain radiates from loin to groin and is severe, the patient being unable to get into a comfortable position. Inflammatory disease of the kidney presents with upper lumbar back pain. The patient may be feverish with rigors, and complain of frequency and dysuria.

Gynaecological

The pain is usually low back pain associated with pelvic discomfort. The patient may also complain of dysmenorrhoea, menorrhagia or post-menopausal bleeding.

EXAMINATION

General

Acute cord compression will cause bilateral leg pain with lower motor neurone signs at the level of the compression, and upper motor neurone signs below. Check for sphincter disturbance. Acute cauda equina compression causes root pain in the legs, saddle anaesthesia and disturbances of bladder and bowel function. In any patient with acute backache the above signs should be sought and, if found, the appropriate urgent referral made to a neurosurgeon or spinal surgeon.

Congenital

Kyphoscoliosis and spina bifida are usually obvious on examination. With spondylolisthesis a 'step' may be palpable in the line of the spinous processes, with a skin crease below. It usually involves L5 slipping on S1, or, less commonly, L4 slipping on L5. Occasionally there are neurological signs in the limbs.

Acquired

Traumatic

This will usually be obvious. Careful positioning of the patient and full neurological examination should be carried out. Always check for associated injuries.

Infective

With acute osteomyelitis there is pyrexia, malaise and local tenderness and spasm. With chronic osteomyelitis, e.g. due to TB, there will be wasting of the paraspinal muscles, spasm and restricted movements. There may be a localised kyphosis or 'gibbus' due to vertebral collapse. A psoas abscess may be present in the groin. Paraplegia may occur. With discitis there will be reduced movement of the spine.

Inflammatory

The patient with ankylosing spondylitis will present with a stiff spine. There will be flexion of the hips and spine. In the advanced case, the patient cannot raise the head to see in front. Check for iritis and plantar fasciitis. Rheumatological disease will also present with problems in other joints.

Neoplastic

With myeloma, in addition to backache there may be pain in the ribs, long bones and skull. Bone tenderness will be present with secondary deposits. Palpate along the spine for tenderness. Check the chest, thyroid, breast, kidney and prostate for malignancy. Check for any neurological signs.

Degenerative

There will be limitation of movement of the spine with osteoarthritis. With acute disc lesion there will be limitation of spine movement, lordosis and neurological symptoms of the lower limbs. Carry out a full neurological examination.

Metabolic

With osteoporosis, usually there will be only localised bone tenderness. There may be evidence of recent vertebral collapse. With osteomalacia, apart from bone pain, there may be proximal myopathy resulting in a waddling gait.

Endocrine

There may be signs of Cushing's disease or prolonged steroid therapy, e.g. cushingoid facies, buffalo hump, proximal myopathy, abdominal striae, etc.

Idiopathic

In Paget's disease check for changes in the skull and long bones (bowing of the tibia). Compressive symptoms due to skull enlargement may result in blindness, deafness or cranial nerve entrapment. There may be signs of high-output cardiac failure due to vascularity of bone. In Scheuermann's disease there will be a smooth, thoracic kyphosis and, below this, a compensatory lumbar lordosis. The chest is flat.

Psychogenic

This is often difficult to assess. Signs may vary from examination to examination. There may be exaggeration of symptoms during the examination. It is best to watch from a distance as the patient leaves the consulting room. The gait, posture and demeanour may suddenly change!

Visceral

Check for epigastric tenderness or mass. Jaundice may be present in pancreatic cancer, and the gall bladder may be palpable (Courvoisier's law). Carry out a digital rectal examination to check for rectal carcinoma.

Vascular

A pulsatile abdominal mass may be palpable. The patient may be shocked. With acute aortic dissection, there may be shock with disparity of pulses in the extremities.

Renal

Check for renal masses or loin tenderness.

Gynaecological

Check for pelvic masses. Carry out bimanual examination.

GENERAL INVESTIGATIONS

■ FBC, ESR
Hb ↓ malignancy, peptic ulceration. WCC ↑ infection, e.g. osteomyelitis. ESR ↑ malignancy, e.g. myeloma or secondary deposits. TB. Ankylosing spondylitis.

- **CRP**
  ↑ infection, inflammation.
- **U&Es**
  May be abnormal in renal disease.
- **LFTs**
  Bilirubin and alkaline phosphatase will be raised in biliary tract obstruction related to carcinoma of the head of the pancreas. Alkaline phosphatase may also be raised in Paget's disease, osteomalacia and secondary deposits in bone. This is bony alkaline phosphatase that is raised and isoenzymes will need checking.
- **CXR**
  Primary tumour, e.g. bronchial carcinoma. Secondary tumours.
- **Spine X-ray**
  Trauma – fractures. Osteoarthritis – narrowed disc spaces and osteophytes. Prolapsed intervertebral disc – mild scoliosis, loss of lumbar lordosis, loss of disc space, Schmorl's node. Spondylolisthesis – decapitated 'Scottie dog' sign. Scheuermann's disease – wedging of vertebra and irregularity of vertebral end plates. Chronic osteomyelitis – erosion of joint surfaces, destruction of bone and intervertebral discs, soft-tissue shadows, e.g. psoas abscess. Myeloma – punched-out lesions. Secondary deposits – osteolytic or osteosclerotic (prostate). Osteoporosis – thinned bones, vertebral collapse. Ankylosing spondylitis – 'bamboo' spine; irregularity, sclerosis and fusion of sacroiliac joints. Paget's disease of bone – 'sclerotic' white vertebrae.
- **US**
  Aortic aneurysm. Renal lesions. Uterine lesions.

SPECIFIC INVESTIGATIONS

- **PSA**
  Prostatic carcinoma.
- **Serum calcium**
  Raised in malignancy, myeloma and bony metastases.
- **Bence Jones protein**
  May be raised in myeloma.
- **Plasma protein electrophoresis**
  Monoclonal gammopathy in myeloma.
- **CT**
  Pancreatic lesions. Aortic lesions. Pelvic lesions.
- **Technetium scan**
  Hot spots with bony secondaries. Occasional hot spots with inflammatory disease.
- **MRI**
  Location of disc lesion.

- In men over 55 years of age with low back pain, consider metastatic prostatic cancer. Perform a digital rectal examination.

- Acute cauda equina compression may cause bilateral sciatica, saddle anaesthesia and disturbances of bladder and bowel function. In any patient with acute backache the above signs should be sought and, if found, urgent referral made to a neurosurgeon.

- Always remember renal and pancreatic disease and aortic aneurysm as a cause of backache.

BREAST LUMPS

A lump in the breast is a common clinical presentation. In every case of a breast lump, in both males and females, carcinoma must be excluded.

CAUSES

DISCRETE LUMPS

MALIGNANT
- Carcinoma
- Phyllodes tumour (some behave in benign fashion)

BENIGN
- Fibroadenoma
- Cyst (in cystic mastitis)
- Duct ectasia
- Sebaceous cyst
- Galactocele
- Fat necrosis
- Lipoma
- Tuberculous abscess
  - (common in parts of the world where TB is endemic)

GENERALISED SWELLING

- Pregnancy
- Lactation
- Puberty
- Mastitis

SWELLINGS BEHIND THE BREAST

- Retromammary abscess from chest disease
- Tietze's disease
- Rib deformities
- Chondroma of the costal cartilages

HISTORY

A diagnosis of carcinoma is suggested by a strong family history, nulliparous state, early menarche, late menopause and history of cystic hyperplasia. The patient may have found a breast lump (carcinoma is painless in 85% of cases) or may have noticed nipple retraction, skin dimpling, axillary swelling. Jaundice may have occurred due to liver secondaries or porta hepatis node involvement. Bone pain may be due to secondary deposits and pathological fractures. Breathlessness may be due to lung secondaries or a pleural effusion. Personality change, fits, headaches suggest cerebral metastases. A patient who presents in pregnancy or lactation may have mastitis, abscess or galactocele. A history of trauma suggests fat necrosis. A patient in the fifth decade with retroareolar pain, nipple retraction and a thick, creamy nipple discharge suggests duct ectasia. The patient presenting between the ages of 15 and 25 years with a non-tender swelling suggests fibroadenoma. A patient with a history of painful breasts may have one of the conditions described under breast pain (p. 54). Enquiries should be made of a past history of TB, as rarely a tuberculous abscess may form within the breast or erode through the chest wall from the lung.

EXAMINATION

Carcinoma

Hard irregular swelling. May be fixed to the skin or fixed deeply. Skin dimpling. Nipple retraction. *Peau d'orange*. Paget's disease of the nipple. Axillary lymphadenopathy. Supraclavicular lymphadenopathy. Hepatomegaly. Pathological fractures – spine, ribs, long bones.

Phyllodes tumour

Mobile mass may become very large.

Fibroadenoma

Smooth, rounded, mobile mass. Breast 'mouse' (so called because it darts about under the examining fingers).

Cyst

Smooth, mobile swelling. May be tender. May be associated with generalised lumpiness of the breast.

Galactocele

Smooth, mobile swelling occurring in the lactating breast.

Fat necrosis

Hard, irregular swelling. May be overlying bruising of the skin or teeth marks! Occasionally the lesion is fixed to the skin and is difficult to distinguish from carcinoma.

Lipoma

Soft, lobulated swelling. Rare on the breast. 'Pseudolipoma' is a bunching of fat between retracted suspensory ligaments of the breast and is associated with an underlying carcinoma.

Duct ectasia

Tender retroareolar area. Retroareolar erythema. Nipple retraction. Thick, creamy nipple discharge.

Sebaceous cyst

Mobile swelling fixed to the skin. May be a punctum. May be infected, with discharge and surrounding redness.

Generalised swellings

Generalised swelling of the breast may occur in pregnancy, lactation and puberty. It may also occur with mastitis, when the breast is enlarged, red, tender and hot.

Swellings behind the breast

These are rare. Tietze's disease is the most common. There will be prominence and tenderness over the second, third and fourth costal cartilages. With retromammary abscess, chest signs may be obvious on percussion and also on auscultation of the chest.

GENERAL INVESTIGATIONS

- **FBC, ESR**
  Hb ↓ widespread malignancy. ↑ WCC breast abscess. ESR ↑ malignancy and TB.

- **LFTs**
  Alkaline phosphatase ↑ with liver secondaries and bone secondaries (isoenzymes).

- **Serum calcium**
  ↑ in bone secondaries.

- **CXR**
  Secondary deposits in lung and rib. Underlying chest disease, e.g. TB or empyema.

SPECIFIC INVESTIGATIONS

- **FNAC**
  Benign versus malignant. Cystic versus solid.

- **Mammography**
  Infiltrating radio-opaque mass or microcalcification indicates malignancy. Dilated retroareolar ducts and skin indentation suggests duct ectasia. Coarse calcification may occur with long-standing fibroadenomas.

- **Open excision biopsy**
  e.g. fibroadenoma, fat necrosis.

- **US**
  US of breast better than mammography in young women. US of liver for metastases. US guided FNA/core biopsy/Mammotome®.

- CT
  Abdomen, chest, brain. Metastases.
- Bone scan
  Metastases.
- BRCA1, BRCA2
  Gene mutations in breast cancer.

- **Skin dimpling and nipple retraction indicate carcinoma until proved otherwise.**
- **Breast lumps after the menopause are most likely to be due to carcinoma.**
- **A lump occurring after trauma may be due to fat necrosis. Re-examine after a few weeks. If it has not resolved, investigation is required.**

BREAST PAIN

Pain in the breast is a common symptom in general surgical practice. Most cases are benign and due to cyclical mastalgia, but occasionally pain may be the presenting symptom of carcinoma.

CAUSES

- Cyclical mastalgia (fibroadenosis, cystic mastitis)
- Non-cyclical mastalgia
- Duct ectasia
- Breast abscess
- Pregnancy
- Lactation
- Carcinoma (15% of lumps are painful)
- Fat necrosis
- Mastitis
- Tietze's disease
- Mondor's disease
- Rib secondaries
- Herpes zoster

HISTORY

Cyclical mastalgia causes soreness, frequently in the upper and outer quadrants of the breast in the week preceding a period. The pain usually disappears after the period and there is freedom from soreness or pain for 2 weeks, when it recommences. Symptoms are common in the 20–45 years age group. Non-cyclical mastalgia may occur and is more common in the fourth and fifth decades. Duct ectasia occurs in the fifth decade. The pain is usually behind the nipple and associated with subareolar erythema and a thick, creamy nipple discharge. Fat necrosis will be suggested by a history of trauma, which occasionally the patient will be embarrassed to admit (often the partner's teeth!). Breast abscess or mastitis will be obvious. It usually occurs during pregnancy or lactation but it may occur in a retroareolar position in a patient with duct ectasia. Breast fullness and soreness is a symptom of early pregnancy. Patients may indicate breast pain where the condition is not actively in the breast but behind it. Tietze's disease (costochondritis of the costal cartilages) will present with pain related to the breast. Mondor's disease (superficial thrombophlebitis of the subcutaneous veins of the chest wall) also presents with pain in the breast. It may be associated with an underlying carcinoma. Rib secondaries may also present with pain behind the breast. Herpes zoster may present with pain radiating round into the breast and precedes the development of a vesicular eruption by 2–3 days.

EXAMINATION

A hard, irregular lump is suggestive of carcinoma (this is discussed in the section on breast lumps). Tenderness and lumpiness, occasionally with a smooth, mobile swelling (cyst), is suggestive of cyclical mastalgia. The tenderness and lumpiness is most often palpated in the upper and outer quadrants of the breast. In the early stages of fat necrosis there may be bruising over the breast and the lump is tender. In the later stages it becomes hard and irregular and may be tethered to the skin. Breast abscess will present with redness, swelling, heat and pain in the breast during pregnancy or, more commonly, lactation. The swelling will be fluctuant and usually there is associated fever. Duct ectasia presents with subareolar erythema, tenderness and occasionally a subareolar lump. Nipple retraction may be present in long-standing cases and there may be a thick, creamy discharge that can be expressed from the nipple. Pregnancy will present with fullness of the breast and increased circumareolar pigmentation. In Tietze's disease there will be tenderness, and occasionally swelling, over the second, third and fourth costal cartilages. In Mondor's disease the veins of the chest wall are felt as red, tender cords, often extending onto the anterior axillary fold. The breast should be carefully checked for an underlying mass, as the condition may be associated with carcinoma of the breast. Herpes zoster will usually present with a characteristic vesicular eruption a few days after the pain.

GENERAL INVESTIGATIONS

- ■ FBC, ESR
  WCC ↑ mastitis and breast abscess. ESR ↑ widespread carcinoma.
- ■ LFTs
  Alkaline phosphatase may be raised with liver or bony secondaries.
- ■ Serum calcium
  May be raised with bone secondaries.
- ■ Swab
  C&S if there is any discharge from an abscess or from the nipple.
- ■ CXR
  Secondaries in lung or ribs. Pleural effusion in carcinoma.

SPECIFIC INVESTIGATIONS

- ■ βHCG
  Positive in pregnancy.

- **FNAC**
  Benign versus malignant. Cystic versus solid.
- **Mammography**
  Carcinoma. Duct ectasia.
- **US**
  US of breast better than mammography in young women.
- **Breast biopsy**
  Benign versus malignant.
- **Bone scan**
  Rib secondaries. Myeloma.

- Always examine the breasts in a patient with breast pain, even if the history strongly suggests cyclical mastalgia.
- Pain is a relatively uncommon presenting symptom of breast cancer but always examine the breasts.
- In women of childbearing age, always consider the likelihood of pregnancy as a cause of breast pain.

CHEST PAIN

Chest pain is a common presenting symptom of disorders that can range from trivial to life-threatening.

CAUSES

CARDIOVASCULAR

- Angina
- Myocardial infarction
- Acute aortic dissection
- Pericarditis

GASTROINTESTINAL

- Reflux oesophagitis
- Peptic ulcer disease
- Oesophageal spasm

PULMONARY

- Pneumonia
- Pneumothorax
- Pulmonary embolism

MUSCULOSKELETAL

- Chest wall injuries
- Herpes zoster
- Costochondritis
- Secondary tumours of the rib

EMOTIONAL

- Depression

HISTORY

Character

The character of angina is tight and crushing, while the pain from aortic dissection has a tearing quality. Oesophageal reflux may be described as a burning pain, and peptic acid-related pain tends to be deep and gnawing.

Location

The pain from angina and oesophageal reflux may be located retrosternally, and they both can radiate to the jaw or down into the left arm. The pain from pericarditis may be centrally located

SECTION A

and radiate to the shoulders (trapezius ridge pain). Pain from aortic dissection often radiates into the back and occasionally into the abdomen (depending on the extent of the dissection). Pulmonary pain can be located anywhere in the thorax.

Precipitating factors

Angina may be precipitated by effort, a defining characteristic. Other known precipitants of angina are emotion, food and cold weather. If angina occurs at rest for more than 20 min it should be treated as a myocardial infarction until proven otherwise. Oesophageal reflux is often related to meals and precipitated by changes in posture, such as bending or lying. Pain originating from pericarditis and pulmonary origin is often pleuritic, i.e. worse on inspiration; however, musculoskeletal pain can also be worse on breathing due to movement of the thorax.

Relieving factors

Both oesophageal spasm and angina may be relieved by GTN, which relaxes smooth muscle. Antacids will relieve the pain of oesophageal reflux but not angina. The pain associated with pericarditis may be relieved by sitting forwards.

Trauma

A history of a blunt or stretching injury immediately suggests the underlying aetiology of chest wall tenderness and it is important to diagnose rib fractures that can result from more severe trauma. Pathological rib fractures that result from minor injuries may be due to bony metastasis or osteoporosis.

Emotion

Occasionally chest pain is a somatic manifestation of patients with depression or anxiety, but it is essential to exclude all organic causes before accepting depression or anxiety as the underlying cause. Moreover a serious aetiology may co-exist.

EXAMINATION

Temperature

Pyrexia can occur with pneumonia, myocardial infarction, pericarditis and herpes zoster infection.

Pulse

Heart rate on its own is not discriminating as pain invariably leads to tachycardia. However, palpating both upper and lower limb pulses may be useful. Occasionally peripheral pulses are absent in patients with aortic dissection.

JVP

The JVP is elevated with congestive cardiac failure and acute right ventricular failure, an occasional complication of inferior myocardial infarction and pulmonary embolism (when more than 60% of the pulmonary vascular supply is occluded).

Palpation of the chest

Chest wall tenderness would imply a musculoskeletal cause. The presence of unilateral tenderness confined to a single or adjacent group of dermatomes would suggest either central (vertebral or spinal origin) or peripheral nerve pathology (herpes zoster infection). The trachea deviates away from the side of a tension pneumothorax, and chest expansion is decreased on the same side for pneumonia and pneumothorax. Dullness to percussion will be noted in an area of consolidation with pneumonia and hyperresonance with pneumothorax (a difficult sign to interpret).

Auscultation of the chest

The unilateral absence of breath sounds is consistent with a pneumothorax; more localised loss occurs over an effusion. Bronchial breath sounds are audible over a segment of consolidation and sometimes above the level of an effusion. Localised areas of crepitations are audible with lobar pneumonia, whereas widespread crepitations suggest multilobar involvement or pulmonary oedema secondary to left ventricular failure (from myocardial infarction).

A friction rub may be auscultated with both pericardial and pleuritic disease, but only a pericardial rub will be present when the patient holds the breath.

Lower limbs

Hemiparesis can occur with aortic dissection, and a hot, swollen, tender calf or thigh may give a clue to an underlying deep vein thrombosis. Measurements of the mid-thigh or mid-calf circumference may demonstrate a larger circumference on the side of a DVT. Less reliably, pain is found on dorsiflexion of the foot (Homans' sign).

GENERAL INVESTIGATIONS

■ FBC
An elevated white cell count will be expected with pneumonia, and to a lesser extent in a myocardial infarction.

■ Serum cardiac markers
Following a myocardial infarction, cardiac troponin rises within 6 hours and remains elevated for up to 2 weeks.

- **ECG**
  Angina or a myocardial infarct will result in ECG changes following the anatomical pattern of coronary vascular insufficiency. Involvement of the left main coronary artery would result in ECG changes of ischaemia or infarction in the anterior (V3–4) and left lateral (V4–6) leads. Involvement of the left anterior descending artery will be reflected in the anterior leads, and insufficiency of the posterior descending artery will produce changes in the inferior leads (II, III, aVF). Changes suggestive of ischaemia or NSTEMI are ST segment depression and T wave inversion. Elevated serum cardiac markers distinguish NSTEMI from angina. ST segment elevation infarcts (STEMI) by definition produce ST segment elevation and Q wave formation in the corresponding leads. Pulmonary emboli usually result in non-specific ECG changes such as tachycardia, right axis deviation, right ventricular strain and atrial fibrillation. Occasionally one may find the S1Q3T3 pattern (S wave in lead I, Q wave and an inverted T wave in lead III), indicative of right heart strain.

- **CXR**
  The line of the pleura with absence of lung markings distal to it is the usual finding for a pneumothorax. Areas of consolidation on a chest film may be confined to a lobe or widespread in bronchopneumonia. The classic wedge-shaped shadow (base is distal) of a pulmonary embolus is rare, and occurs only if pulmonary infarction resulted. Dissection of the aorta may widen its width, causing a bulge to appear at the right mediastinal border. Rib fractures or secondary deposits in ribs may be visible.

SPECIFIC INVESTIGATIONS

- **V/Q scan**
  Will show a mismatch in the majority of pulmonary emboli.

- **Pulmonary angiography**
  Pulmonary emboli will be delineated. It is possible to visualise the site and extent of the embolism and it may also be possible to extract the emboli using a catheter.

- **CT aortography**
  Confirm and assess the extent and site of the dissection of the aorta.

- **Upper GI tract endoscopy**
  Oesophagitis.

- **Oesophageal manometry**
  Abnormal oesophageal pressures.

- It is important to perform a prompt history, examination and initial investigations in patients who present with chest pain as a number of conditions require urgent management.

- If tension pneumothorax is suspected as a cause of chest pain, do not wait for a chest film. Decompress the pneumothorax immediately with a large-bore cannula inserted into the 2nd intercostal space in the midclavicular line.

CLUBBING

Clubbing is the selective bulbous enlargement of the distal segments of fingers or toes due to proliferation of connective tissues.

CAUSES

RESPIRATORY

- Bronchial carcinoma
- Chronic suppurative lung disease
  - Bronchiectasis
  - Lung abscess
  - Empyema
  - Cystic fibrosis
- Interstitial lung disease (fibrosing alveolitis, pulmonary fibrosis)

CARDIOVASCULAR

- Infective endocarditis
  - (in developing countries)
- Congenital cyanotic heart disease

GASTROINTESTINAL

- Cirrhosis
- Ulcerative colitis
- Crohn's disease
- Coeliac disease

OTHER

- Graves' disease (hyperthyroidism)
- Familial

Clubbing is said to be present when there is loss of the normal angle between the base of the nail and the nailfold. In the presence of clubbing, when the fingernails from each hand are placed together, the gap is lost and this is known as Schamroth's sign. Other features are increased curvature of the nailbed (in all directions), sponginess or fluctuation, and expansion of the end of the digit to resemble a drumstick.

HISTORY

A systematic approach to the history is required to determine the cause of clubbing. Respiratory, cardiovascular and gastrointestinal system enquiries should be made in an attempt to determine the underlying cause. A detailed discussion on the diagnosis of congenital cyanotic heart disease (tetralogy of Fallot, transposition of great arteries, total anomalous pulmonary venous drainage) is beyond the scope of this text.

Duration

The duration of clubbing may give an indication of the underlying aetiology. Clubbing present since infancy would suggest a familial trait or congenital cyanotic heart disease. Alternatively, it may be a secondary manifestation of hereditary disorders such as coeliac disease and cystic fibrosis.

Respiratory symptoms

A history of cough, haemoptysis, dyspnoea and weight loss in a chronic smoker should alert the clinician to the diagnosis of bronchial carcinoma. Symptoms of metastasis (bone pain, jaundice) and paraneoplastic involvement (neuropathy, thirst and polyuria from hypercalcaemia) should also be ascertained. With bronchial carcinoma, clubbing may be part of a generalised arthritic manifestation of hypertrophic pulmonary osteoarthropathy.

Cough productive of copious amounts of purulent sputum is usually the main complaint with bronchiectasis. With a chronic lung abscess or empyema, the symptoms are often less specific and may be preceded by a history of pneumonia or aspiration secondary to neurological disorders, dysphagia or alcoholism. Patients may present with a persistent low-grade pyrexia, malaise, weight loss and productive cough. Shortness of breath and a non-productive cough characterise interstitial lung disease.

Gastrointestinal symptoms

Malaise, diarrhoea, abdominal pain and weight loss are experienced by most patients with inflammatory bowel disease and coeliac disease. The presence of aphthous ulceration, fistulae and perianal sepsis are suggestive of Crohn's disease. Predominantly rectal involvement with tenesmus, mucus and blood PR is more characteristic of ulcerative colitis; however, differentiation based on the history alone can be very difficult. Symptoms of coeliac disease tend to be very variable and non-specific, with non-bloody diarrhoea with steatorrhoea.

Heavy alcohol consumption or previous infection with hepatitis B will predispose to cirrhosis of the liver. Patients may complain of jaundice, abdominal distension due to ascites (p. 33), upper gastrointestinal haemorrhage due to varices or bruising from impaired clotting (p. 526). Severely affected individuals may present with encephalopathy or even coma (p. 67).

Family history

A family history of clubbing or cystic fibrosis will suggest a hereditary cause. Approximately 15% of patients with coeliac disease will have an affected first-degree relative.

EXAMINATION

Inspection

The presence of wasting may be accounted for by cachexia of malignancy or chronic lung or gastrointestinal disease. The mucous membranes should be inspected for central cyanosis, which may be a feature of, or sequel to, congenital cyanotic heart disease. Cyanosis may also be noticeable with any of the above causes of severe lung disease. Aphthous ulceration occurs with Crohn's and coeliac disease. A goitre, exophthalmos, ophthalmoplegia and a resting tremor are features of Graves' disease.

With infective endocarditis, splinter haemorrhages, Osler's nodes (raised tender lesions on the pulps of the fingers) and Janeway lesions (flat non-tender macules on the palms and soles) may also be present.

Temperature

Pyrexia is notable in several important causes of clubbing, namely suppurative lung disease, infective endocarditis and active inflammatory bowel disease.

Examination of the chest

Auscultation of the precordium may reveal new or changing murmurs with infective endocarditis. Widespread coarse crepitations of the lungs occur with retained secretions of bronchiectasis. Fine quality end-inspiratory crepitations are suggestive of interstitial lung disease. More localised coarse crepitations and dullness to percussion may be found with a lung abscess. Findings suggestive of pleural effusion (unilateral decreased expansion, dullness to percussion and absent breath sounds) may be due to malignancy. However, when this is associated with pyrexia in an ill patient, it should lead to the consideration of a thoracic empyema.

Abdominal examination

On abdominal examination, signs of chronic liver disease (p. 34) may be present; however, there may be few specific features to suggest inflammatory bowel disease. When this diagnosis is suspected, a sigmoidoscopy should always be performed. Occasionally, right iliac fossa tenderness or a mass may be found in Crohn's disease. The presence of splenomegaly may indicate portal hypertension with liver disease, or enlargement accompanying infective endocarditis.

GENERAL INVESTIGATIONS

■ **FBC**
Hb ↓ carcinomatosis, inflammatory bowel disease, infective endocarditis. WCC ↑ lung abscess, empyema, inflammatory bowel disease.

■ **ESR**
↑ malignancy, inflammatory bowel disease, infective endocarditis.

■ **LFTs**
Liver disease.

■ **CXR**
Should be performed if respiratory symptoms are present. Bronchial carcinoma may manifest as a hilar or peripheral opacity, cavitating mass, collapse of a segment of lung due to luminal obstruction, pleural effusion, elevated hemidiaphragm due to phrenic nerve palsy or destruction of an adjacent rib due to invasion. Lung abscesses present as a spherical shadow with a central lucency or air–fluid level. Bronchiectatic lungs have visibly dilated bronchi and multiple areas of consolidation. With fibrosing alveolitis, hazy shadowing of the lung bases produces a honeycomb appearance.

SPECIFIC INVESTIGATIONS

In view of the diverse nature of causes of clubbing, further investigations should be guided by the history and findings on clinical examination.

■ **Urinalysis**
Blood from microemboli in infective endocarditis.

■ **Blood cultures (three sets)**
Infective endocarditis.

■ **Echocardiography**
Useful in the diagnosis of infective endocarditis, especially in the presence of large vegetations.

■ **Sigmoidoscopy**
Inflammatory bowel disease – characteristic findings include erythematous mucosa, areas of haemorrhage, contact bleeding and ulceration.

■ **Rectal and colonic biopsy**
Ulcerative colitis and Crohn's disease.

■ **Colonoscopy**
Inflammatory bowel disease.

■ **Barium enema**
Inflammatory bowel disease.

■ **Small bowel enema**
Crohn's disease.

■ **Antireticulin and endomysial antibodies**
Coeliac disease.

■ **Jejunal biopsy**
Coeliac disease. May reveal subtotal villous atrophy reversible with a gluten-free diet.

■ **CT thorax**
Should be performed if bronchial carcinoma or thoracic empyema is suspected. Also useful to confirm the diagnosis of bronchiectasis and idiopathic pulmonary fibrosis.

• **Malignancy must be excluded when clubbing develops. Localising features such as respiratory or gastrointestinal disease associated with weight loss and raised inflammatory markers are ominous signs. Investigation is tailored to the presentation.**

COMA

Coma results from sustained impairment of awareness of
self and of the environment. It can simply be defined as a state
of unconsciousness or numerically categorised as a GCS score of <8.

CAUSES

TRAUMA

- Head injury (diffuse axonal injury)
- Extradural haemorrhage
- Subdural haemorrhage

METABOLIC

- Diabetic ketoacidosis
- Hypoglycaemia
- Hypothermia
- Hyperglycaemia
- Hyponatraemia
- Hypernatraemia

ORGAN FAILURE

- Cardiac/circulatory failure
- Respiratory failure
- Liver failure (encephalopathy)
- Renal failure (uraemic coma)
- Hypothyroidism

VASCULAR

- Stroke
- Subarachnoid haemorrhage

INFECTIVE

- Meningitis
- Encephalitis
- Cerebral malaria in developed world
- In endemic areas

TOXIN/DRUG-INDUCED

- Alcohol
- Overdose (opiates, tricyclics, benzodiazepines)
- Carbon monoxide poisoning

CEREBRAL

- Epilepsy
- Brain tumour
- Brain abscess

HISTORY

The history for the comatose patient is usually obtained co-laterally from relatives, friends, witnesses or ambulance crew. Other sources of information are previous hospital notes, records kept by general practitioners, and tablets or prescriptions that have been found at the patient's premises.

Presentation

The circumstances regarding discovery of the patient is usually the first piece of information to be reported. Trauma patients may have been transported from sites of road traffic accidents, fire or have been found assaulted on the street. When teenagers are brought in unconscious from a night club, it is important to exclude alcohol intoxication, epilepsy, hypoglycaemia and the effects of illicit drugs (malignant hyperthermia with 'ecstasy'). Attempted suicides may have an accompanying note, or drug bottles may have been recovered from the scene. Carbon monoxide poisoning occurs with suicide attempts in enclosed areas with running engines or may be a complication in victims involved with fires. Patients who have been brought in from cold environments may also have hypothermia in addition to the primary event.

Onset

When witnessed, information regarding the speed of onset of coma may help in determining a cause. Sudden onset of unconsciousness is characteristic of a seizure or a vascular event.

Trauma

Head injuries are a common cause of coma, but not all causes are due to blunt trauma to the cranium. Diffuse axonal injury results from severe shearing forces on the brain, a sequel to rapid acceleration and deceleration forces. Blunt head injuries may cause extradural haemorrhages as a result of skull fractures with laceration of meningeal arteries. There is usually a history of an injury with transient loss of consciousness, a lucid interval in which the patient feels and appears well, followed by drowsiness, headache, vomiting, progressive hemiplegia and eventually coma. Subdural haemorrhages are a consequence of severe trauma with cortical lacerations or less severe trauma with laceration of bridging veins. Chronic subdural haemorrhages may result even in the absence of trauma; elderly patients with cortical atrophy are predisposed to this type of injury.

In addition to head injury, coma may also complicate any other condition severe enough to result in circulatory or respiratory insufficiency.

Headache

The onset of severe headache prior to coma may be caused by trauma, subarachnoid haemorrhage (classically patients complain of a sudden onset of blinding headache, the worst ever experienced) or meningitis (headache associated with photophobia and neck stiffness). Progressive headache, worse in the mornings and associated with vomiting, may be due to raised intracranial pressure from a cerebral tumour.

Predisposing factors

The history of possible predisposing factors is useful when assessing the comatose patient. The presence of diabetes should lead to the consideration of ketoacidosis (type I diabetics) and hypoglycaemia (oral hypoglycaemic or insulin dosage errors). Patients with known hepatic or renal failure may deteriorate to coma as a result of encephalopathy or uraemia, respectively. Coma may also complicate severe hypothyroidism. Previous suicide attempts or a history of depression should lead to the consideration of drug overdose. Epileptic patients may be in status epilepticus or in a post-ictal recovery state. Pre-existing cardiac or respiratory disease may result in coma as a terminal event.

EXAMINATION

Temperature

Body temperature should be recorded and a series of normal body temperatures will exclude hypothermia and hyperpyrexia as a consequence of heat stroke or illicit drug use.

General examination

A thorough inspection should be performed. This will necessitate removal of clothing, log rolling (to examine the back) and a detailed examination of the scalp for bleeding, haematomas and fractures. The presence of bilateral periorbital haematomas or cerebrospinal fluid rhinorrhoea may indicate an anterior fossa fracture of the skull. Bruising over the mastoid (Battle's sign) or cerebrospinal fluid otorrhoea may be due to a middle cranial fossa fracture. Patients with carbon monoxide poisoning may appear bright red. Patients with myxoedema are characteristically obese, with coarse features, dry skin and brittle hair. The arms should be carefully scrutinised for lacerations and needle puncture sites suggestive of drug abuse and thus the possibility of opiate overdose. A petechial rash may be visible with meningococcal meningitis.

The organ systems should be examined in turn; suspect encephalopathy if signs suggestive of liver disease are present (p. 34) or uraemia with chronic renal failure. The pulse should be examined for arrhythmias, which may precipitate cardiac failure. The JVP may also be elevated. Other causes of JVP distension include tension pneumothorax and cardiac tamponade, both of which may embarrass the circulation and precipitate unconsciousness.

Auscultation of the chest may reveal bilateral crepitations with pulmonary oedema from left ventricular failure, bronchopneumonia, chronic bronchitis or aspiration.

Neurological examination

The neurological examination should begin with the GCS score. Patients who are not involved in trauma should be assessed for neck stiffness which may result from meningitis or subarachnoid haemorrhage. Trauma patients should have the cervical spine assessed for injury before any manipulation is undertaken. The pupils should be examined for size and light reflex. Pinpoint pupils occur with opiate overdoses, small pupils with brainstem lesions and dilated pupils with cocaine or amphetamine use, hypoglycaemia, post-ictal states and brainstem death. A unilateral fixed and dilated pupil occurs with an oculomotor nerve lesion, which may result from pressure exerted from intracranial haemorrhage or tumour. Fundoscopy should be performed to identify loss of retinal vein pulsation or frank papilloedema indicating raised intracranial pressure. A limited neurological examination can be performed on comatose patients; this will include assessment of tone, reflexes and the Babinski response. Unilateral increased tone, hyperreflexia and an up-going plantar response is indicative of a contralateral upper motor neurone lesion, such as a stroke, intracranial haemorrhage or tumour.

GENERAL INVESTIGATIONS

- **FBC**
  ↑ WCC with meningitis. Viral meningitis is associated with lymphocytosis, and neutrophilia is associated with bacterial meningitis.

- **Blood glucose**
  A bedside blood sugar estimation is very useful to exclude hypoglycaemia.

- **Urinalysis**
  Ketones will be present in diabetic ketoacidosis. The urine should also be sent for toxicology analysis if poisoning is suspected.

- **U&Es**
  The urea and creatinine is elevated with renal failure. Disorders of sodium levels will be readily identified.

- **LFTs**
  The bilirubin and transaminases are markedly elevated in liver failure.

- **TFTs**
  $\uparrow$ TSH, $\downarrow$ T_4 with hypothyroidism.

- **Toxicology screen**
  For cases of suspected poisoning and overdose, serum levels of salicylates and paracetamol will be helpful in both diagnosis and treatment. Ethanol levels should also be checked, and carboxyhaemoglobin levels if carbon monoxide poisoning is suspected.

- **ECG**
  An ECG is useful to diagnose arrhythmia and myocardial infarction (p. 60); either disorder may compromise the circulation.

- **CXR**
  May reveal pulmonary oedema or lobar consolidation due to infection or aspiration.

- **X-ray cervical spine**
  Exclude fracture in traumatic causes of coma.

- **CT**
  With a history of trauma or clinical signs which suggest head injury, a CT scan should be requested (this is in preference to a skull X-ray). Additionally, CT will reveal the presence and location of intracranial bleeding and tumours.

SPECIFIC INVESTIGATIONS

- **Lumbar puncture**
  A lumbar puncture is performed in cases of suspected meningitis and the CSF (which may be turbid) is then sent for microscopy and culture.

- **EEG**
  The EEG is indicated when the diagnosis of epilepsy is suspected. Status epilepticus, however, should be diagnosed and treated clinically. The EEG is also useful in the diagnosis of encephalitis.

- Coma is a medical or surgical emergency. The cause must be identified as rapidly as possible in order to improve the prognosis. Early brain imaging is advised once metabolic causes have been excluded.

CONFUSION

Confusion is a behavioural state of reduced mental clarity, coherence, comprehension and reasoning. The causes may be organic or psychiatric (the reader is referred to a textbook of psychiatry for these conditions). The organic causes are listed below.

CAUSES

TOXINS/DRUGS

- Alcohol intoxication/withdrawal
- Drug intoxication

HYPOXIA

- Respiratory disorders
- Cardiac failure

METABOLIC DISORDER

- Hyperglycaemia/hypoglycaemia
- Electrolyte imbalance, e.g. sodium, calcium
- Thiamine (vitamin B_1) deficiency
- Vitamin B_{12} deficiency

SYSTEMIC DISEASE

- Renal failure
- Liver failure
- Thyroid disorders

NEUROLOGICAL

- Head injuries
- Epilepsy (post-ictal)
- Stroke/TIA
- Cerebral metastasis

INFECTION

- Respiratory tract infections
- Septicaemia
- Meningitis/encephalitis
- Urinary tract infection

HISTORY

Onset

Sudden onset of confusion may be precipitated by head injuries, epilepsy, stroke and metabolic disorders. Systemic infection, systemic disease and cerebral metastasis tend to pursue a more gradual onset.

Past medical history

Diabetes is associated with abnormalities of glucose levels with hyperglycaemia resulting from poor diabetic control and hypoglycaemia developing due to drug administration error, missing meals or unaccustomed exercise. A history of thyroid disorder is very relevant and confusion can result from both hyper- and hypothyroidism (myxoedema madness). The presence or carcinoma may precipitate confusion as a result of cerebral metastasis or the development of hypercalcaemia of malignancy. Encephalopathy is a feature of both liver failure and thiamine deficiency. Renal disease can lead to confusion from uraemic encephalopathy or as a result of electrolyte disorders. Hypoxia may result from cardiac failure and respiratory disease.

Drug history

Both the use and abrupt withdrawal of benzodiazepines, barbiturates, steroids and illicit drugs can result in confusion. A drug history is especially important in the elderly, as many drugs may precipitate confusion. Alcohol intoxication and withdrawal (delirium tremens) may cause confusion.

Associated symptoms

Confusion with associated motor weakness may be due to a stroke or cerebral metastasis. Sensory deficits may result from thiamine and vitamin B_{12} deficiencies. The elderly are particularly susceptible to confusion precipitated by respiratory or urinary tract infections and may complain of pyrexia or cough with purulent sputum, or dysuria, frequency, malodorous urine, pyuria and haematuria, respectively. Occasionally, myocardial infarction may present as confusion in the elderly.

EXAMINATION

Temperature

The presence of pyrexia is suggestive of an infective aetiology and a focus for this should be sought.

General

The mental state should be assessed and level of consciousness documented by a GCS score. Careful inspection may reveal scalp lacerations, bleeding or haematoma to suggest the presence of head injury. The antecubital forearm veins may have evidence of needle punctures with intravenous drug abuse.

SECTION A

Systemic examination

Examination of the systems is required to identify general features suggestive of cardiac, respiratory, liver, renal and thyroid diseases.

Neurological examination

The cranial nerves are examined and the presence of nystagmus may be due to acute alcohol intoxication, phenytoin toxicity, barbiturate overdose or cerebellar disease from chronic alcohol abuse. When nystagmus is associated with ocular palsies and ataxia it is suggestive of Wernicke–Korsakoff syndrome, caused by thiamine deficiency. Isolated cranial nerve abnormalities may also result from meningitis. The motor system is examined and unilateral upper motor neurone weakness may be due to stroke or cerebral metastasis. Sensory neuropathy can result from diabetes, renal failure, alcoholism, carcinoma, thiamine and vitamin B_{12} deficiency. With subacute combined degeneration of the cord from vitamin B_{12} deficiency there is predominant involvement of the posterior columns, with loss of vibration, proprioception and light touch. Classically, loss of ankle jerks and an extensor plantar response accompany this.

GENERAL INVESTIGATIONS

- **BM stix**
  ↑ or ↓ glucose.
- **Blood glucose**
  Hypoglycaemia/hyperglycaemia.
- **Oxygen saturation**
  ↓ with cardiac or respiratory disorder.
- **ABGs**
  Hypercapnia with respiratory disease. Hypoxaemia.
- **Infection screen**
  Sputum, urine and blood cultures.
- **Toxicology screen**
  Plasma and urine for alcohol or specific drug/toxin.
- **FBC**
  Macrocytic anaemia with vitamin B_{12} deficiency. WCC ↑ infection and infarction. Thick blood film if malaria is suspected.
- **U&Es**
  ↓ or ↑ sodium, ↑ urea and creatinine with renal failure.
- **LFTs**
  ↑ bilirubin and transaminases with liver failure.
- **Serum calcium**
  ↑ or ↓.
- **TFTs**
  Hypothyroidism (myxoedema). Hyperthyroidism.

- **B_{12} assay**
  ↓ with subacute combined degeneration of the cord.
- **ECG**
  To screen for silent myocardial infarction.
- **CXR**
  Bronchial or lobar consolidation – pneumonia.

SPECIFIC INVESTIGATIONS

- **CT or MRI head**
  Cerebral metastasis. Stroke. Head injuries.
- **EEG**
  Epilepsy.
- **Lumbar puncture**
  Meningitis.

- Acute confusion requires immediate investigation to exclude metabolic causes. A low threshold for brain imaging is mandatory as urgent treatment may be required. Delay in treatment may have devastating consequences, such as in stroke or meningococcal meningitis.

CONSTIPATION

Constipation is a common complaint that results from decreased frequency of abnormally firm motions for a particular patient. It must be related to the patient's normal bowel habit. Acute constipation may be due to acute intestinal obstruction, generalised abdominal disease or sudden alteration in routine, e.g. admission to hospital.

CAUSES

CONGENITAL

- Hirschsprung's disease

ACQUIRED

OBSTRUCTION
- Diverticular disease
- Colonic carcinoma
- Extrinsic compression, e.g. pregnancy, ovarian tumours

PAINFUL ANUS
- Fissure-in-ano
- Perianal abscess
- Strangulated haemorrhoids
- Post-haemorrhoidectomy

ADYNAMIC BOWEL
- Paralytic ileus
- Spinal cord injury

ENDOCRINE
- Diabetes (autonomic neuropathy)
- Myxoedema
- Hyperparathyroidism

DRUGS
- Codeine phosphate
- Morphine
- Tricyclic antidepressants
- Atropine
- Laxative abuse

OTHER
- Dietary changes
- Anxiety/depression
- Irritable bowel syndrome

● Generalised disease
○ Starvation

HISTORY

Congenital

Hirschsprung's disease usually presents with constipation from birth. Gross abdominal distension may eventually occur. The condition may not be picked up until well into the teens or even early adult life.

Acquired

Obstruction

There may be rapid onset of constipation, although the onset is usually gradual with the patient complaining of colicky abdominal pain, bloating, weight loss, lethargy and occasionally spurious diarrhoea. Constipation may occur from pressure from adjacent organs, e.g. with pregnancy, ovarian cyst or large fibroids. Diverticular disease with or without stricture may cause constipation.

Painful anus

Patients may become constipated from any anal disorder that results in pain on defecation. The most common cause is fissure-in-ano, and other causes include strangulated haemorrhoids (the patient often giving a past history of haemorrhoids), perianal abscess and haemorrhoidectomy.

Adynamic bowel

Paralytic ileus may follow abdominal surgery or abdominal inflammatory conditions. It may also arise following spinal fractures or prolonged bedrest, especially in the elderly. The patient's main complaint is usually of a distended abdomen.

Endocrine

Check for a history of diabetes as diabetic autonomic neuropathy *per se* can result in constipation. Myxoedema result, in constipation and there may be associated symptoms of cold intolerance, coarse hair and skin changes. Hypercalcaemia (e.g. hyperparathyroidism) is associated with constipation and symptoms include nocturia, nausea, vomiting, abdominal pain and mental disturbances.

Drugs

Take a careful drug history. Chronic laxative abuse may make the bowel 'lazy' and result in constipation.

Other

Patients with anxiety or depression may complain of constipation. Symptoms of depression include a change in sleep pattern, waking early and having difficulty getting back to sleep. With irritable bowel syndrome, the patient may complain of constipation or diarrhoea, or both alternating. A change in diet alone can also cause constipation, in patients deliberately trying to lose weight or in those with conditions associated with reduced food intake. Generalised disease, which affects the appetite, particularly results in constipation.

EXAMINATION

Obstruction

There will be a distended abdomen with obstructive high-pitched tinkling bowel sounds. The rectum will usually be empty on digital rectal examination. With a diverticular stricture there may be tenderness in the left iliac fossa. With malignancy, a mass may be palpable in the abdomen.

Painful anus

Inspection of the anus may reveal a chronic fissure-in-ano, strangulated haemorrhoids or a perianal abscess. With fissure-in-ano digital rectal examination will be extremely painful, if not impossible. Patients who are post-haemorrhoidectomy may become constipated if appropriate medication has not been given.

Adynamic bowel

The abdomen will be distended and this is often a painless distension. Bowel sounds will be absent. There may be signs of recent surgery. A full neurological examination should be carried out if the cause of the ileus is not apparent.

Endocrine

With diabetes there will usually be other complications of diabetes. In myxoedema, check carefully for other signs, e.g. coarse and dry hair, large tongue, hoarse voice, slow relaxing reflexes.

For any patient with constipation a digital rectal examination must be carried out. The rectum may be completely empty with obstruction, or contain rock-hard faecal masses with functional constipation.

GENERAL INVESTIGATIONS

- **FBC, ESR**
  Hb ↓ anaemia associated with bowel carcinoma. WCC ↑ diverticulitis. ESR ↑ carcinoma.

- **U&Es**
  Urea ↑ with dehydration with obstructive causes.

- **LFTs**
  Albumin ↓ in starvation.

- Sigmoidoscopy
  Tumour – biopsy. Hirschsprung's disease, biopsy – absence of ganglion cells.
- AXR
  Obstruction – dilated bowel.

SPECIFIC INVESTIGATIONS

- Serum calcium
  Hyperparathyroidism.
- TFTs
  $T_4 \downarrow$, TSH $\uparrow$ in myxoedema.
- Blood glucose
  Diabetes – diabetic autonomic neuropathy.
- Barium enema
  Tumours. Diverticular disease.
- Colonoscopy
  Tumours. Biopsy.
- US
  Tumours, ovarian cysts, fibroids, pregnancy.
- MRI
  Spinal trauma. Spinal disease.

- In a patient presenting with constipation, a digital rectal examination is mandatory.
- Constipation is common in the elderly. If it is accompanied by weight loss, rectal bleeding or mucus discharge, carcinoma is a likely diagnosis.
- Hirschsprung's disease does not always present at birth. It may not be picked up until the child is well into their teens. Consider the diagnosis in a child with constipation, a persistently swollen abdomen and an empty rectum on digital examination.

CONVULSIONS

A convulsion is a series of involuntary violent contractions of voluntary muscles.

CAUSES

NEUROLOGICAL

- Epilepsy
- Febrile convulsions

TRAUMATIC

- Head injuries
- Neurosurgery

METABOLIC

- Hypoxia
- Glucose
- electrolyte abnormalities e.g. calcium, sodium
- Uraemia

VASCULAR

- Infarction
- Subarachnoid haemorrhage
- Intracranial haemorrhage

INFECTIVE

- Meningitis
- Encephalitis
- Cerebral abscess

NEOPLASTIC

- Brain tumours

TOXIN/DRUG-INDUCED

- Alcoholism/withdrawal
- Amphetamines, cocaine, antipsychotics, 'ecstasy'

HISTORY

Event

When evaluating patients with convulsions it is also important to exclude the causes of syncope (p. 427). An accurate description from an observer is invaluable for documentation and may help in differentiating the forms of epileptic seizures. A prodrome or aura may be associated with the onset of a seizure.

Precipitating factors

The history should start with precipitating factors, e.g. causes such as trauma, surgery and drug overdose. Flashing lights may precipitate a seizure in patients with a past history of epilepsy.

Headache

Convulsions associated with headaches may be due to trauma, subarachnoid haemorrhage, meningitis or raised intracranial pressure from a tumour. Patients with subarachnoid haemorrhage may also complain of sudden onset of blinding headache. The headache associated with meningitis is often accompanied with neck stiffness and photophobia. In the presence of raised intracranial pressure, the headache tends to be worse in the mornings and on coughing or sneezing. It may be associated with nausea or vomiting. For a fuller description, see p. 207.

Associated neurology

Pre-existing neurological impairment before the onset of convulsions has important implications. A stroke, subarachnoid haemorrhage or intracranial bleed may precipitate neurological impairment preceding a convulsion. Chronic progressive impairment preceding a seizure may be a result of tumour growth. In the post-ictal period, transient motor weakness may accompany epilepsy (Todd's palsy). Permanent neurological deficit can be induced by cerebral anoxia from prolonged seizures.

Past medical and drug history

Co-existing disease such as diabetes will predispose to abnormalities of serum glucose concentrations. A drug history should be obtained and specific enquiries undertaken regarding illicit drug use. Alcohol consumption should be documented. In epileptics, poor drug compliance may lead to seizure control failure.

EXAMINATION

Temperature

The presence of pyrexia usually suggests an infective aetiology, such as meningitis or cerebral abscess. Examination should also be undertaken to look for the primary focus, such as otitis media or mastoiditis. Convulsions may result as a complication of a pyrexia alone, especially in children.

General examination

A general examination is performed to look for the presence of head injury and also any damage resulting as a consequence of the convulsion.

Neurological examination

The primary aim of a neurological examination following a convulsion is to determine the presence of residual neurological deficit. The neurological assessment should include mental state and higher cortical function. If an abnormality is detected the location may be determined by clinical examination to allow focused investigation. However, neurological abnormalities present immediately after a seizure may resolve completely. Todd's palsy may occur post-ictally.

GENERAL INVESTIGATIONS

- **BM stix**
  Rapid assessment for hypoglycaemia and hyperglycaemia.

- **FBC**
  WCC ↑ meningitis, encephalitis, cerebral abscess.

- **U&Es**
  ↑ or ↓ sodium, ↑ urea and creatinine – renal failure.

- **Serum calcium**
  ↑ or ↓ calcium.

- **Blood glucose**
  ↑ or ↓ glucose.

- **ABGs**
  Hypoxia.

- **CT or MRI head**
  Especially in the presence of neurological deficit. Cerebral tumours – alterations in brain density. Skull fractures. Intracranial bleeding – high-density signal during the first 2 weeks. Subarachnoid haemorrhage – high signal (blood) in the subarachnoid space. Strokes – infarction appears normal in the first 24 hours.

SPECIFIC INVESTIGATIONS

- **Toxicology screen**
  Drug use.

- **EEG**
  Epilepsy.

- **Lumbar puncture**
  Meningitis.

• Metabolic causes of convulsions must be excluded immediately. Brain imaging is indicated if the cause is not easily identified as delay in treatment may result in a poor prognosis.

COUGH

Cough is a reflex explosive expiration that prevents aspiration and promotes the removal of secretions and foreign particles from the lung.

CAUSES

ACUTE

- Inhaled foreign body
- Respiratory tract infection

CHRONIC

PRODUCTIVE

- COPD (mucoid/purulent)
- TB (bloodstained)
  - (common where TB is endemic)
- Bronchiectasis (purulent)
- Pulmonary oedema (pink, frothy)
- Lung cancer (bloodstained)
- Pulmonary embolism (bloodstained)

NON-PRODUCTIVE

- Asthma
- Post-nasal drip
- Gastro-oesophageal reflux
- Drugs (ACE inhibitors)
- Sarcoidosis

HISTORY

Onset and duration

The onset of a cough may be acute or chronic (usually defined as a cough that has persisted for more than 3 weeks). Sudden onset of an unrelenting bout of violent coughing may be due to an inhaled foreign body. If this is large enough to occlude the airway, coughing abruptly ceases and is supervened by cyanosis and eventually unconsciousness.

Sputum

The frequency, quantity and appearance of expectorated sputum can be very helpful in the differential diagnosis. Cough continuously productive of purulent sputum is suggestive of chronic bronchitis and bronchiectasis. Expectorated bloodstained sputum tends to be a complaint of patients with bronchogenic carcinoma, pulmonary embolism and TB.

Smoking history

Smoking alone may cause a chronic cough; however, a long smoking history predisposes to bronchogenic carcinoma and chronic bronchitis.

Associated symptoms

Episodic (or even seasonal) wheezing with shortness of breath is common with asthma. This should be differentiated from the monophonic wheeze, which is suggestive of intraluminal obstruction from foreign bodies or tumour.

Most of the respiratory causes of coughing tend to be accompanied by shortness of breath, but sudden onset of dyspnoea may result from aspiration or pulmonary embolism. Shortness of breath that is worse on recumbency is suggestive of pulmonary oedema; however, asthma may also be worse at night. Weight loss can be a prominent feature with lung tumours and TB.

Pleuritic chest pain may be experienced with pulmonary emboli and pneumonia; unrelenting chest pain is more suggestive of bony metastasis from lung cancer. Retrosternal burning chest pain precipitated by posture suggests gastro-oesophageal reflux disease, and the associated cough is due to aspiration of refluxed material. Frequent clearing of the throat due to nasal discharge or a history of allergy with rhinitis may result in post-nasal drip and precipitate coughing.

EXAMINATION

Temperature

The presence of pyrexia usually indicates an infective aetiology; the temperature may also be raised with pulmonary embolism.

Inspection and palpation

With COPD the chest may be barrel-shaped. Patients suffering with lung cancer or TB may appear cachectic. Cyanosis is a feature of pulmonary embolism and COPD. The fingers should be inspected for clubbing (p. 62), which is associated with bronchial carcinoma and bronchiectasis. The JVP is raised in congestive cardiac failure. The supraclavicular nodes may be palpable with respiratory tract infections, TB and lung cancer.

Auscultation

On auscultation, coarse crepitations are a feature of bronchiectasis and pulmonary oedema. Auscultatory features of bronchial carcinoma are non-specific and may manifest as a pleural effusion (dull to percussion, absent breath sounds, decreased vocal resonance) or segmental collapse of the lung. Widespread wheezing is suggestive of asthma, and a fixed inspiratory wheeze may be heard with bronchial luminal obstruction.

GENERAL INVESTIGATIONS

■ **Sputum cultures**
If a productive cough is present, sputum should be sent for cultures. This will include TB-specific cultures and Ziehl–Neelsen staining.

■ **Peak flow**
Bedside determination of peak expiratory flow rate is useful in the diagnosis of asthma (low peak flow).

■ **WCC**
A raised WCC is a non-specific indicator of infection, as it may also be raised with pulmonary embolism.

■ **CXR**
Very useful and may reveal areas of consolidation with infection. Dilated bronchi with persistent areas of infection are suggestive of bronchiectasis. Apical pulmonary consolidation with calcification and hilar lymphadenopathy is characteristic of TB. The presence of pulmonary oedema is appreciated by bilateral patchy shadowing; this may be accompanied by other radiological features of cardiac failure including cardiomegaly, upper lobe diversion of the pulmonary veins, bilateral pleural effusions and Kerley B lines (1–2 cm horizontal lines in the periphery of the lung fields). Bronchial carcinoma may present as a hilar mass, peripheral mass or with collapse and consolidation of the lung due to airway obstruction. Bilateral hilar lymphadenopathy is suggestive of sarcoidosis.

■ **Respiratory function tests**
Formal respiratory function tests can be used to diagnose airway obstruction (asthma, chronic bronchitis and bronchiectasis) and flow volume loops may reveal fixed airway obstruction.

SPECIFIC INVESTIGATIONS

■ **V/Q scan**
Indicated when the diagnosis of pulmonary embolism is suspected.

■ **Pulmonary angiography**
May be indicated in severely ill patients with suspected pulmonary embolism when surgery or thrombolysis is being considered.

■ **CT thorax**
Useful for the diagnosis and staging of lung cancer; it is also specific for the diagnosis of bronchiectasis.

■ **pH studies**
   24-hour pH monitoring may be required when a diagnosis
   of gastro-oesophageal reflux disease cannot be made on the
   history alone.

- Persistent cough, weight loss and hoarseness in a
  smoker are ominous signs. Arrange a CXR to exclude
  malignancy.

- An unrelenting bout of violent coughing of sudden
  onset may be due to an inhaled foreign body. If
  this is large enough to occlude the upper airways,
  coughing may cease abruptly and cyanosis and
  unconsciousness ensue. Cricothyroidotomy may be
  life saving.

- Ask about foreign travel, especially to countries
  where TB is endemic.

CYANOSIS

Cyanosis is the abnormal blue discoloration of the skin and
mucous membranes resulting from the presence of 5 g/dL or
more of reduced haemoglobin in the blood. It is not synonymous
with hypoxaemia, which may be present (e.g. anaemia) without
cyanosis.

CAUSES

CENTRAL CYANOSIS

DECREASED OXYGEN SATURATION
- Severe respiratory disease
- Pulmonary oedema
- Pulmonary embolism
- Congenital cyanotic heart disease

ABNORMAL HAEMOGLOBIN
- Methaemoglobinaemia
- Sulphaemoglobinaemia

PERIPHERAL CYANOSIS
- All causes of central cyanosis
- Cold exposure
- Raynaud's phenomenon
- Arterial occlusion
- Venous occlusion
- Acrocyanosis

HISTORY

Central cyanosis

Onset

Cyanosis due to congenital heart disease causing anatomical right to left
shunts may have been present from birth or the first few years of life.
Immediate onset of cyanosis may be due to pulmonary emboli or cardiac
failure. Acute onset of cyanosis may be precipitated by pneumonia
and asthma. Patients with COPD develop cyanosis over many years.
Accompanying polycythaemia may exacerbate cyanosis in these patients.

Chest pain

Cyanosis associated with pleuritic chest pain may be due to
pulmonary emboli or pneumonia. Dull, aching chest tightness is
experienced by patients who develop cyanosis from pulmonary
oedema as a complication of myocardial infarction.

Dyspnoea

Sudden onset of dyspnoea can occur with pulmonary emboli and pulmonary oedema, while conditions such as asthma may produce a more gradual onset.

Past medical history and drug history

Any co-existing respiratory disease is significant, as cyanosis can result from any lung disease of sufficient severity. Consumption of drugs such as phenacetin and sulphonamides may precipitate methaemoglobinaemia and sulphaemoglobinaemia, respectively.

Peripheral cyanosis

General history

Acrocyanosis is a condition in which the hands are persistently blue and cold; it is not associated with pain. Raynaud's phenomenon is the episodic three-colour change that occurs, with arterial vasospasm (white), cyanosis (blue) and reactive hyperaemia (red). It may be idiopathic or be associated with connective tissue diseases, and drugs such as beta blockers.

Peripheral cyanosis may also result from acute arterial occlusion and is accompanied by pain and mottling of the skin. Iliofemoral deep venous thrombosis can produce a painful blue leg, termed phlegmasia cerulea dolens.

EXAMINATION

Temperature

Pneumonia and pulmonary emboli may be associated with pyrexia.

Inspection

It is often difficult to detect minor degrees of cyanosis. Central cyanosis produces a blue discoloration of the mucous membranes and digits; peripheral cyanosis produces blue discoloration only of the digits. Episodic peripheral cyanosis may be due to Raynaud's disease and this may be associated with small areas of infarction on the fingertips. The presence of clubbing may be due to congenital cyanotic heart disease. Classically, patients with chronic bronchitis appear cyanosed with a poorly expanding barrelled chest. The JVP is elevated with congestive cardiac failure.

Respiratory examination

Poor chest expansion occurs with chronic bronchitis and asthma. Unilateral impairment of expansion may occur with lobar pneumonia; in addition, dullness to percussion is experienced over the area of consolidation. Localised crepitation may be auscultated with lobar pneumonia, but is more widespread with bronchopneumonia, pulmonary oedema and chronic bronchitis.

SECTION A

Air entry is poor with chronic bronchitis and asthma. Bronchial breathing may be auscultated over an area of consolidation, and additional sounds such as wheezing may be heard with asthma.

GENERAL INVESTIGATIONS

- **Oxygen saturation**
  Saturation is usually below 85% with cyanosis.
- **ABGs**
  ↓ pO_2 all severe lung disease.
- **FBC**
  Hb ↑ chronic cyanosis. WCC ↑ pneumonia and pulmonary embolism.
- **ECG**
  Features of myocardial infarction (p. 59–60). Non-specific abnormalities with pulmonary emboli.
- **CXR**
  Pneumonia, pulmonary infarct, cardiac failure (p. 60).

SPECIFIC INVESTIGATIONS

- **Sputum and blood cultures**
  Pneumonia.
- **V/Q scan or CT pulmonary angiography**
  Pulmonary embolus.
- **Echocardiography**
  Cardiac failure.
- **Hb spectroscopy**
  Methaemoglobinaemia, sulphaemoglobinaemia.
- **Digital subtraction angiography**
  Acute arterial occlusion.
- **Duplex Doppler or venography**
  Acute venous occlusion.

- **The sudden development of cyanosis is an emergency and causes for this, such as pulmonary embolus and pulmonary oedema, must be identified immediately.**
- **Arterial occlusion as a cause of peripheral cyanosis must also be recognised and acted on urgently.**

DEAFNESS

Deafness is loss of hearing and may be divided into 'conductive' and 'sensorineural' to facilitate interpretation of clinical examination.

CAUSES

CONDUCTIVE DEAFNESS

CONGENITAL
- Atresia of the meatus

ACQUIRED
- Obstruction
  - Ear wax
  - Foreign body
- Infection
  - Otitis externa
  - Otitis media (including glue ear)
- Trauma
  - Perforation of the tympanic membrane
  - Barotrauma
- Otosclerosis

SENSORINEURAL DEAFNESS

CONGENITAL
- Maternal rubella, toxoplasmosis, CMV infection

ACQUIRED
- Age-related (presbyacusis)
- Ménière's disease
- Infection
  - Mumps
  - Herpes zoster
  - Meningitis
- Trauma
  - Noise-induced
  - Head injuries
- Drugs
  - Aminoglycosides, aspirin, frusemide
- Tumour
  - Acoustic neuroma (vestibular schwannoma)
  - Brain tumours
  - Paget's disease (see p. 45, 47)

HISTORY

Duration

Childhood deafness may be hereditary, result from maternal rubella infection or arise as a complication of childhood infection (meningitis, toxoplasma or CMV infection). The duration of symptoms may coincide with the introduction of ototoxic drugs.

Onset

Sudden onset of deafness can result from foreign bodies in the external auditory canal. Deafness usually occurs only if the foreign body perforates the tympanic membrane or disrupts the chain of ossicles. Sudden onset of deafness may also result from trauma, vascular catastrophes or Ménière's disease. Gradual development of deafness occurs with otosclerosis, tumours and age.

Pain

Deafness associated with ear pain may be a result of otitis externa, otitis media or infection with herpes zoster. Severe pain is experienced with both direct trauma perforating the tympanic membrane and barotrauma, which can result from a slap on the ear or scuba diving.

Precipitating factors

A history of trauma is usually obvious. Sensorineural deafness can result as a complication of mumps or from prolonged exposure to high noise levels.

Associated symptoms

Tinnitus in combination with episodic deafness and vertigo occur with Ménière's disease. When tinnitus occurs with deafness alone, consider otosclerosis, noise exposure, ototoxic drugs and acoustic neuroma.

Drug history

Offending drugs can easily be determined from a drug history.

EXAMINATION

Examination of the ear

On inspection, the vesicles of herpes zoster or presence of otitis externa may be obvious. With otitis externa, the skin appears erythematous with scaling and exudation. Tenderness will be elicited by movement of the pinna or compression of the tragus.

Otoscopic examination will identify ear wax or foreign bodies occluding the external auditory canal. With a patent ear canal, the tympanic membrane may be visualised, traumatic perforations may be seen as a tear of the tympanum accompanied with blood. Injection, erythema or frank perforation of the tympanic membrane can result from otitis media.

Assessment of hearing

Crude tests of hearing can be performed with conversational voice, whispered voice or measuring how far away from the ear the ticking of a watch can be heard.

Rinne's test is performed with a 512-Hz tuning fork; mastoid or BC is compared with AC. AC conduction is normally better than BC. Weber's test is performed holding the base of the struck tuning fork against the centre of the forehead. Normally the sound is heard equally in both ears (see Table).

Deafness	Rinne's test	Weber's test
Sensorineural	AC > BC	Heard in good ear
Conductive	BC > AC	Heard in deaf ear

General examination

A complete neurological examination is performed. Nystagmus may be present with Ménière's disease; rarely acoustic neuromas may affect the facial nerve, producing unilateral facial paralysis; and motor or sensory deficits can result from brain tumours. Examination should also include the nose and throat, as nasopharyngeal sepsis may be a factor predisposing to middle ear infection.

GENERAL INVESTIGATIONS

- Pure tone audiometry
  Allows accurate measurements of hearing levels with bone and air conduction.

- Swab of ear discharge
  In cases of possible infection.

SPECIFIC INVESTIGATIONS

- Speech audiometry
  Impaired speech discrimination in the 50–80% range occurs with conductive deafness, and 0–50% range with sensorineural causes.

- Electric response audiometry
  Assessment of hearing in babies.

- **Impedance tympanometry**
  Increased impedance (reduced compliance) with otitis media with effusion.

- **MRI**
  Acoustic neuroma, brain tumour.

- **Progressive unilateral deafness accompanied by tinnitus, vertigo or neurological symptoms or signs should prompt urgent investigation for an acoustic neuroma.**

DIARRHOEA

Diarrhoea is an increased frequency of abnormally loose motions for a particular patient. The diagnosis of diarrhoea must be related to the patient's normal bowel habit.

CAUSES

INTESTINAL

INFECTIVE ENTERITIS

Non-specific, Bacterial
- *Campylobacter* spp
  - (rare in tropical Africa)
- *Salmonella* spp
  - (rare in tropical Africa)
- *Escherichia coli*
- *Clostridium difficile*
- Staphylococci
- *Shigella* spp
- *Vibrio cholerae*
- *Yersinia enterocolitica*
  - (common in Indian sub-continent)

Viral, Fungal, Protozoal
- *Cryptosporidium* spp
- *Giardia lamblia*
  - (commoner in children worldwide)
- *Entamoeba histolytica*

INFLAMMATORY
- Ulcerative colitis
- Crohn's disease

MALABSORPTION
- Coeliac disease
- Blind loop syndrome
- Short bowel syndrome
- Radiation

NEOPLASTIC
- Carcinoma
- Villous adenoma

OTHER INTESTINAL
- Diverticular disease
  - (rare in rural Africa and Asia)

- Irritable bowel syndrome
- Faecal impaction – spurious diarrhoea
- Ischaemic colitis
- Ileocolic fistula

GASTRIC

- Post-vagotomy (vagotomy rarely performed nowadays)

PANCREATIC

- Chronic pancreatitis
- Cystic fibrosis
- Carcinoma
- Pancreatic resection

ENDOCRINE

- Diabetes
- Thyrotoxicosis
- Carcinoid syndrome
- Zollinger–Ellison syndrome
- VIPoma
- Medullary thyroid cancer

DRUG-INDUCED

- Antibiotics
- Laxatives
- Magnesium-containing antacids
- Cytotoxic agents

OTHER

- Anxiety
- Diet

HISTORY

Infective enteritis

There is usually colicky abdominal pain and diarrhoea. The diarrhoea may be bloody. Cholera presents with cramping abdominal pain, vomiting and severe diarrhoea, described as 'rice water' stools. There may be fever, rapid dehydration, collapse and death. In infective enteritis, check for ingestion of any unusual food or whether anyone else has been affected in the family. Check for a history of foreign travel (traveller's diarrhoea). *C. difficile* is the most important cause of hospital-acquired diarrhoea. Over 80% of infection occurs in those over 65 years of age, affecting particularly those who have been treated with broad spectrum antibiotics. Infection ranges from mild to severe diarrhoea to more, unusually, pseudomembranous colitis.

Inflammatory bowel disease

Both Crohn's disease and ulcerative colitis present with frequent diarrhoea with blood, and occasionally mucus and pus, associated with colicky abdominal pain. The patient may be toxic and febrile, with abdominal pain and distension if toxic dilatation of the colon has occurred.

Malabsorption

In addition to diarrhoea there may be offensive stools, which are fatty and float, i.e. steatorrhoea. Has the patient had any previous surgery for resection of the bowel to suggest short bowel syndrome, or any bypass surgery to suggest blind loop syndrome? Is there any history of abdominal radiotherapy?

Neoplastic

Carcinoma may cause diarrhoea associated with colicky abdominal pain and the passage of blood and mucus PR. The diarrhoea may be spurious, liquefied stools only passing through an area of obstruction, with faecal masses behind the obstruction. Loose watery mucus passed frequently may be associated with a villous adenoma, the patient complaining of weakness associated with hypokalaemia due to the passage of excessive mucus rich in potassium.

Other intestinal

Diverticular disease may cause diarrhoea. The condition usually occurs in the older patient. The patient will also complain of associated colicky abdominal pain and pain usually in the left iliac fossa. Irritable bowel syndrome may cause similar symptoms to diverticular disease but occurs in the younger patient. Faecal impaction may result in spurious diarrhoea, while an ileocolic fistula associated with diverticular disease or rectosigmoid carcinoma is also associated with diarrhoea. Ischaemic colitis usually presents in an elderly patient with colicky abdominal pain, diarrhoea and passage of dark-red blood PR.

Gastric

Check for a history of gastric surgery. Destruction of the pylorus or section of the vagus nerve may result in diarrhoea, often associated with dumping. Vagotomy is rarely, if ever, performed nowadays.

Pancreatic lesions

These may result in diarrhoea or steatorrhoea. Check for a history of cystic fibrosis. The patient may have chronic pancreatitis, in which case there may be chronic back pain associated with epigastric pain and weight loss. Check for a history of pancreatic surgery. Patients with carcinoma of the pancreas may also present with diarrhoea.

Endocrine disorders

Diabetes is associated with an increased incidence of diarrhoea. Check for a history of thyroid disease. The patient may prefer cold weather and complain of sweating, anxiety, tremor and have obvious eye signs. The patient may also have noticed a goitre. Carcinoid syndrome may present as flushing (especially after alcohol, coffee and certain foods), asthma and loud bowel sounds, i.e. borborygmi. Patients with Zollinger–Ellison syndrome may have a past history of recurrent peptic ulceration, with haematemesis or melaena in addition to diarrhoea. VIPoma is rare but presents with severe watery diarrhoea associated with potassium loss, with weakness due to hypokalaemia. Check whether the patient has a goitre, as diarrhoea may be associated with medullary carcinoma of the thyroid. Symptoms and signs of hyperparathyroidism and phaeochromocytoma may also be present (MEN syndrome).

Drugs

Take a careful drug history, especially for recent antibiotics, laxative abuse, the ingestion of magnesium-containing antacids or recent cytotoxic agents.

Other

Anxiety and dietary changes may lead to diarrhoea. A careful history should be taken, particularly looking at any recent changes in diet.

EXAMINATION

Infective enteritis

The patient may be dehydrated or collapsed. Check for tachycardia and hypotension. There may be abdominal tenderness and distension. Digital rectal examination may reveal blood and pus on the examining glove.

Inflammatory bowel disease

There may be little to find except for mild, localised tenderness. In toxic dilatation there will be fever, malaise, abdominal distension, vomiting and localised tenderness. Perforation may occur with peritonitis. An abdominal mass may be palpable with Crohn's disease.

Neoplastic

There may be abdominal distension if obstruction has occurred. There may be a palpable abdominal mass. Digital rectal examination may reveal a carcinoma or a villous adenoma.

Other intestinal

With diverticular disease there may be little to find other than tenderness in the left iliac fossa. The findings are similar in irritable bowel syndrome. With faecal impaction, rock-hard faecal masses may be palpated in the abdomen and may be felt on digital rectal examination. There may be little to find with an ileocolic fistula. With ischaemic colitis there will be tenderness and guarding in the left side of the abdomen. Rectal examination will reveal dark-red blood.

Gastric

Other than a scar and history of gastric surgery there may be nothing else to find on examination.

Pancreatic

There may be epigastric tenderness or a palpable mass in the epigastrium with pancreatic carcinoma.

Endocrine

With thyrotoxicosis there will be tachycardia, sweating, brisk reflexes, eye signs and a goitre. With carcinoid syndrome there may be hepatomegaly and signs of tricuspid incompetence and pulmonary stenosis. In Zollinger–Ellison syndrome there may be little to find on examination. With VIPoma, other than weakness due to hypokalaemia, there may also be little to find on examination. With medullary carcinoma of the thyroid there will be a palpable goitre.

GENERAL INVESTIGATIONS

- **FBC, ESR**
  Hb ↓ bleeding. PCV ↑ dehydration. WCC ↑ infection. ESR ↑ inflammation, tumour.
- **U&Es**
  Urea ↑ dehydration. Potassium ↓ severe diarrhoea, villous adenoma.
- **LFTs**
  Alkaline phosphatase ↑ with liver metastases.
- **Stool culture and microscopy**
  Infective causes. Microscopy for parasites.
- **Sigmoidoscopy**
  Carcinoma, inflammatory bowel disease, villous adenoma, pseudomembranous colitis.
- **Barium enema**
  Tumours, colitis, diverticular disease.
- **Colonoscopy**
  Tumours, colitis (extent and severity), diverticular disease.

SPECIFIC INVESTIGATIONS

- **TFTs**
  $T_4 \uparrow$, TSH $\downarrow$ in thyrotoxicosis.

- **24-hour urine**
  5HIAA $\uparrow$ in carcinoid.

- **US**
  Carcinoid. Liver metastases.

- **Serum gastrin**
  Zollinger–Ellison syndrome.

- **Serum calcitonin**
  Medullary carcinoma of the thyroid.

- **Serum vasoactive intestinal peptide**
  Raised in VIPoma.

- **Faecal fats**
  Malabsorption.

- **Duodenal/jejunal biopsy**
  Malabsorption – coeliac disease.

- **Small bowel enema**
  Crohn's disease.

- Acute diarrhoea in adults is most likely to be due to infection.
- Do not forget to ask about foreign travel.
- It is important to distinguish diarrhoea from steatorrhoea and faecal incontinence.
- Do not be caught out by overflow ('spurious') diarrhoea in the elderly. Always do a PR.
- Chronic diarrhoea in association with weight loss suggests serious underlying disease.

DIZZINESS

Spatial disorientation may be expressed by the patient as dizziness, vertigo or feeling 'light-headed'. True vertigo is not experienced as a sensation of movement but as tilting or sloping of the environment.

CAUSES

EPISODIC

- Ménière's disease*
- BPPV
- Arrhythmia
- Postural hypotension
- Migraine
- Hyperventilation
- Drugs (antihypertensives, antidepressants)
- Hypoglycaemia
- Recurrent posterior circulation TIAs
- Anxiety
- Seizures (partial)
- Carbon monoxide poisoning (e.g. faulty heating)

CONSTANT

ACUTE ONSET

- Labyrinthitis*
- Acute alcohol or drug intoxication
- Head injuries*
- Vestibular neuronitis
- Posterior circulation CVA

GRADUAL ONSET

- Multiple sclerosis
- Aortic stenosis
- Cerebellopontine angle tumour*
- Ototoxicity – aminoglycosides*

HISTORY

General

The causes above are listed according to speed of onset and duration of symptoms. Conditions that are accompanied by additional audiological symptoms, such as tinnitus, are marked with an asterisk.

* Indicates causes accompanied by audiological symptoms.

Precipitating factors

Causes of dizziness that are precipitated by movements of the head include BPPV, labyrinthitis and head injuries. Patients with BPPV complain of short episodes of dizziness accompanying changes in the position of the head. Labyrinthitis may result either as a complication of systemic viral infection or from extension of a cholesteatoma due to chronic suppurative otitis media. A history of trauma is usually obvious. Postural dizziness precipitated by rising from a lying position may be caused by orthostatic hypotension commonly secondary to anti hypertensive drugs.

Associated symptoms

Dizziness may be precipitated by arrhythmia and patients may complain of associated palpitations. It may also be experienced with migraine attacks and patients may complain of associated unilateral throbbing headache, nausea, vomiting and photophobia. Ménière's disease is diagnosed with a history of episodic severe vertigo with continuous tinnitus and hearing loss. Patients with vertebrobasilar insufficiency from cervical spondylosis may complain of dizziness with extension of the neck. With posterior circulation TIAs, sudden onset of dizziness is caused by ischaemia of the lateral brainstem or cerebellum. This may be accompanied by syncope, nausea, vomiting, visual field defects and diplopia. Severe progressive vomiting and ataxia may also result from intracerebral haemorrhage, a neurosurgical emergency. Patients with anxiety disorders may experience attacks of dizziness, tinnitus and tremor, with or without accompanying hyperventilation. Certainly hyperventilation alone is sufficient to precipitate dizziness. Vertigo is a prominent feature of multiple sclerosis when demyelination occurs in the brainstem; this may be accompanied by dysarthria and cranial nerve palsies. Young age would favour the diagnosis of demyelination over ischaemia. Tumours of the cerebellopontine angle tend to present gradually, dizziness may be mild and this may be accompanied by numbness and facial paralysis due to trigeminal and facial nerve involvement. There are no precipitating factors for vestibular neuronitis, the dizziness is not associated with nausea or tinnitus.

Drug history

Numerous drugs have ototoxic effects; perhaps the most commonly known are aminoglycosides and frusemide.

EXAMINATION

Assessment of nystagmus, hearing and positional testing provide the most amount of information when determining the cause of dizziness.

Multidirectional nystagmus results from diffuse cerebellar disease, while unidirectional nystagmus occurs either with ipsilateral cerebellar disease (multiple sclerosis, posterior circulation TIA/CVA) or contralateral vestibular disease (Ménière's, labyrinthitis, acoustic neuroma). On lateral gaze, nystagmus of the abducting eye with failure of adduction of the opposite eye is due to internuclear ophthalmoplegia, classically caused by brainstem demyelination.

Hearing is assessed with Rinne's and Weber's tests (p. 93). Sensorineural hearing loss may be caused by Ménière's, acoustic neuroma and drug-induced ototoxicity. Hearing loss accompanied by trigeminal and facial nerve palsy may be due to tumour effects at the cerebellopontine angle.

Specific positional tests, such as the Hallpike test, are performed to assess the integrity of the vestibulo-ocular and labyrinthine pathways. Patients with BPPV usually complain of vertigo and exhibit delayed nystagmus that fatigues on repeated testing.

A complete neurological examination is then undertaken. Homonymous hemianopia can result from posterior circulation infarcts and brainstem lesions such as demyelination, and stroke may give rise to combinations of ipsilateral cranial nerve palsies and motor or sensory deficits of the face. In addition, pale optic discs due to optic atrophy may be seen in multiple sclerosis. Patients with cerebellar disease will exhibit an intention tremor when performing the finger–nose test. In addition to a broad-based ataxic gait, they may also exhibit nystagmus, dysdiadochokinesia and dysarthria.

When a cardiovascular cause is suspected, the pulse is assessed for irregularities of rhythm, which may suggest atrial fibrillation. The blood pressure is measured both lying and standing to screen for postural hypotension, and potential sites for emboli, such as the cardiac valves and the carotid vessels, are auscultated for murmurs and bruits, respectively. Severe aortic stenosis may lead to dizziness.

GENERAL INVESTIGATIONS

Most causes of dizziness can be diagnosed on history and clinical examination.

- **FBC**
  Hb ↑ predisposes to CVA. WCC ↑ infection.
- **ESR**
  ↑ CVA, malignancy, infection.
- **Urinalysis**
  Raised glucose in diabetes.
- **LFTs**
  May be abnormal in alcohol abuse.
- **Thiamine**
  Reduced in chronic alcohol abuse.

SPECIFIC INVESTIGATIONS

■ **24-hour ECG**
  To screen for arrhythmia.

■ **Audiometry**
  Allows assessment and classification of any accompanying hearing loss.

■ **Carotid Doppler**
  To evaluate patency of the vessel and to screen for the presence of plaque (TIAs).

■ **ECHO**
  To evaluate aortic valve.

■ **CT head**
  Stroke, cerebellar haemorrhage, evaluation of severe head injuries.

■ **MRI**
  Acoustic neuroma and other cerebellopontine angle tumours, demyelination with multiple sclerosis.

■ **EEG**
  To detect seizure activity.

- Dizziness accompanied by other symptoms such as loss of consciousness, palpitations or neurological symptoms should be investigated immediately.

- Dizziness associated with an aortic murmur requires urgent referral. Significant aortic stenosis is a cause of sudden death.

DYSPHAGIA

Dysphagia means difficulty in swallowing and should be distinguished from pain on swallowing. Dysphagia may be associated with ingestion of solids or liquids, or both. Pain on swallowing is odynophagia, which in itself does not interfere with the act of swallowing.

CAUSES

CONGENITAL

- Oesophageal atresia

ACQUIRED

IN THE LUMEN

- Food bolus
- Foreign body

IN THE WALL

- Inflammatory stricture
  - Gastro-oesophageal reflux
  - Caustic stricture
  - Candidiasis
- Carcinoma
- Irradiation
- Scleroderma
- Achalasia
- Plummer–Vinson syndrome
- Chagas' disease
  - (South America)

OUTSIDE THE WALL

- Goitre
- Paraoesophageal (rolling) hiatus hernia
- Mediastinal tumours
  - Bronchial carcinoma
  - Lymphadenopathy
- Pharyngeal pouch
- Enlarged left atrium (mitral stenosis)
- Thoracic aortic aneurysm
- Dysphagia lusoria (rare)

NEUROMUSCULAR DISORDERS

- CVA
- Bulbar palsy
- Guillain–Barré syndrome

- Motor neurone disease
- Myasthenia gravis

HISTORY

Congenital
Oesophageal atresia

This may be associated with maternal polyhydramnios. The newborn baby will show dribbling of saliva, inability to swallow feeds, production of frothy mucus, choking attacks, cyanotic attacks and chest infections.

Acquired
In the lumen

There may be a history of ingestion of a foreign body such as a coin (children) or false teeth (elderly). Occasionally the history may not be forthcoming. In the case of a food bolus it is unusual for this to cause dysphagia without there being some form of underlying stricture.

In the wall

With a caustic stricture there is usually a history of caustic ingestion, except in the psychiatrically disturbed, where the history may not be apparent. There will be sudden onset of pain and dysphagia, which may improve with appropriate treatment only to recur after several months due to a stricture. Patients with inflammatory stricture due to gastro-oesophageal reflux associated with a hiatus hernia will have a history of retrosternal burning pain and acid reflux which is worse on recumbency or bending down. The dysphagia is usually of gradual onset and the patient may localise the site of dysphagia to the level of the lower end of the sternum. Oesophageal candidiasis may cause dysphagia and this usually occurs in the immunocompromised patient. Achalasia is a disorder where there is degeneration of the oesophageal myenteric plexus resulting in loss of peristaltic contraction in the oesophagus and failure of the lower oesophageal sphincter to relax in response to swallowing. It usually presents between 30 and 50 years of age. The dysphagia may be intermittent and then gets progressively worse. It may be worse for liquids than for solids. Fluid regurgitation at night may result in aspiration pneumonitis. With carcinoma, the dysphagia is usually of rapid onset. Initially it is for solids, then for fluids. There may be associated weight loss, anorexia and symptoms of anaemia. There may be a history of achalasia or Barrett's oesophagus. Dysphagia with food sticking at the upper end of the oesophagus in a middle-aged woman may suggest Plummer–Vinson syndrome. This is due to a web in the upper oesophagus (post-cricoid web). The condition is premalignant. A history of radiotherapy to chest or mediastinum may suggest an irradiation stricture. With scleroderma, the patient may have noticed changes in the skin, around the lips, in the fingers (sclerodactyly) or may have a past history of Raynaud's phenomenon. Chagas' disease is extremely rare and is associated with degeneration of the myenteric plexus associated with trypanosomal infection. The symptoms are identical to those of achalasia.

Outside the wall

The presence of a large goitre will be obvious. With the pharyngeal pouch, patients are usually of middle age or elderly. They may have noticed a swelling, usually in the left posterior triangle of the neck. They may also have dysphagia localised behind the manubrium associated with the pouch pressing on the oesophagus. On lying down there is regurgitation of food with coughing. The patient may also have halitosis. With bronchial carcinoma there may be direct pressure on the oesophagus from the tumour or via secondary spread to the mediastinal lymph nodes. There may be a history of bronchial carcinoma or the patient may present with haemoptysis. With dysphagia from mediastinal lymphadenopathy, the patient may have noticed enlarged swellings at other sites, e.g. axilla or groin. Dysphagia from pressure of an enlarged left atrium may be associated with mitral stenosis and there may be a past history of this. With a paraoesophageal (rolling) hernia the dysphagia may be intermittent, due to a full stomach pressing on the adjacent oesophagus. Hiccups may occur due to irritation of the diaphragm.

Neuromuscular

There will usually be a history of Guillain–Barré syndrome, poliomyelitis, motor neurone disease, myasthenia gravis or a CVA.

EXAMINATION

With oesophageal atresia an orogastric tube is passed and it will arrest at the site of the obstruction.

In many cases of dysphagia there will be nothing to find on examination. A goitre is usually an obvious swelling that moves on swallowing. With a pharyngeal pouch there may be a palpable swelling low down in the posterior triangle of the neck (usually left), which gurgles on palpation. With carcinoma there may be signs of weight loss, a palpable liver due to metastases, or cervical lymphadenopathy due to metastases. Koilonychia, angular cheilitis and glossitis are clinical features associated with Plummer–Vinson syndrome. With irradiation stricture there may be changes in the skin consistent with previous radiotherapy. With scleroderma there may be calcinosis of the subcutaneous tissue, Raynaud's phenomenon, sclerodactyly and telangiectasia. With dysphagia due to an enlarged left atrium in mitral stenosis there may be signs of mitral stenosis, e.g. peripheral cyanosis, malar flush, left parasternal heave, tapping apex beat, opening snap and mid-diastolic murmur best heard at the apex. A variety of neurological abnormalities will be associated with dysphagia of neuromuscular origin.

GENERAL INVESTIGATIONS

- **FBC, ESR**
  Hb ↓ associated with carcinoma but may also occur with oesophagitis associated with peptic strictures. Anaemia may also be associated with Plummer–Vinson syndrome. ESR ↑ in malignancy and scleroderma.

- **U&Es**
  Dehydration.

- **LFTs**
  Alkaline phosphatase ↑ in liver secondaries.

- **CXR**
  Foreign body if radio-opaque. Air–fluid level in achalasia. Gastric air bubble in chest in paraoesophageal hernia. Hilar lymphadenopathy. Bronchial carcinoma. Widened mediastinum with aortic aneurysm. Large left atrium (double shadow behind the heart) – mitral stenosis.

- **ECG**
  Left atrial hypertrophy.

SPECIFIC INVESTIGATIONS

- **Barium swallow**
  Pharyngeal pouch (never OGD as it may perforate the pouch), stricture, achalasia, external compression.

- **OGD**
  Foreign body. Food bolus. Candidiasis. Benign versus malignant stricture. Plummer–Vinson syndrome – post-cricoid web. Biopsy – benign lesion versus malignant lesion, absence of myenteric plexus in achalasia.

- **CT**
  Goitre. Mediastinal nodes. Spread of malignancy. Tumour staging. Aortic aneurysm. Dysphagia lusoria (abnormally placed arteries causing external compression).

- Recent onset of progressive dysphagia in the elderly is due to carcinoma of the oesophagus until proved otherwise.

- It is unusual for dysphagia to occur due to a food bolus alone. It is important to screen for any form of underlying stricture or motility disorder.

- Patients with a long history of oesophagitis who develop dysphagia may have a stricture or carcinoma.

- If endoscopy is normal, consider extrinsic compression and arrange a CT scan.

DYSPNOEA

Dyspnoea is the uncomfortable awareness of breathing.

CAUSES

SUDDEN (SECONDS TO MINUTES)

- Pneumothorax
- Chest trauma
- Aspiration
- Anxiety
- Pulmonary oedema
- Pulmonary embolism
- Anaphylaxis

ACUTE (HOURS TO DAYS)

- Asthma
- Respiratory tract infection
- Pleural effusion
- Lung tumours
- Metabolic acidosis

CHRONIC (MONTHS TO YEARS)

- Chronic airflow limitation (COPD)
- Anaemia
- Arrhythmia
- Valvular heart disease
- Cardiac failure
- Cystic fibrosis
- Idiopathic pulmonary fibrosis
- Chest wall deformities
- Neuromuscular disorders
- Pulmonary hypertension

HISTORY

Many cardiac or respiratory diseases of sufficient severity produce dyspnoea. When considering chronic respiratory causes you may relate them anatomically to diseases of the pulmonary vasculature, airways, interstitium and chest wall. When approaching a patient with dyspnoea it is important to ensure that the ABC are attended to before continuing with the diagnostic process.

Onset

The speed of onset is a useful indicator of the disease process. Classification by speed of onset narrows the differential diagnosis in urgent clinical situations.

Precipitating factors

An obvious precipitating factor may be present, such as trauma causing either fractured ribs or a pneumothorax. Aspiration of a foreign body may be determined from the history; however, aspiration of vomit is more difficult as it usually occurs in patients with decreased consciousness levels or who have lost the gag reflex. Dyspnoea on recumbency is caused by cardiac failure; occasionally patients may complain of waking up at night gasping for breath when they slide down the pillows (paroxysmal nocturnal dyspnoea). Dyspnoea associated with asthma may be seasonal (grass pollen) or perennial (house-dust mite faecal proteins), depending on the precipitating allergen. A history of severe allergy should lead to the consideration of anaphylaxis. Stressful events can precipitate asthma attacks but may also cause anxious patients to hyperventilate.

Relieving factors

Dyspnoea resulting from cardiac failure may be relieved by sitting upright, and, when due to asthma, by beta agonists.

Associated factors

Cough productive of (green, yellow, rusty) sputum indicates the presence of a chest infection. This may be the primary cause or it may exacerbate dyspnoea in patients with an existing condition such as asthma, COPD or cardiac failure. Bloodstained sputum may result from a chest infection (especially TB), pulmonary embolism or a tumour. Wheezing may result from asthma or aspiration of a foreign body.

EXAMINATION

Inspection

Cyanosis, which is observed from the fingertips (peripheral) or in the mucous membranes (central), is an indicator of severe underlying disease. Decreased consciousness level may indicate a life-threatening situation. However, it may also be the presenting feature of patients with a metabolic acidosis (diabetic ketoacidosis). Kyphosis severe enough to cause dyspnoea should be evident on general inspection. Patients with COPD may appear barrel-chested and cyanosed or thin and tachypnoeic (with pursed-lip breathing) accompanied by the prominent use of the accessory musculature.

The respiratory rate *per se* may not be very specific but extremes may be indicators of severity of the underlying disease. The respiratory rate should be carefully counted and not just estimated.

The hands should be inspected for clubbing, as it is associated with bronchial carcinoma and idiopathic pulmonary fibrosis (p. 62).

Pulse

A change in rate or regularity of rhythm may indicate an arrhythmia as a precipitating factor (usually in pre-existing heart or lung disease). The rate itself is not, however, very specific to the underlying aetiology.

JVP

Acute elevation of the JVP suggests tension pneumothorax, pulmonary embolism or tricuspid regurgitation (prominent *v* waves). Chronic elevation results from congestive heart failure or any chronic lung disease with right heart failure (cor pulmonale).

Temperature

An elevated temperature may occur with a chest infection and pulmonary embolism.

Trachea

The trachea deviates away from the side of a tension pneumothorax, pleural effusion and any large mass. It deviates to the side of a collapsed segment which can result with obstruction of the bronchial lumen from tumour or foreign bodies.

Expansion

May be reduced on the side of an area of consolidation (infection), pneumothorax and effusion. It may be reduced bilaterally in patients with COPD.

Percussion

The area overlying consolidation, effusion or collapse is dull to percussion. Hyper-resonance is often described on the affected side of a pneumothorax; however, a 'relative dullness' of the unaffected side is the usual initial finding.

Auscultation of the precordium

Auscultation may reveal murmurs associated with valvular heart disease. The presence of a third heart sound is consistent with cardiac failure, and quiet heart sounds may be due to an overexpanded chest from COPD.

Breath sounds

Localised reduction in the intensity of breath sounds occurs over areas with consolidation or collapse of the lung; however, it may be reduced generally with asthma and COPD.

Added sounds

Wheezing may be appreciated in a localised area following intraluminal airway obstruction from an inhaled foreign body or tumour. Generalised wheezing usually occurs with asthma. When a history of pre-existing asthma is not evident, then consider anaphylaxis. Localised crepitations may be auscultated over areas of pulmonary consolidation. Extensive bilateral crepitations occur with idiopathic pulmonary fibrosis (fine inspiratory), pulmonary oedema and bronchopneumonia.

GENERAL INVESTIGATIONS

- **FBC**
  Hb ↓ points to anaemia as the primary cause or as an exacerbating factor of underlying disease. Hb ↑ (polycythaemia) may be seen in chronic lung disease. WCC ↑ usually indicates infection, but it can also occur with other conditions, such as pulmonary embolism.

- **Peak expiratory flow rate**
  This simple bedside test allows you to evaluate airflow limitation. A reduced flow rate may indicate asthma or chronic airflow limitation.

- **ECG**
  Arrhythmias are readily appreciated on the ECG; atrial fibrillation or supraventricular tachycardia may precipitate dyspnoea in patients with pre-existing heart or lung disease. However, an arrhythmia may be a manifestation of the underlying cause, such as myocardial infarction, pulmonary embolism and hypoxia. ST segment elevations occur with myocardial infarction and are also a non-specific finding in pulmonary embolism. Right bundle-branch block may occur in the presence of long-standing lung disease.

- **Pulse oximetry**
  Although low saturation *per se* is not very discriminatory, acute severe impairment of oxygen saturation is associated with pulmonary embolus and pneumothorax. Post-exercise desaturation is helpful if opportunistic pneumonia is suspected.

- **ABGs**
  Useful to quantify severity of the disease and subtype of respiratory failure. Normal levels of oxygenation, however, are not useful to exclude respiratory or cardiac disease. Low levels of bicarbonate indicate metabolic acidosis and should lead to the investigation of the underlying cause, such as diabetic ketoacidosis. An alkalosis (high pH) with low $P\text{CO}_2$ and high $P\text{O}_2$ points to hyperventilation. CO_2 retention may result from

chronic lung disease (type II respiratory failure) or may indicate the need for ventilation with co-existing hypoxia in asthmatics.

- **Serum cardiac markers**
  Cardiac troponin or CK-MB is elevated with myocardial infarction in the setting of acute left ventricular failure.

- **CXR**
  Hyperinflation of the lungs (if the hemidiaphragm is below the seventh rib anteriorly or the 12th rib posteriorly) is a feature of emphysema, and may also result from asthma. Areas of consolidation are seen on a plain film; however, radiographic changes of a chest infection may lag behind in time with the clinical findings. The presence of cardiac failure is appreciated by cardiomegaly, upper lobe diversion of the pulmonary veins, bilateral pleural effusions, Kerley B lines (1–2 cm horizontal lines in the periphery of the lung fields) and patchy pulmonary oedema. A pneumothorax may be diagnosed by identifying the line of the pleura and the absence of lung markings beyond it. Bronchial carcinoma may present as a hilar mass, peripheral opacity or collapse and consolidation of the lung due to airways obstruction.

SPECIFIC INVESTIGATIONS

- **Sputum and blood cultures**
  Should be taken if an infective aetiology (pneumonia, lung abscess) is suspected, preferably before antibiotics are administered.

- **Respiratory function tests**
  Apart from physiological measurements of the lung, spirometry allows classification of restrictive or obstructive lung defects. It can also provide information regarding severity of the disease and the response to inhaled bronchodilators. Flow volume loops can indicate fixed airways obstruction (plateau in the expiration phase), which can result from foreign body or intraluminal tumour. Restrictive pattern of ventilatory impairment is characterised by a normal FEV1 to FVC ratio and a reduced vital capacity. It is characteristic of pulmonary fibrosis, infiltrative lung disease and restriction of chest wall motion. Obstructive pattern of ventilatory impairment is characterised by a reduced FEV1 to FVC ratio and a normal vital capacity. It is characteristic of asthma, COPD, bronchiectasis and cystic fibrosis.

- **Bronchoscopy**
  Bronchoscopy should be performed if aspiration of a foreign body is suspected, the procedure can be both diagnostic and therapeutic. Intraluminal bronchial carcinomas may be visualised and biopsied. Bronchoscopy also allows collection of specimens for culture in the diagnosis of pneumonia.

■ CT thorax/pulmonary angiogram
The majority of pulmonary emboli may be diagnosed by CT
pulmonary angiography. In addition, complete visualisation
of the thorax by CT is useful to evaluate masses of unknown
aetiology, and for staging of bronchial carcinoma. High-
resolution CT is useful to screen for features of idiopathic
pulmonary fibrosis.

■ Echocardiography
An echocardiogram is indicated if cardiac failure or valvular
heart disease is suspected. A large pulmonary embolus can
be diagnosed by a finding of right heart failure and elevated
pulmonary artery pressures. Elevated pulmonary artery
pressures can also be caused by pulmonary hypertension
causing dyspnoea. Although a proportion are idiopathic,
known causes are congenital heart disease, any severe lung
disease and recurrent pulmonary emboli.

- **Cyanosis associated with dyspnoea is an ominous
  sign. Emergency admission and treatment is
  required.**

- **Pneumothorax is commoner in asthmatics. If an
  asthmatic suddenly becomes short of breath,
  consider pneumothorax as a possible diagnosis.**

- **Sudden onset of breathlessness in an elderly patient
  may be due to LVF. This may be the result of a
  myocardial infarction.**

- **Always remember an inhaled foreign body as a
  cause of acute dyspnoea.**

EAR DISORDERS

Ear disorders are common in general practice. Earache is a frequent complaint. It may represent intrinsic ear disease or it may be due to referred pain from the oral cavity or pharynx. Causes of deafness are dealt with on p. 91.

CAUSES

LOCAL

EXTERNAL EAR

- Trauma
- Boils
- Inclusion dermoid
- Malignant disease

EXTERNAL AUDITORY MEATUS

- Otitis externa
- Furuncle
- Malignant disease

MIDDLE EAR

- Acute otitis media
- Chronic otitis media
- Mastoiditis

REFERRED PAIN

- Dental problems
- Pharynx
  - Tonsillitis
  - Pharyngitis
  - Foreign body
  - Quinsy
- Carcinoma of the posterior third of the tongue

NEUROLOGICAL

- Herpes zoster
- Glossopharyngeal neuralgia

HISTORY

Local

External ear

Trauma may cause subperichondrial haematoma. This is usually caused by a shearing blow. The patient will present with bruising and a swelling. If the swelling is not drained, repeated trauma occurs, and this will lead to the condition of 'cauliflower ear', often seen in rugby players. Avulsion of the ear is rare but may occur in major trauma. Occasionally, cellulitis and swelling of the ear occur due to bites, either animal or human. The patient may complain of a swelling on the lobe of the ear. Enquire whether there has been any recent ear-piercing, as inclusion dermoids may result. Ulcers may arise on the pinna as a result of malignant disease, the most common being squamous cell carcinomas and rodent ulcers.

External auditory meatus

The patient may complain of irritation, discharge, pain and occasionally deafness. Inflammation may spread out onto the pinna. There may be a history of poking the ear with a matchstick or hairgrip to remove wax. It may occur in those who swim frequently at public baths. With a furuncle (boil) in the external auditory meatus, the patient will present with extreme pain and throbbing. The pain is made worse by inserting an auriscope into the meatus. There may be a history of a foreign body inserted into the external auditory meatus. The patient is most commonly a child. Seeds or pips may have been inserted into the ear. In adults it is often matchsticks, cotton-wool buds or paperclips that have been inserted to remove wax from the ear. Occasionally an insect gets into the ear. There is usually pain and discharge. Malignant disease of the external auditory meatus is rare. When advanced, it may cause intractable pain, bloodstained discharge, and may invade the middle ear, facial nerve or the temporomandibular joint. The patient may present with a facial palsy.

Middle ear

Acute otitis media usually occurs in children. There may be a preceding history of common cold, tonsillitis, adenoiditis or infectious disease of childhood. In adults there may be a history of sinusitis, trauma, air flight or temporal bone fracture. The patient presents with severe earache, often with deafness, and appears flushed and ill. Chronic otitis media presents with a history of deafness, discomfort in the ear, tinnitus and occasionally problems with the balance. Acute mastoiditis is a complication of otitis media. It is rare nowadays because of antibiotics. Occasionally, children still present with pain, discharge (creamy and profuse) and deafness, with swelling behind the ear.

Referred pain

Check for a history of dental problems. In the elderly there may be carcinoma of the posterior third of the tongue. A classical picture of this used to be the elderly man spitting blood with a piece of cotton wool in his ear. Check for a history of tonsillitis or pharyngitis or difficulty in swallowing due to quinsy. Occasionally a foreign body lodged in the pharynx may be responsible. Other malignant disease of the pharynx may cause referred pain. Check for a history of dysphagia.

Neurological

Herpes zoster of the geniculate ganglion may give rise to lesions of the external auditory meatus, pinna and sometimes the palate. Glossopharyngeal neuralgia presents with very severe pain radiating from throat to tongue and into the ear.

EXAMINATION

Local

External ear

With trauma there may be obvious subperichondrial haematomas. Bites will result in cellulitis and swelling of the ear. Inclusion dermoids usually follow ear-piercing and present as lumps in the lobe of the ear adjacent to the area of piercing. Malignant disease will usually present as an ulcer, either with a typical appearance of a rodent ulcer or with the everted edges of a squamous cell carcinoma.

External auditory meatus

There is often inflammation at the entry to the meatus. The meatus is tender and there is moist debris, oedema and redness of the meatal wall on examination with an auriscope. A furuncle (boil) is extremely painful. Examination with the auriscope will reveal the tense, tender boil or even pus in the external auditory meatus. A foreign body is usually obvious on examination with the auriscope, as is malignant disease.

Middle ear

With acute otitis media the patient is usually flushed and ill, often with a temperature of 39–40°C. Examination of the tympanic membrane shows loss of lustre and disruption of the light reflex. There is redness, fullness and bulging of the drum. There may be signs of perforation with otorrhoea, with a mucoid, purulent or bloodstained discharge. Chronic otitis media shows fluid in the middle ear (glue ear), with discoloration and often retraction of the tympanic membrane. Tuning-fork test will reveal conductive deafness. In acute mastoiditis the child is usually ill with a high pyrexia. There is tenderness over the mastoid process and post-auricular swelling. The tympanic membrane may be red and bulging or perforated with discharge.

Referred pain

Examine for dental problems. Examine the posterior third of the tongue for carcinoma. Inspect the throat with a mirror looking for tonsillitis, pharyngitis, quinsy, foreign body or malignancy.

Neurological

With herpes zoster there will be vesicles in the meatus, on the pinna and sometimes on the palate and fauces. This will have been preceded by severe otalgia. With glossopharyngeal neuralgia there may be a trigger area in the throat in the same way as there is a trigger area that may initiate trigeminal neuralgia.

GENERAL INVESTIGATIONS

The majority of ear disorders can be diagnosed on clinical examination alone.

- ■ **Hb, FBC, ESR**
  Hb ↓ malignant disease. WCC ↑ acute otitis media. Acute mastoiditis. ESR ↑ malignancy and infection.

- ■ **Swab**
  C&S. Otitis externa. Otitis media with discharge. Furuncle. Tonsillitis.

- ■ **Biopsy**
  Malignant disease of the pinna and external auditory meatus. Carcinoma of the posterior third of the tongue.

- ■ **Skull X-ray**
  Opacity and coalescence of the air cells in mastoiditis.

- ■ **CT**
  Malignancy. Mastoiditis.

- • Referred pain to the ear is not uncommon. In the elderly it may represent referred pain from a carcinoma of the posterior one third of the tongue or the nasopharynx.

- • Beware the patient with middle ear infection who develops headache, confusion or neurological signs. Middle ear infection may progress to cause meningitis or cerebral abscess in rare cases.

EYE DISORDERS

Most eye disorders tend to present as the 'red eye'. It is the single most common ophthalmic complaint encountered by general practitioners.

CAUSES

EYELIDS

- Stye (hordeolum)
- Xanthelasma
- Blepharitis
- Meibomian cyst
- Entropion
- Ectropion

EYE

SURFACE

- Trauma
- Foreign body

CONJUNCTIVA

- Conjunctivitis
  - Bacterial
  - Viral
  - Allergic
  - Chlamydial
  - Subconjunctival haemorrhage

SCLERA

- Episcleritis
- Scleritis

CORNEA

- Corneal abrasion
- Corneal ulceration (keratitis)
  - Viral
  - Bacterial
  - Fungal

IRIS AND CILIARY BODY

- Iridocyclitis (uveitis)

INTRAOCULAR

- Acute angle-closure glaucoma

HISTORY

Pain

Most disorders of the eye present with pain. Sudden onset of unilateral eye pain and lacrimation may be due to a foreign body. Patients with infective conjunctivitis tend to complain of a soreness rather than true pain. Patients with blepharitis complain of a foreign body sensation or grittiness, whereas patients with allergic conjunctivitis (hayfever, acute allergy or atopy) tend to complain of itching rather than pain. Severe pain is experienced with corneal abrasions, ulcers, angle-closure glaucoma, herpes zoster ophthalmicus, uveitis and scleritis. Patients with either of the last two conditions experience exacerbation of pain on palpating the globe. A stye is a suppurative inflammation of an eyelash follicle. It is common and extremely painful. A meibomian cyst is an infection of a meibomian gland, which is in the posterior half of the eyelid margin. Following inflammation of a meibomian gland, it may either resolve spontaneously or leave a pea-size swelling known as a chalazion. Entropion is the rolling inwards of the lid margin. The eyelashes irritate the conjunctiva and cornea, causing a painful red eye. The opposite condition is known as ectropion and usually results in a watery eye. Subconjunctival haemorrhages are usually spontaneous and, although they may present with impressive chemosis (soft-tissue swelling), they are not usually painful.

Visual disturbance

Impairment of vision can occur with corneal ulceration, uveitis and acute angle-closure glaucoma. This is usually associated with photophobia. In addition, patients with glaucoma may perceive halos around lights due to corneal oedema.

Discharge

Documenting the presence, amount and colour of any discharge originating from the eye is important. A purulent discharge is associated with bacterial and chlamydial conjunctivitis, and a clear discharge with allergic and viral conjunctivitis.

Past medical history

A history of atopy or hayfever may be present in patients with allergic conjunctivitis. Previous herpes infection on the face may be the only clue with dendritic corneal ulceration. Conjunctivitis, urethritis and arthritis form the triad of Reiter's syndrome caused by *Chlamydia trachomatis* infection. A history of contact lens use is important, as patients may develop sight-threatening infections acutely.

Scleritis is a deeper and more severe inflammatory process than
piscleritis. It tends to be associated with connective tissue diseases,
uch as rheumatoid disease and SLE.

Uveitis is associated with inflammatory bowel disease, psoriasis,
nkylosing spondylitis and sarcoidosis. Orbital congestion may
e seen in patients with thyroid disorders. Xanthelasma are fatty
laques in the skin of the eyelids. Extensive or multiple xanthelasma
ay indicate abnormalities of cholesterol metabolism, diabetes or
rterial disease.

EXAMINATION

isual acuity should be assessed with correcting spectacles or
inhole, and documented with reference to a Snellen chart.
onditions that present with visual impairment are corneal
lceration, uveitis and glaucoma. Patients with these conditions
hould be referred to an ophthalmologist. The eyelids should be
arefully inspected. Swelling of the upper eyelid with redness may
ndicate a stye. There may be a bead of pus apparent at the infected
air follicle. The upper eyelid is everted to inspect for a meibomian
yst and foreign bodies. Papillae (conjunctival elevations with a
essel in the centre) are seen with allergic conjunctivitis, and follicles
collections of lymphocytes) may be visible with viral or chlamydial
nfection. Ectropion and entropion are usually obvious: in the
ormer the lower eyelid is everted and in the latter it is inverted, the
yelashes scratch the conjunctiva and cornea giving rise to a red,
atery eye. A similar effect is produced by trichiasis, which is caused
y irregular pointing lashes. Xanthelasma are fatty plaques in the
kin of the eyelids. They look like masses of yellow opaque fat. They
re not painful or tender.

Inspection is then undertaken to identify the presence of any
oreign bodies on the surface of the eye. Areas of erythema should
e carefully assessed. Diffuse erythema, maximal in the fornices, is
feature of conjunctivitis. Localised areas of segmental erythema
ay be due to episcleritis, but if it is maximal near the limbus it may
e a focal keratitis. Scleritis produces a brawny red discoloration,
hile a deep crimson-red area is observed with subconjunctival
aemorrhage. Marked erythema adjacent to the iris is known as a
iliary flush and occurs with anterior uveitis and glaucoma.

Attention is then focused on to the cornea. Ulceration of the
ornea may not be visible without fluorescein staining. Infection may
xtend to the anterior chamber, and a collection of pus (hypopyon)
an present as a white fluid level. Loss of brightness of the cornea
ccurs with glaucoma due to corneal oedema.

The pupil is examined and the resting position noted. A constricted
upil may result from ciliary spasm with uveitis and it rests in a fixed,
emi-dilated position with glaucoma.

SECTION A

Fluorescein staining should be performed and the eye is then viewed with a blue filtered light: corneal abrasions or ulcerations glow green.

GENERAL INVESTIGATIONS

- **Swab**
  Microscopy and C&S for infective organisms, e.g. stye, bacterial, viral and chlamydial conjunctivitis.
- **Rose bengal staining**
  To assess dead or damaged cells. It is useful in outlining a dendritic ulcer with herpes simplex infection.
- **Blood glucose**
  Infections are often associated with diabetes, as are xanthelasma.

SPECIFIC INVESTIGATIONS

- **Intraocular pressure measurements**
  ↑ glaucoma, uveitis.
- **Corneal scrape**
  For infective lesions.

- **Conjunctivitis is usually bilateral. If unilateral red eye, consider other conditions.**

- **Fluorescein staining should be performed routinely in the assessment of painful disorders of the eye, as corneal ulceration may not be visible without fluorescein staining.**

- **Never use steroid drops if herpetic corneal ulceration is suspected.**

- **If there is a history of foreign body, always check for high-speed injuries, e.g. metal fragments. Urgent specialist referral is required to exclude an intraocular foreign body.**

FACIAL PAIN

Most patients are able to distinguish between pain arising from the cranium, which is termed headache, and that of the face, which is covered here under the heading of facial pain.

CAUSES

LOCAL

SINUS
- Sinusitis
- Carcinoma

EAR
- Otitis media
- Otitis externa

MASTOID
- Mastoiditis

TEETH
- Dental abscess

SKIN
- Herpes zoster
- Post-herpetic neuralgia
- Cellulitis

JOINTS
- Temporomandibular dysfunction

PAROTID GLAND
- Mumps
- Parotitis
- Tumour

GENERAL

- Migraine
- Cluster headache
- Trigeminal neuralgia (*tic douloureux*)
- Temporal arteritis
- Tumour
  - Nasopharyngeal carcinoma
  - (common in Chinese populations)
- Chronic paroxysmal hemicrania

HISTORY

In the majority, facial pain originates from local structures. Therefore when formulating a differential diagnosis, consider the conditions affecting the anatomical structures of the face.

Site

The site of pain is perhaps the most useful feature when discriminating between the causes. Although local tenderness may direct the clinician to the affected site, do not forget to consider referred pain from adjacent structures. Pain in the region of the ear may be referred from the skin, teeth, tonsils, pharynx, larynx or neck. Tenderness over the maxilla may be due to sinusitis, dental abscess or carcinoma.

Character

Patients with trigeminal neuralgia often describe paroxysms of sharp, severe pains in the distribution of the trigeminal nerve or major divisions. Pain associated with infections of structures such as the teeth, mastoid and ear often has a dull, aching quality.

Precipitating factors

Pain precipitated by food or chewing action may be due to a dental abscess, salivary gland disorder, salivary duct disorder, temporomandibular joint disorder or jaw claudication due to temporal arteritis. Pain arising from most structures is aggravated by touch; however, with trigeminal neuralgia, even the slightest stroking of the skin is sufficient to produce intense pain (allodynia).

Associated symptoms

Tears may result when the lacrimal duct is obstructed by nasopharyngeal carcinoma. Complaints of otorrhoea and hearing loss should direct the clinician to infections affecting the ear or mastoid. Nasal obstruction and rhinorrhoea occur with maxillary sinusitis and carcinoma of the maxillary antrum. These may be accompanied by unilateral epistaxis. Swelling of the cheek may be experienced with dental abscesses and maxillary carcinoma. Proximal muscle pain, stiffness and subjective weakness may accompany temporal arteritis due to associated polymyalgia rheumatica. Paraesthesia in the distribution of the trigeminal nerve often precedes the rash of herpes zoster.

EXAMINATION

Inspection

A thorough inspection of the face, salivary glands, ear, nose and throat may produce a wealth of information. This involves the use of specific equipment such as the otoscope and nasal

speculum. Unilateral erythema and vesicles in the distribution of
the trigeminal nerve may be striking with herpes zoster infection
but may not be present in the early stages of the disease. Localised
areas of erythema or swelling may also correspond to the site of
infection, such as the sinus, ear, mastoid and parotid gland. Post-
auricular swelling and downward displacement of the pinna may
be observed with mastoiditis. Maxillary swelling and erythema can
be caused by dental abscess or maxillary carcinoma. With otitis
media, injection or perforation of the tympanic membrane may
be visualised with an otoscope. Nasopharyngeal carcinoma may be
seen on direct inspection of the nose and throat. Facial paralysis
may be seen with infiltration of the facial nerve by tumours of the
parotid gland.

Palpation

Gentle stroking of the skin of the face will precipitate severe
pain with trigeminal neuralgia. Tenderness may be elicited over
the frontal bone with frontal sinusitis, and over the maxilla with
maxillary sinusitis. With dental abscesses, pain is elicited over the
maxilla or mandible. Mastoid tenderness occurs with mastoiditis or
otitis media, and parotid tenderness can result from either mumps
or parotitis. Tenderness along the course of the superficial temporal
artery is suggestive of temporal arteritis. Movement of the pinna
produces pain with otitis externa.

Palpation of the superficial lymph nodes of the neck may reveal
lymphadenopathy in the distribution of the lymph drainage of
structures affected by infection or carcinoma.

GENERAL INVESTIGATIONS

■ **FBC**
Hb ↓ malignancy. WCC ↑ infection.
■ **ESR and CRP**
↑ malignancy and temporal arteritis.
■ **X-rays**
X-rays of the sinuses show mucosal thickening with air–fluid
levels in sinusitis. Occasionally total opacification is seen with
sinusitis and mastoiditis on mastoid films. In carcinoma of the
sinuses there may be complete opacification of the sinus and
destruction of the adjacent bone. CT will reveal the extent of
invasion.

SPECIFIC INVESTIGATIONS

■ **CT**
Carcinoma of the sinuses, nasopharyngeal carcinoma, parotid
conditions. Extent of tumour and degree of invasion will be
apparent.

- **MRI**
  Tumours – extent and invasion.
- **Sialography**
  Parotid conditions, e.g. duct stones, sialectasis.
- **FNAC**
  Parotid tumours.
- **Temporal artery biopsy**
  Temporal (giant cell) arteritis

- Temporal arteritis as a possible cause of facial pain requires emergency investigation and treatment. Other features include jaw claudication, scalp tenderness and visual disturbance associated with a raised ESR and/or CRP. Once blindness occurs it is irreversible.

- Unremitting facial pain should be investigated thoroughly to exclude malignancy.

FACIAL SWELLINGS

Facial swelling is a common presenting complaint. It may be generalised or localised. Many cases are due to trauma or infection but it may be a sign of systemic disease.

CAUSES

TRAUMATIC

- Facial fractures
- Insect bites

INFECTIVE

- Dental infection
- Sinusitis
- Parotitis
- Erysipelas

NEOPLASTIC

- Sinuses
- Parotid
- Jaw
- Mediastinal tumours

VASCULAR

- Superior vena caval thrombosis
- Cavernous sinus thrombosis

ENDOCRINE

- Cushing's syndrome
- Cretinism
- Acromegaly

METABOLIC

- Endocrine
- Renal failure

DRUG-INDUCED

- Steroids

OTHER

- Allergic reactions
- Angioneurotic oedema
- Paget's disease

HISTORY

Traumatic

Usually obvious history of trauma. Swelling may be severe, with bruising and closure of the palpebral fissures. Insect bites may cause swelling due to allergy or infection. The patient may not be aware of an insect bite.

Infective

Erysipelas is an uncommon skin infection caused by streptococci. Pain and redness are apparent usually over the cheek. Pyrexia and malaise may occur. Dental infections are common (see Jaw pain and swellings, p. 245) and are often initially localised, but the side of the face may swell. There is severe associated throbbing pain. Sinusitis presents with constant unilateral pain over the frontal or maxillary sinuses. There is usually puffiness of the skin overlying the sinus. Parotitis presents with pain and swelling over the gland. If this is due to obstruction in the duct, the swelling occurs during eating, when the patient salivates, and regresses afterwards. Bilateral parotitis occurs with mumps.

Neoplastic

Neoplasia may affect the parotids, sinuses and jaw. There is usually localised swelling with carcinoma of the sinuses. The patient complains of a blocked nose and a bloodstained discharge, which may be foul-smelling. With neoplastic lesions of the jaws there is usually deep-seated boring pain in relation to the swelling. Mediastinal tumours compress the superior vena cava and may cause suffusion of the face and facial oedema.

Vascular

Superior vena caval thrombosis may occur. This is rare and there may have been long-term central venous cannulation. There is cyanotic suffusion of the face with facial oedema. Cavernous sinus thrombosis usually presents following a history of infection of the face or in the sinuses. There may be a history of immunosuppression or diabetes. The patient complains of pain in the eye and forehead, with swelling around the eye and a protruding eye. The swelling may eventually involve the whole of the side of the face. Double vision occurs as a result of cranial nerve involvement.

Endocrine

Cushing's syndrome presents with swelling of the face (moon face) with a typical red appearance. Facial swelling is also seen in acromegaly. The patient will usually complain of an increase in shoe size and large hands. There may also be a hoarse voice, protrusion of the jaw and cardiac failure. Cretinism is associated with a puffy swollen face and enlargement and protrusion of the tongue.

Metabolic

Puffiness around the eyelids usually indicates renal failure.

Drugs

History of steroid therapy.

Other

Allergic reactions to drugs, especially antibiotics, or blood transfusions may result in periorbital or facial oedema. Take a careful drug history. Angioneurotic oedema chiefly affects the eyelids and lips. Recurrent attacks of sudden onset of burning and irritation. A family history suggest the diagnosis. Paget's disease often presents with painful enlargement of the skull, femur and clavicles and bowing of the tibia. The patient notices an increase in hat size. The forehead appears enlarged and prominent.

EXAMINATION

Traumatic

Fractures are usually obvious. Check pupillary reaction and test the cranial nerves. Insect-bite puncture wounds may be obvious but often they are not. There is often surrounding cellulitis and oedema.

Infective

Erysipelas presents as a red, tender area with well-demarcated margins raised above the surrounding normal skin. The patient is usually pyrexial. Dental abscesses are usually obvious, with local tenderness and oedema. Sinusitis is largely diagnosed from the history, with localised tenderness and swelling. With parotitis the gland is swollen and tender if infection has occurred, with occasionally redness over the skin. It may be unilateral or bilateral. Examine the orifice of the parotid duct for stone or stenosis.

Neoplastic

Neoplasia of the parotid usually presents as an enlarged, irregular, firm or hard swelling. There may have been a pre-existing pleomorphic adenoma. Test the integrity of the facial nerve, which may be affected by carcinoma. Carcinoma of the maxillary sinus may present with swelling over the sinus. Jaw swellings are considered on p. 245. Superior vena caval obstruction presents with facial oedema and cyanotic suffusion of the face. Examine the chest.

Vascular

Superior vena caval thrombosis presents in a similar way to obstruction. With cavernous sinus thrombosis there will be oedema, redness and swelling around the orbit, spreading onto the face.

Exophthalmos will be present. Test for paresis of cranial nerves III, IV and VI. The patient will usually be pyrexial and ill.

Endocrine

In Cushing's syndrome there will be moon face, and usually other features such as striae, buffalo hump, proximal myopathy. In cretinism there is a broad, flat face, the eyes are wide apart and the tongue protrudes from the mouth. In acromegaly there is a large face with overgrowth of the soft tissues of the face, nose, lips and tongue. The patient will have large hands and a large protuberant jaw (prognathism).

Metabolic

In renal failure the swelling usually occurs around the eyes. There may also be peripheral oedema and hypertension. There is usually a bronze–lemon tinge to the skin in chronic renal failure.

Drugs

Steroid therapy gives an appearance similar to Cushing's syndrome (see above).

Other

In allergic reactions there is often swelling of the eyes, lips and face, with urticaria of other areas on the body. Laryngeal oedema and bronchospasm may occur. Angioneurotic oedema is usually diagnosed from the history. Examination will reveal swellings of the eyelids and lips, with burning and irritation. In Paget's disease there is an enlargement of the skull, with the vault of the skull bulging outwards above the eyes. Deafness may occur. Occasionally there is compression of the cranial nerves. Test the cranial nerves. High output cardiac failure may be present.

GENERAL INVESTIGATIONS

■ **FBC, ESR**
Hb ↓ malignancy. WCC ↑ infection, e.g. sinusitis, cavernous sinus thrombosis. ESR ↑ infection, malignancy.

■ **U&Es**
Urea and creatinine ↑ in renal failure.

■ **Skull X-rays**
Fractures. Sinusitis – opaque sinus. Malignancy – opaque sinus and erosion of bone. Bone tumours. Paget's disease. Pituitary fossa – acromegaly, Cushing's disease.

■ **CXR**
Mediastinal tumour. Primary bronchial carcinoma with inappropriate secretion of ACTH leading to Cushing's syndrome.

■ Swab
C&S – infection, e.g. erysipelas, insect bites.

SPECIFIC INVESTIGATIONS

■ Hand X-ray
Acromegaly.

■ CT
Acromegaly. Cushing's disease. Fractures. Mediastinal tumours.
Carcinoma of the air sinuses. Parotid tumours. Cavernous sinus
thrombosis.

■ Sialography
Parotid conditions, e.g. stone in parotid duct.

■ TFTs
Cretinism.

■ Plasma cortisol
Cushing's syndrome.

■ Glucose tolerance test with growth hormone assay
Acromegaly.

- Localised swelling with complaint of a blocked
  nose or a bloodstained nasal discharge is strongly
  suggestive of carcinoma of the sinuses.

- Parotid swelling with facial palsy suggests a
  malignant parotid tumour with involvement of the
  facial nerve.

- Sudden generalised swelling of the face suggests an
  allergic reaction.

FACIAL ULCERS

Most facial ulcers are serious. Malignant facial ulcers are common
in patients who work outdoors and are exposed to ultraviolet light.
Lesions of the lips have been dealt with elsewhere (p. 299) and will
not be included here.

CAUSES

TRAUMATIC

- Physical
  - (rare in tropical Africa)
- Chemical
  - (rare in tropical Africa)
- Irradiation
- Dermatitis artefacta
- Neuropathy – anaesthetic areas after surgery for trigeminal
  neuralgia
- Bites

NEOPLASTIC

- Basal cell carcinoma (rodent ulcer)
  - (rare in Tropical Africa)
- Squamous cell carcinoma
- Malignant melanoma

INFECTIVE

- Herpes simplex
- Herpes zoster
- Keratoacanthoma
- Syphilis
  - Chancre
  - Gumma
- Leishmaniasis
  - (common in tropical and subtropical areas)

OTHER

- Pyoderma gangrenosum

HISTORY

A history of trauma should be sought. This may be as minor as
scratching a spot. Self-inflicted injury resulting in dermatitis artefacta
may be suspected when other causes have been excluded. Has the

patient had radiotherapy in the past to suggest irradiation causes? Anaesthetic skin is easily traumatised. In the case of the face, anaesthesia may have arisen following surgery to the trigeminal ganglion for trigeminal neuralgia. Syringobulbia is a rare cause of facial anaesthesia. Check for a history of bites, insect, animal or human, which may become infected and ulcerate.

Malignant ulcers are usually on exposed areas of the face. Check the patient's occupation. Malignancy is more common in outdoor workers exposed to ultraviolet light. Most rodent ulcers occur above a line drawn from the angle of the mouth to the lobe of the ear. Their incidence increases with increasing age. Malignant ulcers are usually painless unless they become infected. They may be pigmented and there may be a history of a change in a pre-existing mole to suggest malignant melanoma. These changes include: change in size; change in colour, with deepening pigmentation; bleeding or ulceration; itching; inflammatory 'halo'; satellite nodules; palpable regional lymph nodes.

Infection may be due to herpes simplex, which may spread from around the lips or nose. The patient will complain of an itchy, burning red area on which vesicles form and then crust over and ulcerate. Herpes zoster may arise in the distribution of the trigeminal nerve. Pain precedes malaise and fever by a few days. Vesicles develop later and may ulcerate. Syphilis is rare and may give rise to either a chancre or gumma (see Lip lesions, p. 299). Leishmaniasis is spread by sandflies and there would be a history of travel to India, Africa, the Middle East or the Mediterranean. There would be a history of bite leaving an itchy papule, leading to an ulcer. Keratoacanthoma may be due to a virus. It resembles a squamous cell carcinoma, from which it needs to be carefully distinguished. It occurs in adults as a rapidly growing lump with a central core filled with keratin. It usually takes 2–3 weeks to grow and often resolves spontaneously over several months. A history of inflammatory bowel disease will suggest pyoderma gangrenosum.

EXAMINATION

Benign ulcers

These usually have a sloping edge. Check the face for normal sensation to pain and temperature.

Malignant ulcers

Basal cell carcinomas (rodent ulcers) usually have a raised, rolled, pearly margin. They may become very large and erode deeply and locally. They do not metastasise and therefore local lymph nodes should not be enlarged unless the lesion becomes infected. Squamous cell carcinoma presents as an ulcerated lesion with an everted edge. Metastasis occurs to local lymph nodes and these may be palpable. Care should be taken to distinguish a squamous cell carcinoma from a keratoacanthoma, which is a benign, fast-growing, self-limiting papule surmounted by a keratin plug (it resembles a small volcano with a crater). Malignant melanomas vary in colour from pinkish-brown to black. They may develop a purplish hue due to a rich blood supply. There may be a brownish-pink 'halo' around the lesion or there may be 'satellite' nodules. The local lymph nodes may be enlarged. Early metastases may occur to the liver and therefore patients should be examined for hepatomegaly.

Infective

The characteristic lesions of herpes simplex will be seen around the lips and nose. In immunosuppressed patients, these lesions may coalesce and become infected. Ophthalmic herpes zoster will be recognised by its characteristic distribution in the ophthalmic division of the trigeminal nerve. It may affect the cornea. A syphilitic chancre begins as a macule, becoming a painless, hard ulcer, which is very infectious. It develops rapidly and is associated with enlargement of the local lymph nodes. A gumma occurring on the face is uncommon. It appears as a punched-out ulcer with a wash-leather base. Cutaneous leishmaniasis (oriental sore) develops at the site of a sandfly bite, commencing as an itchy papule from which the crusts may separate, leaving an ulcer with deep perpendicular edges. Pyoderma gangrenosum presents with a nodule or pustule, which ulcerates with tender, reddish, blue necrotic edges.

GENERAL INVESTIGATIONS

■ FBC, ESR
WCC ↑ infected ulcer. ESR ↑ malignancy, syphilis.

■ LFTs
Alkaline phosphatase may be raised with liver secondaries, e.g. malignant melanoma.

■ Swab
C&S from infected ulcer. Dark-ground illumination microscopy for *Treponema pallidum*.

■ Biopsy
Benign versus malignant. Keratoacanthoma versus squamous cell carcinoma. In the case of malignant melanoma, excision biopsy is required.

SPECIFIC INVESTIGATIONS

■ VDRL
Syphilis.

■ Aspiration of lesion
Leishmaniasis – protozoal organism may be seen by microscopy in aspirates from fluid at the edge of the ulcer.

■ **Viral culture**
Herpes simplex, herpes zoster (rarely needed – diagnosis usually obvious clinically).

■ **Antibody titres**
Herpes simplex, herpes zoster (rarely needed – diagnosis usually obvious clinically).

- **Facial ulcers in the elderly and those with outside occupations are likely to be malignant. Rodent ulcers are the most common.**

- **Ophthalmic herpes zoster will be recognised by its characteristic distribution in the ophthalmic division of the trigeminal nerve. Corneal ulceration may occur. Urgent treatment is required.**

FAECAL INCONTINENCE

Faecal incontinence implies loss of voluntary control of passage of faeces from the anus. Faecal soiling of the clothes occurs, which is socially embarrassing for the patient. Any disease process that interferes with rectal sensation or affects function of the anorectal musculature may produce incontinence. However, incontinence may still occur with normal sphincters and pelvic floor, for example in severe diarrhoea.

CAUSES

NORMAL SPHINCTERS AND PELVIC FLOOR

- Severe diarrhoea, e.g. infection, inflammatory bowel disease
- Faecal impaction

ABNORMAL SPHINCTERS AND/OR PELVIC FLOOR

CONGENITAL
- Anorectal anomalies, meningomyelocele

ACQUIRED
Traumatic
- Iatrogenic
  - Internal sphincter surgery, e.g. anal dilatation or sphincterotomy
  - Fistula-in-ano surgery
  - Obstetric – traumatic childbirth
- Pelvic fractures
- Impalement

Neurological
- Multiple sclerosis
- Spinal injuries
- Spinal tumours
- Peripheral neuropathy
- Stroke
- Dementia

Other
- Rectal prolapse
- Extensive anorectal carcinoma
- Fistula-in-ano
- Radiotherapy
- Lymphogranuloma venereum

HISTORY

Is there a history of trauma, e.g. pelvic fractures, impalement injuries? Probably the commonest cause of faecal incontinence is gastroenteritis. The history will be obvious. A history of inflammatory bowel disease may be elicited. Other important factors to elicit in the history are recent anorectal surgery; recent difficult childbirth – long duration of labour, forceps delivery, forceful delivery, perineal tears, episiotomy; predisposition to peripheral neuropathy, e.g. diabetes mellitus, vitamin B_{12} deficiency, alcoholism or medication. A history of constipation may suggest faecal impaction. A history of a recent stroke, dementia or neurological illness will usually be obvious.

EXAMINATION

Soiling of the underwear may be apparent at examination. Digital rectal examination will demonstrate any reduction in anal tone and the inability to sustain a voluntary contraction. It may be possible to feel the defect in the anorectal ring. Faecal impaction may well also be obvious on digital rectal examination. Is there any evidence of trauma or infection? Rectal prolapse may be apparent or descend during straining. Look for evidence of a fistula-in-ano or extensive anorectal cancer. Full neurological examination will often be necessary.

GENERAL INVESTIGATIONS

- **FBC, ESR**
  Macrocytic anaemia may be associated with vitamin B_{12} deficiency (peripheral neuropathy).

- **LFTs**
  Deranged in alcoholism, which may be a cause of peripheral neuropathy.

- **Blood glucose**
  Neuropathy of diabetes mellitus.

- **Sigmoidoscopy**
  Biopsy.

- **Proctoscopy**
  Biopsy.

SPECIFIC INVESTIGATIONS

- **Endoanal US**
  May show defect in anorectal musculature.

- **Anorectal manometry**
  May demonstrate cause of incontinence.

- ■ EMG
- ■ MRI
  Defects in anorectal musculature. Pelvic malignancy. Spinal tumours.

- Faecal incontinence is common in frail elderly people.
- Faecal incontinence is a feature of many neurological diseases. Up to 50% of patients with multiple sclerosis may experience faecal incontinence.
- Faecal incontinence is a symptom or sign rather than a disease. Onset of faecal incontinence in an otherwise well patient may be an indication of developing neurological disease.

FINGER LESIONS

Lesions of the fingers are common. The fingers are important tactile organs and hand function may be impaired. Painful finger lesions are dealt with on p. 143.

CAUSES

CONGENITAL

- Absent digit
- Extra digit
- Syndactyly (fusion of digits)
- Camptodactyly

ACQUIRED

TRAUMATIC/DEGENERATIVE

- Dupuytren's contracture
- Implantation dermoid
- Trigger finger
- Mallet finger
- Swan-neck deformity
- Boutonnière deformity
- Heberden's nodes
- Mucous cyst

METABOLIC

- Tophaceous gout
- Ectopic calcification (chronic renal failure)

CONNECTIVE TISSUE DISEASE

- Calcinosis in CREST syndrome

NEOPLASTIC

- Subungual melanoma
- Enchondroma

HISTORY

Congenital

These lesions will be recognisable at birth. They may be associated with other congenital abnormalities.

Acquired

Traumatic/degenerative

Dupuytren's contracture In the early phases the patient may merely complain of a nodule in the palm near the base of the ring finger.

Eventually the patient complains of being unable to extend fully the MCP joint at the ring, and later, the little finger. It affects the patient's grip. The patient complains of difficulty dressing – either poke themselves in the eye while brushing hair or catch the finger on trouser pocket. There may be a family history. Check also for a history of epilepsy, cirrhosis or diabetes.

Implantation dermoid   Cysts occur where skin is forcibly implanted into the subcutaneous tissue as a result of injury. There is likely to be a history of injury, often minor, e.g. pinprick. Implantation dermoid used to be common in women who sewed – hence the use of protective thimbles. The patient complains of small painful swellings on the finger tips.

Trigger finger   The patient complains that the finger 'jumps' or 'clicks' as it moves. It may get stuck in the flexed position. There is not usually a history of injury.

Mallet finger   This results from injury to the extensor tendon of the terminal phalanx. There is usually a history of injury. It occurs if the tip of the finger is forcibly flexed during active extension (stubbed), e.g. catching a cricket ball. The finger adopts a position in which the distal phalanx is flexed.

Swan-neck deformity   The patient complains of deformity of the distal finger.

Boutonnière deformity   This is the opposite of swan-neck deformity. Again, the patient merely complains of a deformity of the distal finger.

Heberden's nodes   The patient complains of swelling close to the distal finger joints, i.e. swelling and deformity of the knuckles. There may be a history of osteoarthritis elsewhere.

Mucous cyst   The patient complains of a swelling over the dorsum of the DIP joint. It may discharge.

Metabolic

Tophaceous gout   There may be a history of gout. Deposits of uric acid occur in joints or soft tissues and the patient complains of swellings on the fingers.

Ectopic calcification   The patient complains of hard, whitish, subcutaneous swellings. There may be a history of hyperparathyroidism, hypercalcaemia, or chronic renal failure.

Connective tissue disease

CREST syndrome   The patient complains of white deposits in the pulps of the fingers.

Neoplastic

Subungual melanoma   This occurs as a pigmented lesion beneath the nail. There is no history of trauma as with a subungual haematoma, which may also appear pigmented when the bruise organises. Unlike subungual haematoma, a melanoma does not grow out with the nail. Eventually the melanoma may lift the nail and ulcerate.

Enchondroma   The patient notices a bony, hard swelling along the finger. It may occur beneath the nail and result in deformity of the nail (subungual exostosis).

EXAMINATION

Congenital

Congenital anomalies of the fingers will be obvious at birth. With camptodactyly there is painless flexion deformity at the PIP joint of the little finger. Check for other associated congenital anomalies.

Acquired

Traumatic/degenerative

Dupuytren's contracture   Examination may reveal only a firm painless nodule in the palmar fascia near the base of the ring finger. Puckering of skin of the palm may be obvious. Eventually the MCP joint and PIP joint become flexed. The DIP joint remains extended. Garrod's knuckle pads on dorsum of PIP joints. Check for signs of diabetes or liver disease. Occasionally the condition is associated with Peyronie's disease of the penis.

Implantation dermoid   Examination reveals small firm spherical swellings in the subcutaneous tissues of the finger tips.

Trigger finger   The patient may be able to demonstrate how the finger sticks and then snaps out in extension. Thickening of the tendon and the tendon sheath may be felt over the head of the metacarpal bone.

Mallet finger   The distal phalanx of the affected finger remains flexed at about 20° when the patient tries to straighten the finger.

Swan-neck deformity   There is hyperextension of the PIP joint and flexion of the distal interphalangeal joint.

Boutonnière deformity   This is the opposite of swan-neck deformity. Flexion of the PIP joint occurs, with hyperextension of the DIP joint. It develops when the PIP joint pokes through a rupture of the centre of the extensor expansion.

Heberden's nodes   These are bony swellings on the dorsal surface of the fingers just distal to the DIP.

Mucous cyst   Swelling on the dorsum of the DIP joint. Discharge may be apparent. May be groove in nail due to pressure on nailbed.

Metabolic

Tophaceous gout   Swellings, often multi-lobulated, occur on the fingers. They contain toothpaste-like infiltrates of uric acid crystals.

SECTION A

Ectopic calcification   Firm to hard, yellow–white deposits of calcium occur in the subcutaneous tissues.

Connective tissue disease

CREST syndrome   Small, hard, subcutaneous nodules in the finger pulps and on the dorsal aspects of the fingers.

Neoplastic

Subungual melanoma   A subungual melanoma is seen as a brown lesion with an indistinct edge. Occasionally it may be quite extensive and have lifted the nail.

Enchondroma   This is a painless, hard swelling on the bone. The surface of it is usually smooth. It may occur under the nail and lift the nail.

GENERAL INVESTIGATIONS

The diagnosis of most of these lesions is made on clinical examination alone.

■ FBC, ESR
  Hb ↓, ESR ↑ in disseminated malignancy from subungual melanoma.

■ Blood glucose
  Diabetes (Dupuytren's).

■ LFTs
  Cirrhosis (Dupuytren's).

■ Serum calcium
  Hypercalcaemia – ectopic calcification. Hyperparathyroidism.

■ Serum uric acid
  Gout.

■ Rheumatoid factor
  Rheumatoid arthritis – swan-neck deformity. Boutonnière deformity.

■ Finger X-ray
  Heberden's nodes. Enchondroma. Mucous cyst – degenerative/osteoarthritic changes in the DIP joint. Ectopic calcification. Calcinosis. Erosion of phalangeal bone with tophaceous gout.

■ Biopsy
  Excision biopsy for malignant melanoma.

• Subungual melanoma needs to be carefully distinguished from subungual haematoma. Check for a history of trauma. A subungual haematoma grows out with the nail. A subungual melanoma does not.

FINGER PAIN

A painful finger is a common presenting symptom. This may vary from an obvious local lesion to part of a generalised disease, e.g. rheumatoid arthritis. Impairment of the function of even a single finger may grossly impair the overall function of the hand.

CAUSES

TRAUMATIC

- Subungual haematoma
- Fractures

INFLAMMATORY/INFECTIVE

- Paronychia
- Pulp space infection
- Tendon sheath infection

NEOPLASTIC

- Glomus tumour
- Bone tumour
- Secondary deposits in bone

DEGENERATIVE

- Rheumatoid arthritis

VASCULAR

- Chilblains
- Small vessel disease
  - Raynaud's phenomenon
  - Buerger's disease
  - Diabetes
  - Emboli

METABOLIC

- Gout

AUTOIMMUNE

- Scleroderma

NEUROLOGICAL

- Carpal tunnel syndrome
- Cervical lesions

HISTORY

Traumatic

There will be a history of trauma, often a crushing injury. Subungual haematoma results from 'trapping' of the nail. It is extremely painful, as a bruise comes up between the nail and the nailbed.

Inflammatory/infective

Paronychia

This presents as a painful, tender spot close to the nail. It throbs and may keep the patient awake. There may be a history of picking the skin around the nail. Pus may exude from the side of the nail.

Pulp space infection

This occurs in the pulp space of the fingertip. There may be a history of penetrating injury, e.g. a prick with a sharp object. There is pain, redness and swelling and the finger throbs.

Tendon sheath infection

There may be a history of a direct puncture wound or there may be a preceding pulp space infection, which has extended into a tendon sheath. The patient presents with a red, tender and painful finger held in slight flexion at the IP and MCP joint.

Neoplastic

Glomus tumour

This is a rare lesion but is very painful. The patient complains of severe pain every time the nail is touched, the most common site being below the nail.

Primary and secondary bone tumours

These are rare in the phalanges. Pain and swelling occurs and there may be a history of a primary tumour, e.g. breast, bronchus, thyroid, kidney or prostate.

Degenerative

Rheumatoid arthritis

Women are more commonly affected than men. The usual symptoms are pain, swelling and stiffness of the fingers. General malaise may occur. The patient may complain of deformities of the fingers.

Vascular

Chilblains

The simplest vascular problem that affects the fingers is chilblains. Women are more affected than men. The patient complains of a swelling on the side or backs of the fingers, which develops rapidly after exposure to cold. The lesion is painful and itches. The lesions are usually multiple and occur most commonly in winter.

Small vessel disease

Ischaemia results in pain, discoloration, ulceration or frank gangrene. The patient may complain of sudden onset of a cold, painful finger, or frank gangrene may be apparent. There may be a history of Raynaud's phenomenon, Buerger's disease, diabetes or scleroderma. There may be cardiac disease, peripheral vascular disease or a cervical rib to suggest embolism. With Raynaud's phenomenon there are often the characteristic changes of sudden onset of pallor induced by exposure to the cold, followed by cyanosis, followed by sudden vasodilatation with a painful, tingling, red digit.

Metabolic

Gout

Gout usually affects the first MTP joint but may affect any joint. The patient will complain of sudden onset of pain, swelling and redness in relation to a joint. There may be a previous history of gout. There may be a family history. An attack may be precipitated by trauma, starvation, infection, diuretics, cytotoxic or immunosuppressive drugs. Gouty tophi may be present.

Autoimmune

Scleroderma

Females are affected more than males. There may be thickening of the fingers. The patient may also complain of Raynaud's phenomenon and splits and ulcers of the fingertips. There may be a change in facial appearance and the patient may complain of dysphagia.

Neurological

Carpal tunnel syndrome

The patient will complain of pain, paraesthesia in the thumb, index and middle fingers. Worse in bed at night. Relieved by hanging arm out of bed.

Cervical lesions

The patient may complain of pain or tingling in the fingers. There may be a history of cervical spondylosis or other previous problems with the cervical spine.

EXAMINATION

Traumatic

Deformity, redness and swelling to suggest a fracture will be obvious. 'Trapping' of the nail or a blow to it will cause a collection of blood under the nail. The diagnosis is usually obvious from the history and the patient will be in considerable pain.

Inflammatory/infective
Paronychia

The skin at the base and side of the nail is red, shiny and bulging. A bead of pus may be seen discharging from under the nail.

Pulp space infection

There is swelling and redness over the pulp of the finger. A pus-filled blister may be seen. If the tension is not rapidly relieved it may either discharge into the tendon sheath or may cause pressure necrosis and osteomyelitis of the distal part of the terminal phalanx.

Tendon sheath infection

The finger is acutely painful and held in slight flexion. It is red and swollen and exquisitely tender along the line of the tendon sheath.

Neoplastic
Glomus tumours

These are rare. They are angioneuromyomas. If the tumour occurs under the nail (most common site), there is a small purple-red spot below the nail.

Primary and secondary tumours

These are rare. There is palpable bony swelling, which may or may not be tender.

Degenerative
Rheumatoid arthritis

The finger joints enlarge and become fusiform. Joint deformities occur, with ulnar deviation at the wrist and hyperextension of the proximal interphalangeal joints. There is wasting of muscles of the hand.

Vascular
Chilblains

These usually occur on the dorsum and side of the fingers. The skin over the swelling is reddish-blue. The swellings are oedematous and may burst and ulcerate. There are usually chilblains on the ankles and feet as well as on the fingers.

Small vessel disease

In ischaemic patients there may be pallor, cyanosis or even frank gangrene of a finger. Ischaemic ulcers may be apparent on the fingertips. The pulp of the fingers may be wasted. Palpate for a cervical rib. Check the pulse for atrial fibrillation (emboli).

Metabolic
Gout

Acute inflammation of a joint occurs, the skin being tense, shiny, hot and red over the joint. The presence of gouty tophi locally or elsewhere, e.g. on the ears, suggests the diagnosis.

Autoimmune
Scleroderma

The skin of the hands has a thickened, white, waxy appearance. The fingers appear swollen with thickened skin, while the pulps of the fingers may be wasted. Small subcutaneous nodules, which are hard, may be palpable. These are due to calcinosis. Look for other signs of scleroderma, e.g. the skin of the face looks tight and shiny and is puckered around the mouth. There may be multiple telangiectasia over the face. Evidence of weight loss due to dysphagia may be present.

Neurological
Carpal tunnel syndrome

Wasting of the thenar muscles. The reduction of sensation in distribution of the median nerve in the hand occurring in advanced cases. Pressure over the carpal tunnel may reproduce symptoms.

Cervical spondylosis

Check sensation in the fingers. Check also the range of neck movements and the reflexes in the upper limbs.

GENERAL INVESTIGATIONS

- **FBC, ESR**
  Hb ↓ anaemia of chronic disease, e.g. rheumatoid arthritis. WCC ↑, e.g. tendon sheath infection. ESR ↑, e.g. rheumatoid arthritis.
- **U&Es**
  Urea and creatinine raised in chronic renal failure, which may be associated with gout or scleroderma.
- **Rheumatoid factor**
  Rheumatoid arthritis.
- **Blood glucose**
  Diabetes.
- **ECG**
  Atrial fibrillation – emboli.
- **Hand X-ray**
  Rheumatoid arthritis. Bone lesions. Pulp space infection – pressure necrosis with osteomyelitis of the distal part of the terminal phalanx.

- **CXR with thoracic inlet**
  Cervical rib – Raynaud's phenomenon, emboli.

- **Cervical spine X-ray**
  Cervical spondylosis with referred pain.

SPECIFIC INVESTIGATIONS

- **Serum uric acid**
  Gout.

- **Autoantibody screen**
  Autoimmune disease.

- **Cold agglutinins**
  Raynaud's disease.

- **Echocardiography**
  Cardiac disease – embolism.

- **Arteriography**
  Arterial lesions. Mural thrombus from aneurysms leading to emboli. Peripheral vascular disease.

- **Referred pain to the fingers is not uncommon. This is usually due to cervical spondylosis or carpal tunnel syndrome. Always carry out a full neurological examination.**

- **Infection of the fingers and restriction of movement may represent a tendon sheath infection. Antibiotics and urgent referral are required.**

FOOT DEFORMITIES

These are not common. The deformity will often be apparent at birth but occasionally does not present until the child starts walking. A deformity of the foot and ankle is normally referred to as 'talipes'. Other terms may qualify the word talipes, e.g. varus (inverted heel), valgus (everted heel) and equinus (foot plantarflexed). Deformities of the toes are dealt with under toe lesions (p. 442).

CAUSES

- Talipes equinovarus (congenital clubfoot)
- Metatarsus adductus (intoeing)
- Pes planus (flatfoot)
- Pes cavus (high-arch foot)
  - Idiopathic
  - Neuropathic
  - Spastic dysplasia
  - Spina bifida
  - Spina bifida occulta
  - Poliomyelitis
  - Charcot–Marie–Tooth disease (hereditary motor and sensory neuropathy)
  - Friedreich's ataxia
- Acquired talipes

UPPER MOTOR NEURONE LESION
- Spastic paresis
- Cerebrovascular accident

LOWER MOTOR NEURONE LESION
- Spina bifida
- Poliomyelitis
- Amyotrophic lateral sclerosis
- Cerebellar lesions
- Friedreich's ataxia

MUSCULAR DISEASE
- Muscular dystrophy
- Volkmann's ischaemic contracture

TRAUMA
- Fractures
- Burns

HISTORY

Talipes equinovarus

Apparent at birth. The child is born with clubfoot. Picked up on routine post-natal examination.

Metatarsus adductus

Common cause of intoeing in children. Only the forefoot is adducted and not the hindfoot.

Pes planus

All children are flatfooted and the arches are not fully developed until the age of 10. The parents may notice an abnormality of gait and perhaps rapid and uneven wear and tear of the shoes. Pain is rare.

Pes cavus

There is accentuation of the longitudinal arch of the foot. There may be pain and discomfort. Again, the condition may be noted by the child's parent. There may be no specific cause. Alternatively, there may be a history of spina bifida, spina bifida occulta, poliomyelitis, or rarely Friedreich's ataxia, for which there will be a family history, Charcot–Marie–Tooth disease begins at puberty with foot drop and weakness in the legs.

Acquired talipes

There are a variety of causes of upper and lower motor neurone lesions giving rise to acquired talipes. Check for a history of spastic paresis, cerebrovascular accident, spina bifida, poliomyelitis. There may be a family history of Friedreich's ataxia. The patient may be known to have muscular dystrophy. With Volkmann's ischaemic contracture there will be a history of ischaemia of the calf muscles, e.g. from supracondylar fracture of the femur with popliteal artery damage.

Trauma

There will usually be an obvious history of trauma or of burns causing contractures.

EXAMINATION

Talipes equinovarus

This will usually be apparent in the newborn. There is an equinus deformity, i.e. the hindfoot is drawn up with a tight Achilles tendon; varus deformity – the sole faces inwards; and adduction of the forefoot – the inner border of the forefoot is concave and points upwards.

Metatarsus adductus

The hindfoot is normal with a normal sized heel. The forefoot is adducted.

Pes planus

The longitudinal arch is flattened and the medial border of the foot rests on the ground.

Pes cavus

The high arch is clearly visible. The toes are clawed due to hyperextension of the MTP joints and flexion of the IP joints. The patient cannot straighten the toes. Callosities usually develop under the metatarsal heads. Check for spina bifida, spina bifida occulta (hairy patch over lumbar spine), poliomyelitis. With Charcot–Marie–Tooth disease there will be foot drop and also atrophy of the peroneal muscles. With Friedreich's ataxia there will be other signs, e.g. ataxia, dysarthria and nystagmus.

Acquired talipes

Check for upper motor neurone and lower motor neurone lesions. Friedreich's ataxia (see above). Volkmann's ischaemic contracture will demonstrate firmness and wasting of the calf muscles together with clawing of the foot.

Trauma

The deformity will depend on the type and severity of trauma. Scarring and contractures of burns will be obvious.

GENERAL INVESTIGATIONS

The diagnosis of nearly all the above conditions is made on history and clinical examination.

■ Foot X-rays
   May help with assessment.

• **Foot deformities are rare. Orthopaedic or neurological referral is usually required.**

FOOT PAIN

Pain in the foot is a common presenting complaint. The majority of causes are related to either postural problems or arthritis.

CAUSES

TRAUMATIC

- Fractures
  - March fracture

INFECTIVE

- Cellulitis
- Osteomyelitis
- Pyogenic arthritis

INFLAMMATORY

- Rheumatoid arthritis
- Plantar fasciitis
- Reiter's disease
- Osteochondritis of the navicular bone (Köhler's disease)
- Osteochondritis of the metatarsal head (Freiberg's disease)

VASCULAR

- Ischaemia
- Ulcers

METABOLIC

- Gout

DEGENERATIVE

- Osteoarthritis
- Flatfoot
- Other foot deformities (p. 149)

OTHER

- Corns and callosities
- Metatarsalgia
- Morton's metatarsalgia
- Plantar warts
- Referred pain, e.g. disc lesions, neuropathies

HISTORY

Traumatic

History of trauma, e.g. heavy object falling on foot, crush injuries. Fatigue or march fractures may occur with prolonged walking, e.g. as in soldiers marching. Severe pain may result. It usually affects the second metatarsal.

Infective

Cellulitis may occur following a puncture wound, e.g. standing on nail, insect bite. The history will usually be apparent. The patient will present with a painful, red, swollen foot. Osteomyelitis is rare but may follow blood-borne infection, e.g. with salmonella, or local infection, especially in diabetics. There will be pain, tenderness, swelling and redness over the affected bone. Pyogenic arthritis is rare but presents with a painful, red, swollen joint.

Inflammatory

The foot is commonly involved in rheumatoid arthritis. Deformities are multiple and severe eventually. There are usually signs of rheumatoid arthritis elsewhere. Plantar fasciitis causes pain under the heel. The patient is often middle-aged. It may also be associated with Reiter's disease. The pain is often worse on standing after a period of rest. Osteochondritis may affect the second metatarsal head (Freiberg's disease) or the navicular bone (Köhler's disease). Pain, tenderness and swelling occur in relation to the particular bone.

Vascular

There may be a history of intermittent claudication progressing to ischaemic rest pain. The patient complains of severe pain in the foot, usually in bed at night, which is relieved by hanging the foot out of bed. The patient may also complain of ulcers and discoloration of the foot. Gangrene may be apparent. Check for a history of smoking, diabetes.

Metabolic

Gout classically affects the first MTP joint but other joints of the foot may be affected. There is acute onset of pain, redness and swelling. There may be a previous history. Attacks may be precipitated by trauma, surgery, infection or drugs, e.g. diuretics. There may also be a history of leukaemia, polycythaemia, and cytotoxic or immunosuppressive therapy.

Degenerative

Osteoarthritis, flatfoot, or other foot deformities (p. 149) may cause foot pain. Hallux rigidus, i.e. primary osteoarthritis of the MTP joint of the great toe, causes pain and stiffness.

Other

Metatarsalgia causes pain under the metatarsal heads. It is most common in middle-aged women. Excessive standing triggers the symptoms. Morton's metatarsalgia is caused by a digital neuroma. It most often affects the nerve running between the third and fourth metatarsal heads. It is commonest in women aged 40–50 years. Sharp intermittent pains shoot into the toes, usually occurring only when shoes are worn. Plantar warts are painful. The patient will usually have noticed the wart. They are common in the region of the metatarsal head, great toe and heel. Corns and callosities over pressure points may be painful. They are often associated with deformities of the foot. Referred pain to the foot may occur due to spinal lesions. A history of backache or weakness in the limb may be relevant.

EXAMINATION

Traumatic

Pain, tenderness, swelling, deformity or crepitus will be present with fractures. With march fractures there may be localised tenderness and oedema on the dorsum of the foot.

Infective

Cellulitis, osteomyelitis and pyogenic arthritis will be associated with fever, malaise, and swelling, redness and tenderness of the foot.

Inflammatory

Rheumatoid arthritis may be associated with signs elsewhere, e.g. hands. In the foot there may be pes planus, hallux valgus, clawing of the toes, and subluxation at the MTP joints. With plantar fasciitis there is usually localised tenderness over the undersurface of the os calcis. With Reiter's disease there may be urethritis and conjunctivitis. Freiberg's disease and Köhler's disease present with swelling and tenderness over the relevant bone.

Vascular

Look for signs of ischaemia, e.g. pallor, paraesthesia, loss of pulses, ulcers, gangrene.

Metabolic

With gout there will be swelling, redness, and tenderness of the first MTP joint. Gouty tophi may be present elsewhere.

Degenerative

Osteoarthritis presents with pain and stiffness, e.g. hallux rigidus. Flatfoot and other deformities may be apparent (p. 149).

Other

In metatarsalgia there is tenderness under the metatarsal heads. Callosities may be present under the metatarsal heads. In Morton's metatarsalgia, squeezing the forefoot may produce the symptoms. Plantar warts (verruca plantaris) are usually obvious. They present as flat, hyperkeratotic lesions which seem to have been pushed into the skin of the sole of the foot. In contrast to callosities, pressure over them causes pain. If referred pain is suspected, a full neurological examination should be carried out.

GENERAL INVESTIGATIONS

- FBC, ESR
  Hb ↓ anaemia of chronic disease, e.g. rheumatoid arthritis. WCC ↑ infection, e.g. cellulitis, osteomyelitis. ESR ↑ rheumatoid arthritis.

- Blood glucose
  Diabetes.

- Foot X-ray
  Fractures (march fractures may not be apparent until callus forms, therefore the need for repeat X-ray). Osteomyelitis – normal in early stages, osteoporosis, subperiosteal new bone, sequestration. Rheumatoid arthritis. Osteoarthritis. Osteochondritis – dense fragments of bone. Foot deformities.

SPECIFIC INVESTIGATIONS

- Serum uric acid
  Gout.

- Blood culture
  Osteomyelitis.

- Bone scan
  Osteomyelitis.

- CT
  Spinal lesions – referred pain.

- MRI
  Spinal lesions – referred pain.

- Duplex Doppler
  Vascular disease.

- Arteriography
  Vascular disease. Site of disease. Small vessel versus large vessel disease.

- Sudden onset of pain in the foot in an arteriopathy or in a patient with atrial fibrillation is likely to be due to ischaemia. Examine the pulses. Urgent referral is usually required.

- Systemic illness and fever with localised severe bone pain may suggest osteomyelitis or septic arthritis. Risk factors include diabetes and immunosuppression. Urgent investigation is required.

- Pain with no obvious signs, especially lack of localised tenderness, may suggest neuropathy or an L5/S1 nerve lesion.

FOOT ULCERS

Ulcers on the feet are common. The majority of them are of vascular or neuropathic origin.

CAUSES

VASCULAR

LARGE VESSEL DISEASE
- Arteriosclerosis
- Embolism

SMALL VESSEL DISEASE
- Diabetes
- Buerger's disease
- Raynaud's disease
- Embolism
- Vasculitis, e.g. SLE, rheumatoid arthritis, scleroderma

NEUROPATHIC

PERIPHERAL NERVE LESIONS
- Diabetes
- Peripheral nerve injuries
- Leprosy
- In endemic areas
- Alcoholism

SPINAL CORD LESIONS
- Spina bifida
- Tabes dorsalis
- Syringomyelia

NEOPLASTIC
- Squamous cell carcinoma
- Malignant melanoma

TRAUMATIC
- Ill-fitting footwear

INFECTIVE
- Madura foot
- Endemic in Africa, India

HISTORY

Vascular

Ischaemic ulcers are common in the elderly. They are painful and do not bleed much. They show no signs of healing. There is often a history of intermittent claudication and rest pain. Check for a history of diabetes. In the younger patient, diabetes, Buerger's disease or Raynaud's disease may be responsible. Check for a history of cardiac disease, which may suggest embolism leading to ischaemic ulceration. Proximal arterial disease, e.g. aneurysm, may also cause emboli.

Neuropathic

These are painless ulcers occurring over pressure points. Patients may give a history of neuropathy. They may describe a feeling as though they are walking on cotton wool. Check for a history of diabetes and peripheral nerve lesions. Spinal cord lesions may also be present. In diabetes, ulceration may be associated with both ischaemia and neuropathy.

Neoplastic

Malignant ulcers may occur on the foot. Squamous cell carcinoma is rare but malignant melanoma is not infrequent, especially on the sole of the foot. The patient may have noticed the pigmented lesion, which has changed, with bleeding, itching and ulceration. The patient may also have noticed a lump in the groin, suggesting lymph node secondaries.

Traumatic

Foot ulcers may be caused by minor trauma, e.g. ill-fitting shoes. However, there is usually a history of an underlying predisposing condition, e.g. poor circulation, steroid therapy, neuropathy.

Infective

Pure infective ulcers on the foot are rare. Infections may occur with *Nocardia* species in tropical countries causing Madura foot. Check for a history of foreign travel.

EXAMINATION

Vascular

Ischaemic ulcers are found on the tips of the toes and over the pressure areas. The edge is usually punched out and healing does not occur. The base may contain slough or dead tissue. Occasionally tendons are seen in the base of the ulcer. Pulses may be absent. Check for atrial fibrillation, which may be associated with embolism as a cause of ischaemic ulceration.

Neuropathic

Neuropathic ulcers are deep, penetrating ulcers. They occur over pressure areas but the surrounding tissues are healthy and have good circulation. The ulcers themselves are painless. Examine the surrounding tissues for blunting of sensation, e.g. absence of pinprick sensation. Pulses are usually present. Carry out a full neurological examination looking for peripheral nerve injuries or evidence of spinal cord lesions.

Neoplastic

Squamous cell carcinomas have an everted edge, often with necrotic material in the base of the ulcer. The edge of the ulcer is hard. Check for inguinal lymphadenopathy. Ulcers associated with malignant melanoma tend to vary from brown to black, although they may be amelanotic. Bleeding and infection may make the surface of the tumour appear wet, soft and boggy. Check for inguinal lymphadenopathy and hepatomegaly.

Traumatic

Traumatic ulcers tend to occur either at pressure points, due to ill-fitting footwear, or at a site of injury. They usually have sloping edges and granulation tissue developing in the base. Always check the circulation, as most traumatic foot ulcers readily heal unless there is an abnormality of the circulation.

Infective

Infective ulcers by themselves are rare. Secondary infection may occur on any type of ulcer. With Madura foot there may be ulceration and bone destruction with little systemic illness.

GENERAL INVESTIGATIONS

- **FBC, ESR**
  Hb ↓ malignant disease. WCC ↑ infection. ESR ↑ malignancy.
- **Blood glucose**
  Diabetes.
- **Swab**
  Microscopy – fungal infection. C&S.

SPECIFIC INVESTIGATIONS

- **Antibody screen**
  Connective tissue disease.
- **Doppler studies**
  Ischaemic ulceration.
- **Arteriography**
  Ischaemic ulceration. Large versus small vessel disease.

- ■ Nerve conduction studies
  Neuropathic ulcers.
- ■ CT
  Spinal cord lesions.
- ■ MRI
  Spinal cord lesions.
- ■ Biopsy
  Benign versus malignant.

- A painful ulcer is likely to be infective or have an arterial aetiology.
- A painless ulcer is likely to be neuropathic.
- Neuropathic ulcers are deep and penetrating and likely to occur over pressure areas.
- Deep ulcers involving deep fascia, tendon and periosteum are likely to have an arterial component.

GAIT ABNORMALITIES

Disorders of gait may be structural or neurological. When assessing gait, it is important to observe the whole patient and not merely the feet.

CAUSES

STRUCTURAL

- Pain – antalgic gait
- Length discrepancies – short leg gait
- Weak hip abductors – Trendelenburg or waddling gait
- Femoral anteversion – intoe gait

NEUROLOGICAL

- Stroke – hemiplegic gait
- Parkinson's disease – festinant gait
- Peripheral neuropathy – sensory ataxia
- Cerebellar disease – cerebellar ataxia
- Peroneal nerve palsy – foot drop gait
- Cerebral palsy – scissoring gait
- Frontal lobe lesions – apraxic gait

HISTORY

Duration

An abnormality of gait that has been present since birth is usually due to a structural cause or cerebral palsy. Discrepancies of length may originate from disorders affecting joint articulation, bone length or from soft-tissue contractures surrounding the joints. Most of the neurological causes of gait abnormalities result from acquired lesions of the central or peripheral nervous systems.

Associated symptoms

Pain is the underlying cause for the antalgic gait and patients will be able to direct you to the site of origin of the pain. Loss of motor function such as paralysis of dorsiflexion of the foot causes the foot drop gait, more extensive paralysis of the arm and leg with the hemiplegic gait may occur with stroke. Paraesthesia, sensory loss or impairment of joint position sense is suggestive of peripheral neuropathy. Patients with sensory apraxia suffer from proprioceptive impairment and have great difficulties walking in the dark when visual cues are lost. A concomitant resting tremor is associated with Parkinson's disease and an intention tremor results from cerebellar disease.

Past medical and drug history

A previous history of trauma to the lower limb is very significant; fractures of the long bones predispose to length abnormalities on healing. Fractures of the fibular neck may disrupt the common peroneal nerve causing foot drop. Frontal lobe contusions may result from severe head injuries. Diabetes, carcinoma and vitamin B deficiencies are associated with peripheral neuropathies. Alcoholism, multiple sclerosis and drugs such as phenytoin are associated with cerebellar impairment. Direct questioning should be undertaken for previous strokes and Parkinson's disease.

EXAMINATION

The clinical examination is divided into three sections. The initial examination of a gait disorder is to determine a structural or neurological cause. If a structural lesion is suspected then it is followed by an orthopaedic examination. Conversely a neurological examination is performed if a neurological lesion is suspected. Once the disorder of gait is defined, the clinical examination should then be tailored to determine the underlying cause.

The asymmetrical gait

The gait is first assessed for symmetry. Apart from the hemiplegic gait, the remaining unilateral gait disorders are structural. The normal gait consists of several phases; there are the swing, heel strike, stance and toe-off phases. The antalgic gait or painful limp is characterised by a decrease in time spent in the stance phase. The Trendelenburg gait is characterised by a downward tilt of the pelvis when the leg is lifted forwards. It may be caused by a painful hip disorder, weakness of the contralateral hip abductors, shortening of the femoral neck or subluxation of the hip joint. With a hemiplegic gait, the leg swings in an outward arc and then back to the midline. A foot drop gait often results in the knee being lifted higher on the affected side.

The symmetrical gait

When analysing the symmetrical gait, observe movement of the whole patient. The stooped posture with small shuffling steps and reduced arm swing is characteristic of Parkinson's disease. Patients with apraxia have disjointed movements akin to 'walking on ice', the aetiology is frontal lobe disorder most commonly due to cortical degeneration. Attention is then brought to the movement of the legs, scissoring of the gait due to crossing of the midline when lifting the leg forwards is associated with cerebral palsy. The movements of the feet are then noted, lifting of the knees with slapping of the foot as it contacts with the ground is descriptive of the foot drop gait. The foot is rotated inwards with femoral anteversion. The base of the gait is then analysed, a broad-based gait is characteristic of cerebellar disease and sensory ataxia. With cerebellar disease, patients are unsteady standing with their eyes open, while with sensory ataxia patients are able to stand with their eyes open but not shut (positive Romberg's test).

Orthopaedic examination

An examination of the hip, knee and ankle is required. Measurements are undertaken to determine real and apparent length of the lower limbs. The real length is the distance between the anterior superior iliac spine and the medial malleolus, and the apparent length is the distance between the xiphisternum and the medial malleolus. Any discrepancies will require individual measurements of the femur and tibia to determine the site of shortening. Thomas' test is performed to identify the presence of fixed flexion deformities of the hip that can give rise to apparent shortening. The resting position of both feet can be inspected and internal rotation due to femoral anteversion may be apparent.

Neurological examination

The mask-like facies and resting pill-rolling tremor of Parkinson's disease may be apparent on inspection and examination of the limbs will reveal cog wheel or lead pipe rigidity. Patients with cerebellar disease will exhibit an intention tremor when performing the finger–nose test; in addition to their broad-based ataxic gait they may also exhibit nystagmus, dysdiadochokinesia and dysarthria. With frontal lobe disorders primitive reflexes such as the grasping (the hand of the examiner is grasped when placed or stroked along the patient's palm), sucking (sucking action is produced on stroking on side of the mouth) and palmomental reflexes (gentle stroke of the thenar eminence produces dimpling of the chin) are released. Examination of the sensory system may reveal loss of light touch, vibration and proprioception in a glove and stocking distribution with peripheral neuropathy. Unilateral upper motor neurone weakness, hyperreflexia and clasp knife rigidity are features of cortical strokes.

Specific examination

Once the diagnosis of a gait disorder is made, a specific examination is now undertaken to determine the underlying aetiology. For example, with apraxic gait due to frontal lobe disorder, a mental state examination is performed to screen for dementia, and fundoscopy is performed to screen for papilloedema, which may be indicative of raised intracranial pressure from a brain tumour.

GENERAL INVESTIGATIONS

The diagnosis of the majority of gait abnormalities is made on clinical history and examination.

SPECIFIC INVESTIGATIONS

■ Local X-rays
Structural causes.

■ Nerve conduction studies
Peripheral neuropathy. Peroneal nerve palsy.

■ CT/MRI scans
CNS causes, e.g. stroke, space-occupying lesions.

- When evaluating abnormalities of gait it is important to assess the patient in a safe environment, if necessary with an assistant to hand to prevent falls or injury.

- Always observe the whole patient and not only the legs. The cause may be central.

- Onset of ataxia without an obvious cause requires an urgent neurological referral.

GOITRE

A goitre is an enlargement of the thyroid gland. It can result from physiological causes such as puberty (due to increased demand for thyroid hormone) which require no treatment to frank malignant disease requiring urgent diagnosis and treatment.

CAUSES

SIMPLE (NON-TOXIC) GOITRE

- Simple hyperplastic goitre
- Multinodular goitre

TOXIC GOITRE

- Diffuse goitre (Graves' disease)
- Toxic nodule
- Toxic multinodular goitre

AUTOIMMUNE

- Hashimoto's thyroiditis

NEOPLASTIC GOITRE

BENIGN
- Adenoma

MALIGNANT
- Papillary
- Follicular
- Anaplastic
- Medullary
- Lymphoma

INFLAMMATORY

- de Quervain's thyroiditis
- Riedel's thyroiditis

HISTORY

Simple hyperplastic goitre

The patient presents with a swelling in the neck. Physiological causes include puberty and pregnancy. Iodine deficiency is the most common cause but is rare in the UK, where iodide is added to table salt.

Multinodular goitre

This is the commonest cause of goitre in the UK. It is more common in women. The usual presentation is a lump in the neck which moves on swallowing, but with a very large gland the patient may complain of dyspnoea or dysphagia.

Toxic goitre

The patient presents with a lump in the neck. He or she may indicate a preference for cold weather, and may also complain of excessive sweating, tiredness, anxiety, increased appetite, weight loss, diarrhoea, palpitations and tremor.

Autoimmune

Hashimoto's disease presents with a firm goitre. It needs to be distinguished from lymphoma. Eventually the patient becomes hypothyroid, and will complain of intolerance to cold weather, tiredness, a change in voice (hoarseness), weight gain, constipation, and dry skin and dry hair.

Neoplastic goitre

The patient may present with diffuse enlargement of the thyroid or may have noticed a well-defined swelling in the area of the thyroid gland. Papillary carcinoma occurs in the younger patient (under 35 years) and, in addition to the goitre, the patient may have noticed lymph node swelling in the neck. Follicular carcinoma occurs in middle age (40–60 years). The patient may also complain of bone pain due to metastases. Anaplastic carcinoma occurs in the elderly. Anaplastic carcinoma may present with stridor, dyspnoea and hoarseness. There may be gross lymph node involvement. Medullary carcinoma can present at any age. Check for a family history of medullary carcinoma and symptoms related to phaeochromocytoma and hyperparathyroidism (associated MEN syndrome). Lymphoma of the thyroid is rare and may develop in pre-existing autoimmune (Hashimoto's) thyroiditis.

Inflammatory (rare)

The patient may present with a painful swelling of the thyroid associated with malaise or myalgia (de Quervain's thyroiditis). A hard mass associated with dysphagia or dyspnoea may suggest Riedel's thyroiditis.

EXAMINATION

Simple hyperplastic goitre

The patient is usually euthyroid and the goitre is smooth.

Multinodular goitre

The gland is usually smoothly nodular. Occasionally only one nodule may be felt – the dominant nodule in a multinodular goitre. Check for tracheal deviation when the gland is large, and percuss for retrosternal extension.

Toxic goitre

Palpation of the gland may reveal a diffuse goitre, a multinodular goitre or a solitary nodule. Check for exophthalmos, lid lag, lid retraction, warm moist palms and tremor. Check for atrial fibrillation. Examine for pretibial myxoedema. Reflexes are brisk. The goitre may have a palpable thrill or a bruit may be heard on auscultation.

Autoimmune

Hashimoto's disease presents with a diffusely enlarged, firm gland. Eventually there may be signs of hypothyroidism. These signs include a pale, waxy skin, periorbital oedema, dry thickened skin and hair, slow pulse, large tongue, peripheral oedema and slow relaxing reflexes. Carpal tunnel syndrome may be present.

Neoplastic goitre

There may be a solitary thyroid nodule (papillary carcinoma) or a more diffuse mass (follicular carcinoma). Anaplastic carcinoma is hard and irregular and invades locally. Check for tracheal deviation. Cervical lymphadenopathy may be present with a papillary carcinoma, when the glands are usually mobile and discrete, and is invariably associated with anaplastic carcinoma, where the glands may be hard and matted. Check for recurrent laryngeal nerve palsy – has the patient got a hoarse voice or is unable to produce an occlusive cough?

Inflammatory

Subacute thyroiditis (rare). There will be a painful, swollen gland. In Riedel's thyroiditis there is a woody, hard goitre, which infiltrates into adjacent muscle. It must be carefully differentiated from anaplastic carcinoma.

GENERAL INVESTIGATIONS

- FBC, ESR
  Hb ↓ in disseminated malignancy. ESR ↑ in thyroiditis.
- TFTs
  T_4 ↑, TSH ↓ in toxic goitre. T_4 ↓, TSH ↑ in hypothyroidism.
- Thyroid antibodies
  Thyroid antibodies will be demonstrated in Hashimoto's disease.
- CXR
  Secondary deposits in thyroid carcinoma (follicular, anaplastic).

- ■ Thoracic inlet X-ray
  Tracheal compression.

- ■ US
  Cystic versus solid. Position of gland.

- ■ CT scan
  Position of gland. Compression/invasion of local structures.

- ■ Radioisotope scan
  Hot versus cold nodule. Cold nodules may be malignant.

- ■ FNAC
  Benign versus malignant.

- ■ Laryngoscopy
  Involvement of recurrent laryngeal nerve.

SPECIFIC INVESTIGATIONS

- ■ Serum calcitonin
  Calcitonin ↑ in medullary carcinoma.

- ■ PTH
  Raised in MEN syndrome.

- • Dysphagia or dyspnoea in association with a goitre requires urgent referral and may require urgent thyroidectomy.

GROIN SWELLINGS

These are common clinical problems, especially hernias. They are therefore common in clinical examinations.

CAUSES

ABOVE THE INGUINAL LIGAMENT

- Sebaceous cyst
- Lipoma
- Direct inguinal hernia
- Indirect inguinal hernia
- Imperfectly descended testis
- Lipoma of the cord
- Hydrocele of the cord
- Hydrocele of the canal of Nuck

BELOW THE INGUINAL LIGAMENT

- Sebaceous cyst
- Lipoma
- Femoral hernia
- Lymph nodes
- Saphena varix
- Femoral artery aneurysm (true or false)
- Imperfectly descended testis
- Neuroma of the femoral nerves
- Synovioma of the hip joint
- Obturator hernia
- Psoas abscess

HISTORY

Sebaceous cyst

The patient will complain of a mobile lump on the skin. It may be red and inflamed and discharging.

Lipoma

The patient will present with a soft, painless swelling.

Hernias

A patient with a groin hernia will present with a lump that disappears on recumbency or may be pushed back (reducible). The patient may present with a tense, tender lump that will not reduce and is accompanied by signs and symptoms of intestinal obstruction. Femoral hernia is more common in females. With hernias there is occasionally a history of sudden straining or trauma, following which a lump may become manifest.

Imperfectly descended testis

An imperfectly descended testis may present as a groin swelling. The patient, or, if a child, the mother, will have noticed absence of a testis from the scrotum. Enlargement and pain may indicate malignant change which is more common in an imperfectly descended testis.

Lipoma of the cord

The patient will have noticed a soft swelling in the groin. This is often mistaken for a hernia.

Hydrocele of the cord

This may present as a lump in the inguinal region which does not reduce.

Hydrocele of the canal of Nuck

This is similar to a hydrocele of the spermatic cord but presents in the female. It represents a cyst forming in the processus vaginalis.

Lymph nodes

Lymph nodes may present as swellings below the inguinal ligament. They may be discrete and firm; tender and red; or matted to form a mass. The patient may have noticed a lesion on the leg. Care must be taken to elicit a full history with inguinal lymphadenopathy, as the nodes drain not only the tissues of the leg but also the penis, the scrotal skin, the lower half of the anal canal, the skin of the buttock and the skin of the lower abdominal wall up to and including the umbilicus. In the female they drain the labia, the lower third of the vagina, and the fundus of the uterus via lymphatics accompanying the round ligament down the inguinal canal. A careful history should therefore be taken of any anorectal disease, e.g. bleeding PR, or gynaecological disease, e.g. bleeding PV to suggest a carcinoma of the uterus.

Saphena varix

A saphena varix is normally associated with varicose veins lower down the leg. The patient will present having noticed a small, soft, bluish mass in the lower part of the groin.

Femoral artery aneurysm

A pulsatile expansile mass suggests a femoral aneurysm. Check for a history of arterial surgery at the groin or arteriography via the femoral artery, which may suggest the presence of a false aneurysm.

Imperfectly descended testis

An imperfectly descended testis may descend into the upper thigh but its descent is arrested by the attachment of Scarpa's fascia to the deep fascia of the thigh.

Neuroma of the femoral nerve

This is rare and may be associated with anaesthesia or paraesthesia on the anterior aspect of the thigh and inability to extend the knee.

Synovioma of the hip joint

This is rare. The patient complains of a lump deep in the groin which may interfere with hip movement.

Obturator hernia

This is rare. The sac passes through the obturator canal and may present in the groin deep to pectineus. A lump is rarely palpable due to the overlying pectineus. The diagnosis is not usually made until obstruction or strangulation occurs.

EXAMINATION

Sebaceous cyst

This is attached to the skin and a punctum is usually seen at the point of attachment. Sebaceous cysts are firm, spherical and mobile on the underlying tissue. They may be hot, red and tender when inflamed.

Lipoma

The lump will be soft, lobulated, mobile, being fixed neither to the skin nor to the underlying tissue. They may be distinguished from hernias in that they are not reducible and do not have a cough impulse.

Hernias

A hernia may be reduced and has an expansile cough impulse. They may be irreducible. Irreducible hernias may be: (1) incarcerated – imprisoned in the sac because of adhesions between contents and the wall of the sac; (2) obstructed – small bowel is caught in the sac and intestinal contents cannot pass on; (3) strangulated – the arterial blood supply is cut off and gangrene of the contents ensues. In the last case the lump would be tender, the overlying skin may be red and the patient will be pyrexial with a tachycardia. There will be signs of intestinal obstruction.

It is important to distinguish between an inguinal and a femoral hernia. An inguinal hernia lies above and medial to the pubic tubercle, a femoral hernia below and lateral. An inguinal hernia may be either direct or indirect. An indirect hernia comes down the inguinal canal from the deep inguinal ring. A direct hernia comes through the posterior wall of the canal through Hesselbach's triangle (base – inguinal ligament; lateral border – inferior epigastric artery; medial border – the lateral border of rectus abdominis muscle). Distinction between direct and indirect hernia is made by reducing the hernia and exerting pressure over the deep inguinal ring, asking the patient to cough. If the hernia sac appears medial to the fingers, it is direct. If the hernia appears only after removing the pressure over the deep inguinal ring then it is indirect.

Imperfectly descended testis

An imperfectly descended testis may be in an ectopic position (root of the penis, upper thigh or perineum) or along the normal line of descent. An imperfectly descended testis cannot be felt in the inguinal canal – it is usually too flabby and atrophic and cannot be palpated through the tough overlying external oblique aponeurosis. However, should it become malignant then the hard and irregular testis can be palpated in the inguinal canal. An imperfectly descended testis may also be palpable in the upper thigh below the inguinal ligament. The scrotum will be empty on that side. The testis cannot descend more than a few centimetres into the upper thigh as its descent is prevented by the attachment of Scarpa's fascia to the deep fascia of the thigh below the inguinal ligament. An imperfectly descended testis may also be palpable at the root of the penis or in the perineum.

Lipoma of the cord

This can be confidently diagnosed only at surgery, although there will not be an expansile cough impulse as with a hernia.

Hydrocele of the cord

This is rare. There will be a smooth, palpable swelling along the line of the cord. It does not have a palpable expansile cough impulse. If gentle traction is exerted on the testis, a hydrocele of the cord will be felt to move down the canal. It may transilluminate.

Hydrocele of the canal of Nuck

A swelling, similar to a hydrocele of the cord in the male, occurring in the female is called a hydrocele of the canal of Nuck. Findings will be similar to those of a hydrocele of the cord in the male, except there is nothing to exert traction on!

Femoral hernia

This is more common in females. It lies below and lateral to the pubic tubercle. There will be an expansile cough impulse. It may be reducible. Strangulation of a femoral hernia is not uncommon, particularly one of the Richter's type. A tense, tender, irreducible swelling will be found below and lateral to the pubic tubercle.

Lymph nodes

Lymph nodes are palpable below the inguinal ligament. Classically they are arranged into groups: (1) superficial, with subdivision into horizontal and vertical groups; and (2) deep. In practice it is difficult to distinguish between the groups. Lymph nodes in the groin may be palpable as discrete nodules or they may be hard, irregular and matted together. This type is usually associated with malignant disease. Tender, fluctuant lymph nodes with erythema of the overlying skin are usually associated with lymphadenopathy due to an infective condition. It is important to examine all sites that are drained by these nodes, namely: (1) the skin of the leg, including examination under the toe nails; (2) the skin of the buttock; (3) the skin of the lower abdominal wall up to and including the umbilicus; (4) the skin of the scrotum, penis and glans penis; (5) the labia and lower third of the vagina; (6) the lower half of the anal canal; (7) the fundus of the uterus. It is therefore necessary not only to examine superficial structures but also to carry out a digital rectal examination and a bimanual vaginal examination.

Saphena varix

This is a soft, compressible dilatation at the termination of the saphenous vein. It has a cough impulse and disappears on recumbency. A fluid thrill is felt if the veins lower down the leg are percussed.

Femoral artery aneurysm

A femoral artery aneurysm presents as an expansile pulsatile mass in the line of the femoral artery. Look for a scar in relationship to it, which may suggest a false aneurysm.

Imperfectly descended testis

An imperfectly descended testis may be palpable in the upper thigh below the inguinal ligament. The scrotum will be empty on that side. The testis cannot descend more than a few centimetres into the upper thigh as its descent is prevented by the attachment of Scarpa's fascia to the deep fascia of the thigh below the inguinal ligament.

Neuroma of the femoral nerve

This is rare. It will be palpable along the course of the nerve (lateral to the femoral artery). Test the integrity of the femoral nerve (sensation on the anterior aspect of the thigh; extension of the knee joint).

Synovioma of the hip joint

This is rare. There may be a palpable thickening deep in the groin in relation to the hip joint. Hip joint movements may be limited.

Obturator hernia

This is rare. In a very thin patient a lump may be felt deep in the medial aspect of the groin. More commonly, obturator hernias present with intestinal obstruction and the diagnosis is made at laparotomy.

Psoas abscess

This is rare. It used to be associated with spinal TB, a cold abscess of a vertebral body discharging down the psoas sheath and presenting as a soft fluctuant swelling below the inguinal ligament. Most psoas abscesses nowadays are related to perforation of a hollow viscus retroperitoneally, e.g. the right colon into the psoas sheath.

GENERAL INVESTIGATIONS

The diagnosis of most groin swellings is made on history and physical examination.

- **FBC, ESR**
  Hb ↓ lymph node tumours. WCC ↑ infection in the lymph nodes, strangulated hernia. ESR ↑ lymph node tumours, infection, e.g. TB spine.
- **US**
  Lipoma, imperfectly descended testis, femoral artery aneurysm, psoas abscess.
- **Hip X-ray**
  Osteoarthritis with synovioma.
- **AXR**
  Intestinal obstruction associated with obstructed/strangulated hernia.

SPECIFIC INVESTIGATIONS

- **Duplex Doppler**
  Aneurysm. False aneurysm. Saphena varix.
- **Thoracolumbar spine X-ray**
  TB spine (psoas abscess).
- **CT scan**
  Psoas abscess. TB spine.
- **MRI scan**
  Psoas abscess. TB spine. Cord compression.
- **Herniography**
  Inguinal or femoral hernia.
- **FNAC**
  Lymph node pathology.
- **Biopsy**
  Lymph node pathology.

- An acutely painful and irreducible lump suggests a strangulated hernia. Urgent surgical treatment is required.

- Femoral hernia is more common in women and is at higher risk of strangulation.

- Undescended testis has a high risk of malignancy.

- If the cause of the swelling is thought to be lymphadenopathy, examine all regions that drain to the inguinal lymph nodes.

GUM DISORDERS

Disorders of the gums are common, especially bleeding from the gums. Most disorders that cause bleeding are due to local infective disease but may be a manifestation of systemic disease.

CAUSES

BLEEDING

- Dental disease
- Infection
  - Bacterial
  - Viral
  - Fungal
- Blood dyscrasias
- Iatrogenic
  - Anticoagulants
  - Chemotherapy
  - Radiotherapy

HYPERTROPHY

- Infection associated with dental disease
- Drugs
  - Phenytoin
  - Nifedipine
  - Ciclosporin

RETRACTION

- Chronic periodontal disease
- Ageing

OTHERS

- Malignancy (ulcers)
- Lead poisoning
- Arsenic poisoning

HISTORY

Periodontal disease is probably the most common factor causing bleeding from the gums. Poor hygiene is usually obvious from the condition of the teeth. Infection will cause the patient to complain of red, inflamed gums, which bleed spontaneously or on brushing the teeth. Patients may have a history of recent malignancy for which they have undergone either chemotherapy, with associated blood dyscrasia, or local radiotherapy. There may be a history of painful lesions in the mouth to suggest herpes simplex. Rarely infectious mononucleosis may cause gingivostomatitis. The patient may present with a pyrexial illness with malaise, lethargy and lymphadenopathy. Abnormalities of the bone marrow, e.g. malignant infiltration, or aplastic anaemia will result in agranulocytosis and thrombocytopenia. Agranulocytosis causes reduced resistance to infection; thrombocytopenia is associated with a bleeding tendency. There may be a generalised illness with malaise and lethargy associated with lymphadenopathy, bruising and spontaneous bleeding from other orifices. There may be a history of haemophilia or von Willebrand's disease. Rarer conditions include scurvy (subclinical vitamin C deficiency may occur in the elderly) and hereditary haemorrhagic telangiectasia. Check for a family history of bleeding disorders. A full drug history should be taken. Check whether the patient is on phenytoin, nifedipine or ciclosporin. Check for occupational exposure to chemicals, especially arsenic and lead.

EXAMINATION

Local

Inspect the gums for signs of inflammation and bleeding. Is it only the gums that are involved or does the condition affect the whole of the oral cavity? Check the condition of the teeth, looking for dental caries or periodontal disease. Is there any evidence of gingival hyperplasia? In gingival hyperplasia, the gum hypertrophy predominantly involves the interdental papillae. Is there any localised ulceration of the gum to suggest neoplasia? Is there any evidence of gum retraction? This occurs commonly in ageing but may be associated with chronic periodontal disease. Arsenic and lead are rare causes of gingival bleeding. The gingiva become inflamed, swollen and bleed easily, and, in the case of lead, there is a characteristic blue line at the gingival margin. Other signs of lead poisoning may be present, particularly pigmentation of the skin, vomiting, diarrhoea and hyperkeratosis of the soles of the feet and the palms of the hands. Peripheral neuropathy may be present with arsenic poisoning.

General

Conduct a general examination of the patient. Is there any evidence of systemic disease? Check for lymphadenopathy, hepatosplenomegaly and generalised bruising. Check for telangiectasia.

GENERAL INVESTIGATIONS

■ **FBC, ESR**
Hb ↓ malignancy, malnutrition. WCC ↑ infection. WCC ↓ blood dyscrasias, chemotherapy. ESR ↑ malignancy, infection. Platelets ↓ thrombocytopenia.

■ **Swab**
C&S. Infected ulcers.

SPECIFIC INVESTIGATIONS

■ **Clotting screen**
Dyscrasias, anticoagulants.

■ **Vitamin C level**
Scurvy.

■ **Biopsy**
Malignant ulcers.

- Take a careful drug history. Iatrogenic causes of gum soreness and bleeding are easy to overlook.
- Petechiae of the soft palate in conjunction with gingivitis raises the possibility of acute leukaemia.
- If blood dyscrasia is a possible diagnosis, carry out a full blood count.

GYNAECOMASTIA

Gynaecomastia is enlargement of the male breast. There is an increase in the ductal and connective tissue elements of the breast. The condition should not be confused with fat in the mammary region, which may occur in obese patients and in old age with weight loss. In most cases, gynaecomastia is a result of an increase in the oestrogen–androgen ratio. In many cases the actual mechanism is unknown or the cause is idiopathic.

CAUSES

PHYSIOLOGICAL

- Neonates
- Puberty
- Old age

PATHOLOGICAL

- Drugs
  - Oestrogens
  - Cyproterone
  - Spironolactone
  - Cimetidine
  - Digitalis
  - Griseofulvin
  - Amphetamines
  - Tricyclic antidepressants
  - Cannabis
- Chronic liver disease (especially alcohol)
- Renal failure
- Carcinoma of the male breast
- Hyperthyroidism
- Hypogonadism
  - Klinefelter's syndrome
  - Agenesis
- Testicular tumours
- Other tumours
  - Bronchial carcinoma (inappropriate secretion of hormones)
  - Pituitary tumours (e.g. prolactinoma)
- Malnutrition
- Idiopathic

HISTORY

In newborn babies gynaecomastia is associated with placental oestrogens and may be associated with a milky discharge from the nipple (witch's milk). Is the patient pubertal? A minor degree of gynaecomastia occurs in a majority of boys prior to puberty. This often regresses but occasionally remains and is a source of embarrassment. Senescent gynaecomastia occurs in the sixth or later decades.

Most cases of gynaecomastia present as painless, or tender, enlargement of one or both breasts. The majority of pathological causes of gynaecomastia are related to drugs. A careful drug history should be taken. Is there a history to suggest hypogonadism, e.g. undescended testes, bilateral torsion, Klinefelter's syndrome (XXY – tall, female distribution of fat around breast and pelvis, normal male hair distribution, atrophic testes). Has the patient noticed any testicular swelling? Check for a history of alcoholism or hepatitis which might suggest liver failure. Is the patient in chronic renal failure? This will usually be apparent as he will have been on some form of dialysis. Are there any signs of hyperthyroidism? Has the patient noticed any visual disturbance to suggest a pituitary tumour involving the optic chiasma?

EXAMINATION

Local

One or both breasts may be involved. Enlargement may be considerable, resembling a female breast, but this is rare; it is usually small and localised behind the areolar. The swelling may be soft or hard. In the younger male the hard enlargement is usually confined to a disc of tissue behind the areolar and this usually occurs around puberty. Hard irregular enlargement in an elderly man should raise the diagnosis of carcinoma. Soft or diffuse enlargement is usually associated with drugs.

General

Examine the axillary and supraclavicular lymph nodes. Examine the testes – atrophic or enlarged (tumour). Check for signs for hyperthyroidism, liver failure or renal failure. The patient may have a CAPD tube or an arteriovenous fistula for treatment of chronic renal failure.

GENERAL INVESTIGATIONS

- **FBC, ESR**
  Hb ↓ anaemia – liver failure. ESR ↑ liver disease.

- **U&Es**
  Renal failure.

- **LFTs**
  Liver failure.
- **TFTs**
  Hyperthyroidism.
- **CXR**
  Primary tumour (bronchial carcinoma with inappropriate secretion of hormones).

SPECIFIC INVESTIGATIONS

- **FNAC**
  Carcinoma.
- **Mammography**
  Carcinoma.
- **Chromosome analysis**
  Klinefelter's syndrome.
- **βHCG**
  Testicular tumour.
- **AFP**
  Testicular tumour.
- **Basal serum prolactin**
  Prolactinoma.
- **CT head**
  Pituitary tumour.

- Unilateral gynaecomastia in an adult male may be due to breast carcinoma, especially if there is a hard mass behind the areola.

- In a patient with gynaecomastia always examine the testes. There may be an underlying testicular tumour. If there is any doubt, carry out an ultrasound scan.

- Gynaecomastia associated with headache and visual disturbance may be caused by a pituitary tumour, e.g. prolactinoma. In a smoker with gynaecomastia and clubbing of the fingers, bronchial carcinoma is a likely diagnosis.

- Always take a full drug history, especially recreational drugs.

SECTION A

HAEMATEMESIS

Haematemesis is the vomiting of blood. This may be frank blood or blood altered by the action of gastric acid and digestive enzymes, i.e. 'coffee grounds'. Haematemesis is usually caused by lesions proximal to the duodenojejunal junction.

CAUSES

SWALLOWED BLOOD

- Epistaxis
- Haemoptysis

OESOPHAGUS

- Reflux oesophagitis
- Oesophageal varices
- Oesophageal carcinoma

STOMACH

- Peptic ulceration
- Acute gastric erosions
- Mallory–Weiss syndrome
- Carcinoma
- Leiomyoma (gastro-intestinal stromal tumour-GIST)
- Hereditary haemorrhagic telangiectasia
- Vascular malformations

DUODENUM

- Peptic ulceration
- Duodenal diverticulae
- Aortoduodenal fistulae
- Invasive pancreatic tumours
- Haemobilia

BLEEDING DISORDERS

- Liver disease-associated
- Thrombocytopenia
- Haemophilia

DRUGS

- Anticoagulants
- Aspirin

- NSAIDs
- Steroids

OTHERS

- Uraemia
- Connective tissue disorders

HISTORY

Swallowed blood

Check for a recent history of epistaxis or haemoptysis.

Oesophagus

There may be a history of excess alcohol consumption or a history of other liver disease to suggest oesophageal varices. A history of retrosternal burning pain and heartburn would suggest oesophagitis. The bleeding associated with varices is often torrential; that associated with oesophagitis is minor. Check for a history of dysphagia, which can result from carcinoma.

Stomach

History of epigastric pain to suggest peptic ulceration. There may be a history of steroid or NSAID medication. Mallory–Weiss syndrome usually occurs in the younger patient who has had a large meal with much alcohol followed by a forceful vomit. The first vomit contains food, the second contains blood. Acute gastric erosions may occur with stressful illnesses, e.g. major surgery, acute pancreatitis, burns (Curling's ulcer), head injuries (Cushing's ulcer). It is unusual to get a large bleed with a carcinoma. Anaemia is a common presentation, although there may be 'coffee grounds' vomit. Leiomyoma causes a moderate haematemesis. There is usually no preceding history. There will also be no preceding history with vascular malformations. Hereditary haemorrhagic telangiectasia is rare. The patient may present with a history of the condition, or it may be apparent from the telangiectasia around the lips and oral cavity.

Duodenum

Melaena tends to be a more common symptom than haematemesis with duodenal lesions. There may be a history of chronic duodenal ulceration, although often presentation may be acute with little background history. Bleeding from invasive pancreatic tumours is rare. The patient will present with malaise, lethargy, weight loss and vomiting. Haemobilia is rare. Aortoduodenal fistula is rare and usually follows repair of an aneurysm with subsequent infection of the graft. There is massive haematemesis and melaena.

Bleeding disorders

The patient may present with a history of a bleeding disorder, e.g. haemophilia. There may be a history of spontaneous bruising or bleeding from other orifices.

Drugs

There may be a history of anticoagulant, steroid or NSAID therapy. Always question the patient carefully to see whether he or she has bought any proprietary, 'across the counter' preparations that may contain aspirin or NSAIDs.

Others

Uraemia may cause bleeding. Other symptoms such as dyspnoea, nausea, malaise, peripheral oedema or coma may be present. Rarely gastrointestinal bleeding may be a presenting symptom of a connective tissue disease.

EXAMINATION

Depending upon the severity of the bleed, there may be shock. The patient will be cold, clammy, with peripheral vasoconstriction; there will be a tachycardia and hypotension.

Swallowed blood

Check for blood around the nose. Examine the chest for a possible cause of haemoptysis.

Oesophagus

There may be little to find on examination except clinical signs of anaemia and weight loss, unless the cause is oesophageal varices. In the latter case there may be jaundice, abdominal distension due to ascites, spider naevi, liver palms, clubbing, gynaecomastia, testicular atrophy, caput medusae, splenomegaly or hepatomegaly.

Stomach

There may be little to find on examination. There may be an epigastric mass with a carcinoma, or a palpable left supraclavicular node (Virchow's node). There may be epigastric tenderness. With hereditary haemorrhagic telangiectasia there may be telangiectasia on the lips and mucous membrane of the mouth.

Duodenum

Again, there may be little to find on examination other than epigastric tenderness. In the rare case where duodenal bleeding comes from an invasive pancreatic carcinoma, there may be a palpable mass in the region of the pancreas.

Bleeding disorders

There may be signs of bruising or bleeding from other orifices.

Drugs

The signs will depend on the severity of the bleed and the site of the lesion produced.

Others

There may be signs of uraemia, e.g. pallor, bronze colour of the skin, pulmonary oedema, peripheral oedema, pericarditis, cardiac tamponade, hypertension, retinopathy. Rarely haematemesis may be associated with connective tissue diseases, e.g. polyarteritis nodosa. Other manifestations of polyarteritis nodosa may be apparent, e.g. neuropathies, cardiac disease, skin lesions.

GENERAL INVESTIGATIONS

- **FBC, ESR**
  Hb↓ anaemia due to chronic bleeding, e.g. from carcinoma. ESR ↑ connective tissue disease.

- **U&Es**
  Urea and creatinine will be raised in uraemia. Urea may be raised due to absorption of blood from the bowel.

- **LFTs**
  Liver failure, oesophageal varices, haemobilia.

- **Clotting screen**
  Liver disease. Bleeding diatheses. Anticoagulants.

- **OGD**
  Will demonstrate most lesions, e.g. varices, oesophagitis, peptic ulcer, gastric erosions, Mallory–Weiss tear, carcinoma and rarer causes of bleeding. Biopsy may be carried out where necessary.

SPECIFIC INVESTIGATIONS

- **Angiography**
  Vascular malformations. Also may diagnose rarer distal duodenal causes, e.g. vascular malformations.

- **US**
  Aortic aneurysm.

- **CXR**
  Chest lesion.

- **CT**
  Aortic graft infection.

- When assessing a patient with haematemesis it is important to secure intravenous access with a large-bore cannula and to send blood for cross-matching as soon as possible.

- Always take a careful drug history, especially of 'over-the-counter' drugs.

- Tachycardia may be the only physical sign of a significant GI bleed, especially in the younger patient.

HAEMATURIA

Haematuria is the passage of red blood cells in the urine. Care must be taken to distinguish it from other causes of discoloration of urine. All patients with haematuria must be fully investigated. If haematuria has initially been diagnosed on dipstick testing it must always be confirmed by microscopy.

CAUSES

KIDNEY

- Glomerular disease
- Carcinoma
- Stone
- Trauma (including renal biopsy)
- Polycystic kidney
- TB
  - (common in some parts of the world where TB is endemic)
- Embolism
- Renal vein thrombosis
- Vascular malformation

URETER

- Stone
- Neoplasm

BLADDER

- Carcinoma
- Inflammatory, e.g. cystitis, TB, schistosomiasis
- Stone
- Trauma

PROSTATE

- Benign prostatic hypertrophy
- Carcinoma

URETHRA

- Trauma
- Stone
- Urethritis
- Neoplasm

GENERAL

- Anticoagulant therapy
- Thrombocytopenia
- Strenuous exercise
- Haemophilia
- Sickle cell disease
- Malaria
  - (common where malaria is endemic)

RED URINE

- Haemoglobinuria
- Myoglobinuria
- Acute intermittent porphyria
- Beetroot
- Senna
- Phenolphthalein
- Rifampicin

HISTORY

Is there pain associated with haematuria to suggest infection or inflammation? Painless haematuria is usually associated with tumour or TB. Total haematuria (throughout the stream) suggests bleeding from the upper urinary tract or bladder. Initial haematuria (at the start of the stream) suggests bleeding from the urethra or the prostate. Terminal haematuria (at the end of the stream) suggests bleeding from the bladder or prostate. Check for a family history of polycystic kidney disease. There may be a history of TB elsewhere. Has there been any recent foreign travel (schistosomiasis)? Is there any pain in the loin to suggest kidney disease, or a history of ureteric colic to suggest passage of a stone or clot down the ureter? Bladder disease may be accompanied by suprapubic pain, frequency and dysuria. Check for symptoms of prostatism, i.e. difficulty in starting, poor stream and nocturia. Urethral injury will normally be apparent. It may occur following pelvic fractures or falling astride an object. Is the patient on anticoagulants? Is there any history of blood dyscrasia? Is there evidence of sickle cell disease or exposure to malaria? Strenuous exercise may cause haematuria. Has there been a recent renal biopsy? Discoloration of urine may be due to a variety of causes. Haemoglobinuria may occur with haemolysis and myoglobinuria following crush injuries or ischaemia of muscle. Check for ingestion of any substance that may change the colour of the urine. Acute intermittent porphyria is extremely rare and is accompanied by abdominal pain. If the urine from a patient is allowed to stand in the light it will become purplish-red.

EXAMINATION

Anaemia, weight loss, signs of chronic renal failure. Abdominal examination may reveal a palpable mass, e.g. hypernephroma, distended bladder. Rectal examination may reveal smooth enlargement of the prostate (benign prostatic hypertrophy) or a hard, craggy prostate (carcinoma). Feel along the course of the urethra, e.g. stone or neoplasm. Examine the chest, e.g. TB, secondary deposits from carcinoma of the kidney. Check for any localised bone tenderness, e.g. secondary deposits from carcinoma of the prostate or hypernephroma.

GENERAL INVESTIGATIONS

- **FBC, ESR**
  Hb ↓ gross haematuria, malignancy. Hb ↑ polycythaemia associated with hypernephroma. WCC ↑ infection. Platelets ↓ blood dyscrasias. ESR ↑ malignancy, TB.

- **Urine microscopy**
  Red cells (excludes haemoglobinuria and ingestion of substances that cause discoloration of urine). White cells in infection. Organisms in infection. Cytology.

- **U&Es**
  Renal failure.

- **Clotting screen**
  Anticoagulant therapy. Blood dyscrasias.

- **CXR**
  Metastases (cannonball metastases with hypernephroma). TB.

- **KUB**
  Renal calculus.

SPECIFIC INVESTIGATIONS

- **PSA**
  Prostatic carcinoma.

- **Sickling test**
  Sickle cell disease.

- **IVU**
  Stone. Tumour. TB.

- **US**
  Cystic versus solid. Stone. Urinary tract obstruction.

- **CT**
  Tumour (confirmation and degree of invasion). Cyst. Obstructive uropathy.

- **Cystoscopy**
  Infection. Tumour. Stone.

- **Ureteroscopy**
  Tumour. Obstruction.
- **Selective renal angiography**
  Vascular malformation. Tumour.
- **Renal biopsy**
  Glomerular disease. Tumour.
- **Prostatic biopsy**
  Carcinoma of the prostate.

- Painless haematuria suggests malignancy and requires urgent investigation.
- Dipstick testing must always be confirmed by microscopic examination of an MSU.
- A patient with microscopic haematuria associated with abnormal red cell morphology and proteinuria should be referred to a nephrologist rather than a urologist in the first instance.

HAEMOPTYSIS

Haemoptysis is the expectoration of blood or bloodstained sputum. With massive haemoptysis, the main priorities are to secure the airway and initiate emergency resuscitative measures before establishing a diagnosis.

CAUSES

RESPIRATORY

- Bronchial carcinoma
- Pneumonia
- TB (worldwide)
- Chronic bronchitis
- Bronchiectasis
- Pulmonary oedema
- Goodpasture's syndrome
- Wegener's granulomatosis

VASCULAR

- Pulmonary embolism
- Pulmonary hypertension – mitral stenosis
- Hereditary haemorrhagic telangiectasia

SYSTEMIC

- Coagulation disorders

HISTORY

Onset

Sudden onset of haemoptysis can occur with pulmonary embolism and acute respiratory tract infections; the remaining conditions tend to pursue chronic recurrent courses. Although the amount of blood expectorated is not very useful as a discriminating feature, small amounts of blood sufficient to stain the sputum pink are characteristic of pulmonary oedema.

Acute onset of cough with haemoptysis may occur with respiratory tract infections and pulmonary embolism. Associated sputum production may be purulent and long-standing with chronic bronchitis and bronchiectasis. This is accompanied by flecks of blood when lung carcinoma, TB or mitral stenosis is present.

Dyspnoea

A long history of dyspnoea may be associated with chronic lung disease or mitral stenosis. Acute onset of dyspnoea that occurs with pulmonary embolism may be accompanied by pleuritic chest pain. Dyspnoea that is associated with pulmonary oedema may have a variable speed of onset and is often worse on recumbency.

Weight loss

Progressive weight loss is suggestive of TB or bronchial carcinoma, especially with a background of heavy smoking. Night sweats may be an additional accompanying feature of TB.

Other sites of bleeding

Other bleeding sites should be excluded as haematuria may be due to Goodpasture's syndrome. Epistaxis and haemoptysis occur together with Wegener's granulomatosis and hereditary haemorrhagic telangiectasia. Epistaxis *per se* may occasionally be confused with haemoptysis when expectorated sputum is mixed with blood originating from the nasal passages.

Past medical and drug history

A careful history is taken to identify a generalised coagulation disorder. This may be congenital, such as haemophilia, or acquired, such as with the use of anticoagulant drugs or in DIC. Previous rheumatic fever predisposes an individual to mitral stenosis. Consider Goodpasture's syndrome and Wegener's granulomatosis in the presence of co-existing renal disease.

EXAMINATION

Inspection

Cachexia is a prominent feature of carcinoma, TB and chronic lung disease. Loss of the nasal bridge and saddling of the nose may be apparent in patients with Wegener's granulomatosis. The presence of clubbing (p. 62) is associated with bronchial carcinoma, chronic bronchitis and bronchiectasis. The malar flush characteristic of mitral facies may be present with mitral stenosis. Small dilated blood vessels present on the mucous membranes are features of hereditary haemorrhagic telangiectasia. The JVP may be elevated with a large pulmonary embolus or accompanying congestive cardiac failure secondary to mitral stenosis. The chest may be hyperexpanded with decreased inspiratory movement in chronic bronchitis.

Palpation

During an acute episode, tachycardia is very common. This may be due to the effort of coughing, anxiety or blood loss. The presence of an irregularly irregular heartbeat of atrial fibrillation is associated with mitral stenosis. Moreover, patients with atrial fibrillation are usually on anticoagulant therapy. Supraclavicular lymphadenopathy may be present with pulmonary infections or carcinoma. The calves should be palpated and measured for tenderness and increased girth from deep venous thrombosis, which may give rise to pulmonary emboli.

Percussion and auscultation

Localised crepitations and bronchial breathing may be audible with lobar pneumonia. Generalised coarse crepitations are suggestive of bronchiectasis, pulmonary oedema and chronic bronchitis. Breath sounds tend to be decreased in intensity with chronic bronchitis. Patients with bronchial carcinoma may present with a number of clinical features from the primary tumour, such as wheezing due to large airway obstruction, pulmonary collapse, pleural effusion and superior vena cava obstruction. On auscultation of the mitral area, the loud first heart sound and mid-diastolic rumbling murmur of mitral stenosis is accentuated on expiration with the patient in a left lateral position.

GENERAL INVESTIGATIONS

- **Sputum analysis**
  Sputum should be collected for microscopy, culture and cytology. Infective organisms may be isolated or cytological features of malignancy may be present. When TB is suspected, serial cultures should be taken from sputum, urine, bronchial washings or lung biopsy specimens during bronchoscopy. Polymerase chain reaction amplification techniques may also be performed on cultured specimens to provide a more rapid diagnosis.

- **ECG**
  Sinus tachycardia may be noted with violent coughing, anxiety and blood loss. $S_1Q_3T_3$ is indicative of right heart strain with pulmonary embolism, although non-specific ST abnormalities are more common.

- **FBC**
  Hb ↓ with chronic haemoptysis resulting in iron deficiency anaemia. Acute bleeding may not be associated with changes in the blood count until 24 hours later. WCC ↑ may be due to acute bleeding or respiratory tract infection. Monocytosis may be a feature of TB. Platelets ↓ with blood dyscrasias.

- **U&Es**
  The presence of impaired renal function with deranged urea and creatinine estimations may be due to glomerulonephritis from Goodpasture's syndrome or Wegener's granulomatosis.

However, pre-renal failure may also be precipitated by acute blood loss and volume depletion.

- **Clotting screen**
  A clotting screen is performed to identify any impairment that may prolong the PT or APTT.

- **CXR**
  Bilateral patchy areas of consolidation may be seen on a chest film with bronchopneumonia and pulmonary oedema. Opacification of an entire lobe suggests lobar pneumonia, although pulmonary emboli may have a similar appearance due to the wedge-shaped shadowing of a pulmonary infarct. Recurrent fluffy shadowing may be seen with Goodpasture's syndrome and Wegener's granulomatosis, due to repeated intra-alveolar haemorrhage. The primary focus of tuberculous infection is usually in the middle to upper zones of the lung. This may resolve, with variable amounts of calcification, whereas post-primary TB tends to present with the classical apical shadow. The chest film may be normal with uncomplicated chronic bronchitis; however, with bronchiectasis, visibly dilated bronchi with persistent consolidation may be prominent. With bronchial carcinoma, numerous features may be seen on a chest radiograph, such as a peripheral mass, a hilar mass, collapse of a lobe or pleural effusion. The double right heart border and tenting of the left heart border are all features of enlargement of the left atrium with mitral stenosis. When pulmonary hypertension is present, there may be dilatation of the central pulmonary arteries with right ventricular enlargement.

- **Bronchoscopy**
  Fibreoptic bronchoscopy is useful for locating the site of bleeding. In addition, biopsies of the bleeding site may be sampled for pathological analysis. Multiple arteriovenous malformations will be visible with hereditary haemorrhagic telangiectasia.

SPECIFIC INVESTIGATIONS

- **Mantoux test**
  When TB is suspected an initial dilute Mantoux test (1 in 10 000) may be performed in individuals who have not received BCG immunisation.

- **Urinalysis**
  May reveal the presence of protein and red cell casts with glomerulonephritis due to Goodpasture's syndrome and Wegener's granulomatosis.

- **Antiglomerular basement antibodies**
  Characterises Goodpasture's syndrome.

- **c-ANCA**
  Wegener's granulomatosis is associated with elevated levels.

- **Renal biopsy**
  Will aid in confirming the diagnosis in both Goodpasture's syndrome and Wegener's granulomatosis.

- **Tissue biopsies**
  Majority of lung cancers are diagnosed on CXR; a smaller proportion are diagnosed by cytology. Definitive tissue diagnosis can be made by biopsies from bronchoscopy, mediastinoscopy, CT-guided biopsy or surgical resection.

- **CT thorax/pulmonary angiogram**
  Very useful adjunct to the diagnosis of bronchiectasis in cases where the diagnosis cannot confidently be made on the clinical grounds and a chest film. It may also be useful in the staging of lung carcinomas. The CT pulmonary angiogram is currently the investigation of choice to screen for pulmonary embolism.

- **Echocardiography**
  Allows assessment of left ventricular function with pulmonary oedema. It may also aid in the diagnosis of pulmonary embolism, as right heart failure can occur with large emboli. The integrity of the cardiac valves can be assessed, and valve stenosis with restriction of movement of the mitral valve leaflets can be visualised in mitral stenosis.

- **Haemoptysis in a smoker is an indication for a CXR, especially if associated with other features, e.g. dyspnoea, clubbing.**

- **Always consider TB, especially in the elderly, immigrants and the immunocompromised (from whatever cause).**

- **With massive haemoptysis the main priorities are to secure the airway and initiate emergency resuscitative measures before establishing a diagnosis.**

HALITOSIS

Halitosis is a frequent or persistent unpleasant odour to the breath. It is usually due to poor dental hygiene. It may have a significant impact, both personally and socially, on those who suffer from it. Rarely it may be the symptom of a serious underlying condition.

CAUSES

- Poor oral hygiene
- Smoking
- Diet, e.g. onions, garlic, spices
- Gingivitis
- Excess alcohol intake
- Dental abscess
- Dry mouth, e.g. starvation, salivary gland disease
- Acute and chronic sinusitis
- Acute tonsillitis
- Nasal foreign body
- GORD
- Abdominal sepsis, e.g. foetor of acute appendicitis
- Drugs, e.g. disulfiram
- Psychogenic halitosis
- Pharyngeal pouch
- Bronchiectasis
- Liver failure
- Renal failure (uraemia)
- Necrotic oral/nasopharyngeal cancer

HISTORY

History of toothache, poor diet, smoking, alcohol. Painful gums, bleeding from gums. Acute necrotising ulcerative gingivitis (Vincent's angina) is rare but presents with swollen gums with small ulcers which may spread to the buccal mucosa and the patient will complain of bleeding from the gums, together with a constitutional upset with fever and malaise. Heartburn (GORD), dysphagia (pharyngeal pouch). Dysphagia may occur due to a pharyngeal pouch pressing on the oesophagus. It may gurgle on palpation and regurgitation of food may occur on lying down with subsequent development of aspiration pneumonia. Sinusitis may present with a nasal discharge and facial pain over the sinus. Cough, sputum and recurrent chest infections may indicate bronchiectasis. Dry mouth may be a part of prolonged starvation with chronic or acute illness or disease of the salivary glands, e.g. Sjögren's syndrome. There may be a history of diabetes, renal failure or liver failure. Is the halitosis worse in the morning and gets better during the day? Is the patient otherwise well?

EXAMINATION

A worse odour through the mouth suggests an oral aetiology. A worse odour through the nose suggests either sinusitis or a foreign body. Nasal odours are usually more pungent than oral odours. The tongue may be coated, especially the posterior one-third. Check for gingivitis, periodontal disease and dental abscess. Gingivitis presents with red swollen and bleeding gums. In acute necrotising ulcerative gingivitis, in addition to the swollen, bleeding gums there may be yellowish ulcers which may also be seen on the buccal mucosa and occasionally on the tonsils. There is usually tender lymphadenopathy. Examine the salivary glands. Carry out a full examination of the oral cavity. Ulcers with hard everted edges which bleed on contact are likely to be neoplastic. Look for signs of liver failure.

GENERAL INVESTIGATIONS

- **Swab**
  C&S infections.
- **FBC**
  Infective causes.
- **U&Es**
  Chronic renal failure.
- **LFTs**
  Liver failure.
- **CXR**
  Chest infection. Bronchiectasis.

SPECIFIC INVESTIGATIONS

- **Antinuclear antibodies**
  Sjögren's syndrome
- **Rheumatoid factor**
  May be positive in Sjögren's syndrome.
- **Skull X-ray**
  Sinusitis – sinus opacity.
- **OGD**
  GORD.
- **Barium swallow**
  Pharyngeal pouch.

- **Laryngoscopy**
  Nasopharyngeal carcinoma.

- **Biopsy**
  Benign versus malignant.

- **CT**
  Nasopharyngeal carcinoma. Carcinoma of the maxillary antrum.
  Assess extent of disease.

- Most (85%) cases halitosis are due to poor oral hygiene.

- In the absence of an obvious cause, always fully examine the head and neck, including the oral cavity and nasal airway. Check for lymphadenopathy.

- Remember alcohol abuse. Check for signs of liver failure.

- In the patient who complains of halitosis, in the absence of obvious bad breath, consider psychogenic halitosis, especially if there is a history of depression.

HALLUCINATIONS

An hallucination is an apparent sensory perception of an external object when no such object is present. It is to be differentiated from an illusion, which is a real perception that is misinterpreted.

CAUSES

- Fever (especially children and the elderly)
- Drugs (and drug withdrawal)
  - Marijuana
  - Cocaine
  - LSD
  - Ecstasy
  - Solvent sniffing
  - Amphetamines
  - Tricyclic antidepressant overdose
- Alcohol
  - Alcoholic hallucinations
  - Delirium tremens (alcohol withdrawal)
- Extreme fatigue
- Psychiatric disorders
  - Schizophrenia
  - Psychotic depression
  - Post-traumatic stress disorder
  - Mania
- Sensory deprivation (e.g. blindness or deafness)
- Hypoxia
- Severe metabolic disturbances (e.g. diabetic ketoacidosis, hypothyroidism)
- Severe medical illness
  - Liver failure
  - Renal failure
- Neurological disease
  - Temporal lobe epilepsy
  - Cerebral tumour
  - Post-concussional state
  - Dementia
  - Narcolepsy
- Others
  - Bereavement reaction

HISTORY

Obtain a clear history of the hallucination. Common hallucinations include hearing voices when no-one has spoken; seeing patterns, lights, beings or objects that are not there; feeling a crawling sensation on the skin. Hallucinations related to smell or taste are rare. Pure olfactory hallucinations are strongly suggestive of temporal lobe epilepsy. Enquire about recreational drugs. Auditory hallucinations are more common in psychotic conditions such as schizophrenia. Acute onset of febrile illnesses may be associated with hallucinations, especially in children and the elderly. Enquire about alcohol abuse or alcohol withdrawal. Hallucinations may be 'normal', e.g. hearing the voice of a loved one who has recently died, being part of a bereavement reaction.

EXAMINATION

Check the temperature. Look for signs of infection. Look for signs of liver failure and kidney failure. Carry out a full neurological examination to exclude the possibility of a cerebral space-occupying lesion. A full mental state examination should be undertaken for possible psychiatric disorder.

GENERAL INVESTIGATIONS

- **Urinalysis**
  UTI, hyperglycaemic ketoacidosis.

- **FBC**
  WCC ↑ infection. MCV ↑ alcohol excess.

- **U&Es**
  Metabolic disturbances. Renal failure

- **LFTs**
  Liver failure.

- **Blood sugar**
  Hyperglycaemic ketoacidosis.

SPECIFIC INVESTIGATIONS

- **ABGs**
  Hypoxia. Severe metabolic disturbances.

- **Toxicology screen**
  Drug abuse.

- **EEG**
  Temporal lobe epilepsy.

- **CT scan**
  Cerebral space-occupying lesion. Dementia.

- Hallucinations in children with febrile illness are common.
- Pure olfactory hallucinations are strongly suggestive of temporal lobe epilepsy.
- Tactile hallucinations strongly suggest acute alcohol withdrawal.

HAND DEFORMITIES

Impairment of hand function can lead to severe disability.

CAUSES

CONGENITAL

FAILURE OF FORMATION
- Absent digit
- Radial club hand

FAILURE OF SEPARATION
- Syndactyly (fusion of digits)
- Camptodactyly

DUPLICATION
- Extra digit

PRIMARY MUSCLE CONTRACTURES
- Arthrogryposis multiplex congenita

ACQUIRED

- Dupuytren's contracture
- Rheumatoid arthritis
- Trauma (mal-united fracture)
- Burns
- Volkmann's ischaemic contracture
- Brachial plexus lesions
- Peripheral nerve lesions
- Spinal cord lesions
  - Poliomyelitis
  - Syringomyelia
- Multiple chondromas (Ollier's disease)

HISTORY

Congenital

These lesions will be recognisable at birth. Arthrogryposis multiplex congenita is due to non-differentiation of mesenchymal tissues, often together with a neurogenic element, the combination producing gross contractures.

Acquired

Trauma and burns

There will be a clear history of previous trauma and burns.

Dupuytren's contracture

In the early phases there will be little deformity, the patient merely complaining of thickening in the palm near the base of the ring finger. Eventually the patient will complain of being unable to straighten the ring and little fingers. The grip is also affected. Check for a history of epilepsy, cirrhosis or diabetes.

Rheumatoid arthritis

By the time the hand is deformed the patient is usually well aware of the diagnosis. There is pain and swelling of the joints with weakness of the hand, together with gross deformity.

Volkmann's ischaemic contracture

This is shortening of the long flexor muscles of the forearm due to ischaemia. There may be a history of trauma, e.g. supracondylar fracture of the humerus, a tight plaster restricting blood flow, or arterial disease, e.g. embolism. Movements of the fingers are painful and limited. There may be pins and needles in the hand due to pressure on nerves. Eventually a claw hand results.

Spinal cord lesions

By the time deformity of the limb has resulted, the diagnosis will usually be apparent. There may be a history of poliomyelitis.

Brachial plexus lesions

There will usually be a history of trauma, although occasionally invasion of the brachial plexus from tumours may occur.

Peripheral nerve lesions

There is usually a clear history of trauma to suggest a nerve lesion. Check for any possible causes of peripheral neuropathy, e.g. diabetes, uraemia, connective tissue disease, leprosy.

Ollier's disease

This results in deformities of the limb. There are irregularly distributed areas of cartilage and bone. The patient will complain of deformity of joints and bones and possible shortening of the limb, and will have noticed nodules along the line of bone.

EXAMINATION

Congenital

Congenital anomalies will be obvious at birth. They may be associated with congenital anomalies elsewhere.

Acquired

Trauma and burns

A variety of deformities may be seen, depending upon the degree and type of trauma. With burns, scarring of the skin will be obvious.

Dupuytren's contracture

Examination will reveal a firm nodule in the palmar fascia near the base of the ring finger. Puckering of the skin is usually present around the nodule. The MCP joint and the PIP joint are flexed, the DIP joint being extended. The ulnar digits (ring and little finger) are most commonly affected.

Rheumatoid arthritis

There is thickening of the joints, especially the MCP joint and PIP joints. The joints become fusiform in shape. There is ulnar deviation of the fingers. The wrist joint develops a fixed flexion deformity with some ulnar deviation. Swan-neck and boutonnière deformities of the fingers will be apparent. Ultimately, tendon rupture occurs and this leads to a variety of deformities.

Volkmann's ischaemic contracture

The skin of the hand is pale and the hand clawed and wasted. Extension of the fingers is limited but improves if the wrist is flexed. Eventually, the forearm muscles feel hard and taut due to fibrosis.

Spinal cord lesions

In the case of poliomyelitis, there is usually a clear history and the limb usually looks reddish-blue, wasted and deformed. Syringomyelia may cause a variety of hand deformities. With upper motor neurone lesions there may be fixed flexion of the wrist and fingers with adduction of the thumb.

Brachial plexus injuries

Upward traction on the arm may damage the lowest root (T1) of the brachial plexus, which is the segmental supply of the intrinsic muscles of the hand. The hand becomes clawed (Klumpke's paralysis). Check for a possible associated Horner's syndrome due to traction of the cervical sympathetic chain.

Peripheral nerve lesions

With ulnar nerve lesions it is appropriate to check for damage to the medial epicondyle. Also check for any evidence of recent lacerations at the wrist. With division at the wrist all the intrinsic muscles of the fingers (except for the radial two lumbricals – median nerve) are paralysed and the hand appears clawed. The clawing is less for the index and middle fingers because the lumbricals are intact. In late cases, wasting of the interossei is clearly seen on the dorsum of the hand. There is sensory loss over the medial 1½ fingers. If the nerve is injured at the elbow the flexor digitorum profundus to the ring and little fingers is paralysed so that the clawing of these two digits is not so pronounced.

In median nerve lesions at the wrist the thenar eminence becomes wasted due to paralysis of opponens pollicis and sensation is lost over the lateral 3½ digits. Fine movements, e.g. picking up a small object, are clumsy. With lesions at the elbow, wrist flexion is weak and the forearm muscles wasted. Ulnar deviation occurs at the wrist, as the wrist flexion depends upon flexor carpi ulnaris and the medial half of flexor digitorum profundus. Often the hand is held with the medial two fingers flexed and the lateral two fingers straight.

Ollier's disease

Multiple lumps (chondromas) are located on the bones. Often associated with limb shortening. Only one limb or one bone may be involved.

GENERAL INVESTIGATIONS

Most of the conditions described above will be obvious on clinical examination.

■ FBC, ESR
  Hb ↓ in anaemia of chronic disease, e.g. rheumatoid arthritis.

■ CRP
  ↑ in inflammatory disease

■ Rheumatoid factor
  Rheumatoid arthritis.

■ LFTs
  Cirrhosis (Dupuytren's contracture).

■ Blood glucose
  Diabetes. Peripheral neuropathy, Dupuytren's contracture.

■ Arm X-ray
  Local fractures, e.g. evidence of previous supracondylar fracture of the humerus with subsequent Volkmann's ischaemic contracture.

■ Hand X-ray
  Rheumatoid arthritis. Ollier's disease – multiple translucent areas in the bones of the hand. Evidence of mal-united fracture following trauma.

■ MRI
  Spinal lesions, e.g. syringomyelia.

■ Nerve conduction studies
  Brachial plexus and peripheral nerve lesions.

• The hand is a sophisticated mechanism from both motor and sensory considerations. Every attempt should be made to prevent hand deformities occurring as a result of trauma and infection. All hand injuries and infections should be referred to a specialist hand surgeon as expert care is necessary from the outset to preserve or restore function.

HEADACHE

When assessing a patient with headache it is important to exclude life-threatening causes first.

CAUSES

ACUTE HEADACHE

- Trauma
- Cerebrovascular
  - Subarachnoid haemorrhage
  - Intracranial haemorrhage/infarction
- Systemic infection
- Meningitis
- Acute angle-closure glaucoma

CHRONIC OR RECURRENT HEADACHE

- Tension headache
- Migraine
- Cluster headaches
- Drugs, e.g. glyceryl trinitrate, nifedipine, substance withdrawal (especially alcohol)
- Cervical spondylosis
- Psychological (including anxiety and depression)
- Raised intracranial pressure
  - Tumour
  - Hydrocephalus
  - Cerebral abscess
  - Benign intracranial hypertension
- Temporal arteritis
- Pre-eclampsia
- Paget's disease of bone
- Severe hypertension
- Carbon monoxide poisoning

HISTORY

Onset

Sudden onset of severe pain is usually due to a vascular cause, especially subarachnoid haemorrhage from a ruptured berry aneurysm. Cluster headache and migraine intensify over minutes and may last several hours, while meningitis tends to evolve over hours to days. Progressive severe headaches that develop over days or weeks should lead to the consideration of raised intracranial pressure from tumour or chronic subdural haemorrhage. The onset of headache may be preceded by an aura with migraine.

Site

Classically, headache from migraine is unilateral. Temporal arteritis leads to more localised pain over the superficial temporal arteries that can be accompanied by jaw claudication. Ocular pain is experienced with glaucoma, and retro-orbital pain with cluster headaches.

Character

The intensity of pain contributes little when discriminating between the causes; however, the character of the pain may be useful. Patients with tension headache often complain of a tight band-like sensation; this is in contrast to the pain experienced with raised intracranial pressure, which is often reported to have a bursting quality. Migraine-related and temporal arteritis headaches have a throbbing character.

Precipitating factors

Headache originating from raised intracranial pressure is precipitated by changes in posture, coughing or sneezing, and is often worse in the mornings. Photophobia may be experienced by patients suffering with migraine, meningitis or glaucoma. They may prefer to lie in a darkened room when headaches arise. Certain foods such as cheese, red wine and chocolate are known to precipitate migraine. It is very common for headache to be precipitated by systemic illnesses such as a cold or influenza. Headache precipitated by touch occurs with superficial temporal artery inflammation from temporal arteritis. A drug history may elucidate the relationship between the administration of drugs with headache as a side-effect, such as glyceryl trinitrate and nifedipine. Alternatively, headache can also result from substance withdrawal in substance-dependent patients.

Associated symptoms

Neck stiffness (meningism) is experienced with both meningitis and subarachnoid haemorrhages. Visual disturbances in the form of haloes occur with glaucoma. Flashing lights and alternations in perception of size may be reported by patients suffering with migraine, and this may be accompanied by photophobia, nausea and vomiting. Transient neurological deficits may also occur. However, progressive neurology associated with headache is more suggestive of an intracranial space-occupying lesion, such as haemorrhage, abscess and tumour. Unilateral visual loss may result as a complication of temporal arteritis, and this may be accompanied by proximal muscle pain, stiffness and weakness or tenderness. Conjunctival infection is experienced with both glaucoma and cluster headaches, along with lacrimation, which is a feature of the latter. With normal pressure hydrocephalus in adults, headaches are associated with dementia, drowsiness, vomiting and ataxia.

EXAMINATION

Temperature

Pyrexia may indicate the presence of systemic infection, meningitis or vasculitis.

Inspection

An assessment of the conscious state should be undertaken and quantified on the GCS. Impairment of consciousness is a sign of a serious underlying aetiology, such as meningitis, subarachnoid haemorrhage and raised intracranial pressure. Inspection of the eyes may reveal conjunctival infection with glaucoma and cluster headaches during an acute attack. With acute angle-closure glaucoma the cornea is hazy and the pupil fixed and semi-dilated. Petechial haemorrhages classically occur with meningococcal meningitis.

Palpation

Tenderness along the course of the superficial temporal artery, with absent pulsation, is consistent with temporal arteritis.

Neurological examination

A detailed neurological examination is performed to identify the site of any structural lesion. Unilateral total visual loss can be precipitated by temporal arteritis due to ischaemic optic neuritis. Visual field defects (hemianopia) can be caused by contralateral lesions in the cerebral cortex. Fundoscopy is performed to identify papilloedema from raised intracranial pressure.

Transient hemiplegia can occur with migraine, but progressive hemiplegia is more indicative of a space-occupying lesion, such as a tumour or intracranial haemorrhage. Neck stiffness is a feature of both meningitis and subarachnoid haemorrhage. With meningitis, Kernig's sign (pain on extending the knee with the hip in a flexed position) may be present.

GENERAL INVESTIGATIONS

- **FBC**
  WCC ↑ meningitis, cerebral abscess and systemic infection.

- **ESR and CRP**
  ↑ temporal arteritis, infection, intracranial bleeding.

- **U&Es**
  Hypertensive headaches with renal disease.

- **Alkaline phosphatase**
  Elevated in Paget's disease.

- **Radiology**
  Cervical spine X-rays identify cervical spondylosis and cranial X-rays may reveal Paget's disease.

SPECIFIC INVESTIGATIONS

In most cases, the diagnosis can be made on clinical assessment. Features in the history and examination may guide specific investigations.

- **Blood cultures**
  With meningitis, systemic infection.

- **CT/MRI**
  Visualisation of the anatomical structures in the cranium is very useful in the presence of neurological deficit. Cerebral tumours may be visualised as high or low-density masses. Intracranial bleeding can be identified as areas of high density during the first 2 weeks. An extradural haematoma presents as a lens-shaped opacity, and subdural haematoma presents as a crescent-shaped opacity. After 2 weeks, intracranial haematomas become isodense and more difficult to visualise. Following subarachnoid haemorrhage, blood may be visualised in the subarachnoid space. Occasionally the offending aneurysm or arteriovenous malformation may be imaged. Enlargement of the ventricles may be an indication of hydrocephalus. Contrast-enhanced CT or MRI will increase the sensitivity to diagnose cerebral abscesses.

- **Lumbar puncture**
  A lumbar puncture may be undertaken following the exclusion of raised intracranial pressure when there is suspicion of meningitis or subarachnoid haemorrhage. The opening pressure is recorded and the CSF obtained is inspected for consistency and colour. The consistency of the CSF is turbid with meningitis, and yellow staining of the CSF (known as xanthochromia) occurs with subarachnoid haemorrhage, owing to breakdown of haemoglobin from red blood cells. The CSF is then sent for microscopy, culture, cytology and biochemical analysis for glucose and protein. An abnormal increase in white cells may be seen on microscopy with meningitis. With bacterial or tuberculous meningitis, the glucose is low and protein content high. With viral meningitis the glucose content is normal and protein content mildly elevated. A lumbar puncture may also be helpful in cases of benign intracranial hypertension.

■ **Temporal artery biopsy**
Inflammation and giant cells may be seen with temporal arteritis. A normal biopsy does not, however, exclude the disease, as there may be segmental involvement of the temporal artery.

■ **Intraocular pressure measurements**
Tonometry will reveal high intraocular pressures with glaucoma.

- Although extremely common, headache should always be investigated if there is any concern regarding sinister pathology, such as CVA or malignancy.

- Temporal arteritis must be treated immediately with high-dose corticosteroids to avoid complete and irreversible blindness.

HEMIPLEGIA

Hemiplegia is paralysis of one side of the body; it usually arises from unilateral lesions above the midcervical spinal cord.

CAUSES

VASCULAR

- Cerebrovascular ischaemia
- Cerebral or spinal infarction
- Intracerebral haemorrhage
- Cerebral vasculitis

TRAUMATIC

- Subdural haematoma
- Extradural haematoma

OTHER

- Epilepsy (Todd's paralysis)
- Multiple sclerosis
- Brain tumour
- Cerebral abscess

HISTORY

Onset

The speed of onset of hemiplegia is useful when trying to determine the underlying aetiology. Sudden onset hemiplegia is usually due to a cerebrovascular event such as a TIA, infarct or intracerebral haemorrhage. Hemiplegia developing over minutes or hours after trauma can be due to an evolving extradural or subdural haemorrhage. Although a history of trauma is usually evident, chronic subdural haematomas in the elderly may result from tearing of bridging veins without apparent trauma. Subacute hemiplegia may also result as part of a spectrum of neurological deficits caused by demyelination from multiple sclerosis. Gradual onset of hemiplegia is usually due to a tumour, although a cerebral abscess or chronic subdural haemorrhage may pursue a similar time course.

Precipitating factors

A history of trauma may be evident with extradural and subdural haemorrhages. Cerebral abscesses may result from haematogenous dissemination of bacteria from a distant site of infection, such as the lung, or more commonly from adjacent infections, such as middle ear, mastoid and paranasal sinus infections. Transient hemiplegia may also result from an epileptic seizure and this phenomenon is known as Todd's paralysis. Unfortunately, the precipitating factor for the seizure may be underlying structural abnormalities such as a cerebral abscess or tumour.

Associated symptoms

Owing to the multifocal nature of demyelination, patients with multiple sclerosis may present with a host of associated symptoms, such as areas of motor deficits, sensory deficits, diplopia and monocular blindness from optic neuritis. Space-occupying lesions such as extradural haematoma, brain tumour and cerebral abscesses may also present with symptoms of raised intracranial pressure, such as headaches, classically worse in the morning, and with coughing or sneezing, nausea, vomiting and drowsiness.

EXAMINATION

The neurological examination is the key to determining the location of the lesion. Cortical lesions impinging on the motor area of the frontal lobe produce total contralateral paralysis. Similar effects can result from lesions of the internal capsule. Midbrain lesions tend to produce ipsilateral neurological deficits of the face and contralateral deficits of the limbs. Multifocal neurological deficits may be produced by demyelination or cerebral metastasis.

After determining the site of the lesion, the examination should be continued to determine the cause. Pyrexia should alert the clinician to the presence of infection, which may be caused by a cerebral abscess. The presence of facial myokymia, which is rippling of the muscles on one side of the face, is reported to be very suggestive of multiple sclerosis; cervical involvement may produce Lhermitte's sign, which is paraesthesia of the hands and feet on flexion of the neck.

Examination of the ear, mastoid and sinuses is useful to locate the site of primary infection, which may give rise to a cerebral abscess. Distant sites of infection that may precipitate cerebral abscesses are the lungs and emboli from infective endocarditis. The fingers are examined for nailfold infarcts with endocarditis and the precordium is auscultated for new or changing murmurs. The pulse is assessed for irregularity from atrial fibrillation, which is a predisposing factor for cerebral emboli. The blood pressure is measured, as hypertension is an additional risk factor for stroke. Carotid bruits from atherosclerotic plaques may be the only examination feature present with TIAs.

GENERAL INVESTIGATIONS

- FBC
  WCC ↑ infection, infarction.

- **ESR**
  ↑ infection, infarction, vasculitis.
- **U&Es, magnesium, calcium and glucose**
  Abnormal electrolytes and glucose level may precipitate a seizure.

SPECIFIC INVESTIGATIONS

- **Blood cultures**
  For suspected cerebral abscess.
- **CT head**
  Intracerebral haemorrhage, cerebral infarction, head injuries, tumour and abscess.
- **MRI head and cervical spine**
  Abscess, tumours, focal demyelination and periventricular plaques with multiple sclerosis.
- **EEG**
  Epilepsy.
- **Lumbar puncture**
  Exclude raised intracranial pressure first. With multiple sclerosis there is raised CSF IgG, and oligoclonal bands are present on electrophoresis.

- Sudden onset hemiplegia is an emergency and requires immediate investigation. A CT scan should be performed expeditiously to identify cerebral bleeds or infarction.

HEPATOMEGALY

Hepatomegaly is enlargement of the liver. The most common causes in the UK are cirrhosis, cardiac failure and secondary malignancy.

CAUSES

HEPATITIS/INFECTION

ACUTE
- Alcohol
- Viruses
- Bacteria
- Protozoans
- Parasites

CHRONIC
- Chronic active hepatitis

CONGESTION
- Congestive cardiac failure
- Constrictive pericarditis
- Budd–Chiari syndrome

INFILTRATION
- Fatty liver
- Amyloid

BILIARY TRACT DISEASE
- Extrahepatic obstruction, e.g. carcinoma of the pancreas, bile duct stricture
- Sclerosing cholangitis
- Primary biliary cirrhosis

MALIGNANCY
- Metastases
- Hepatoma
- Myeloproliferative disorders
- Myelofibrosis
- Leukaemia

METABOLIC
- Glycogen storage diseases
- Haemochromatosis
- Wilson's disease (hepatolenticular degeneration)

OTHERS

- Cryptogenic cirrhosis
- Riedel's lobe

HISTORY

Hepatitis/infection

Predisposing factors include a history of contact with hepatitis, blood transfusion, drug abuse, homosexuals, haemophiliacs, health workers, the institutionalised (e.g. homes, prison) and travel abroad to endemic areas. Amoebiasis occurs worldwide, and hepatitis B is prevalent in the tropics and Mediterranean areas. Hydatid disease is more common in sheep-rearing countries, e.g. Australia, Africa, Wales. Leptospirosis can result from swimming in rat-infested waters. History of alcohol abuse predisposes to alcoholic cirrhosis. Chronic active hepatitis should be considered with a history of alcohol, hepatitis B or hepatitis C. In the majority of hepatitis/infection cases, the patient presents with general malaise, pyrexia, weight loss and jaundice.

Congestion

History of congestive cardiac failure, may be evident and the patient often complains of upper abdominal pain caused by a tender liver due to stretching of the liver capsule. With constrictive pericarditis there is often a history of TB but it may follow any cause of pericarditis, e.g. acute renal failure. Budd–Chiari syndrome is hepatic vein thrombosis. A history of taking the contraceptive pill may be contributory. Tumour may also cause Budd–Chiari syndrome. It presents insidiously with portal hypertension, jaundice and cirrhosis.

Infiltration

There is usually a history of alcohol abuse with fatty infiltration. Secondary amyloidosis follows chronic infection, e.g. rheumatoid arthritis, bronchiectasis, inflammatory bowel disease.

Biliary tract disease

There may be a history of biliary tract obstruction, e.g. carcinoma of the pancreas or stricture of the common bile duct. Sclerosing cholangitis causes jaundice and fevers and is associated with inflammatory bowel disease. Primary biliary cirrhosis is of unknown aetiology. Some 90% of the patients are female. It presents with obstructive jaundice, pruritus and hepatosplenomegaly. The patient will complain of dark urine and pale stools.

Malignancy

The chief cause is metastases from a known malignancy, which may have been treated, e.g. gastrointestinal tract or bronchus.

Hepatoma is rare. With hepatoma there may be a past history of hepatitis B infection, use of the contraceptive pill, aflatoxin exposure, or use of anabolic steroids. Myeloproliferative disease presents with tiredness, lethargy and spontaneous bruising.

Metabolic

Glycogen storage disease is rare. There is usually hepatomegaly from birth. The early features of haemochromatosis include fatigue, arthralgia and hepatomegaly. Skin pigmentation, diabetes and cardiac failure occur later.

Others

Cryptogenic cirrhosis presents with hepatomegaly without an obvious cause. Riedel's lobe is usually an incidental finding and asymptomatic. Riedel's lobe is an extension of the right lobe of the liver below the costal margin. It is a normal anatomical variation.

EXAMINATION

Remember that a liver edge that is palpable is not always enlarged and may have been pushed down by pulmonary hyperinflation, e.g. emphysema. The upper border of the liver should therefore be identified by percussion and is usually at the level of the eighth rib in the midaxillary line. The edge of the liver can be sharp or rounded and its surface smooth or nodular.

Regular generalised enlargement without jaundice

Cirrhosis
Congestive cardiac failure
Reticulosis
Budd–Chiari syndrome
Amyloid.

Regular generalised enlargement with jaundice

Viral hepatitis
Biliary tract obstruction
Cholangitis.

Irregular generalised enlargement without jaundice

Secondary tumours
Macronodular cirrhosis
Polycystic disease of the liver
Primary tumours.

Irregular generalised enlargement with jaundice

Cirrhosis
Widespread liver secondaries.

Localised swellings

Riedel's lobe
Hydatid disease
Amoebic abscess
Primary carcinoma.

General

Carry out a general examination of the patient. Look for signs of liver failure: jaundice, flapping tremor, ascites, spider naevi, liver palms, clubbing, gynaecomastia, testicular atrophy, caput medusae, peripheral oedema, leuconychia, Dupuytren's contracture, xanthoma, mental changes, coma, bruising. Look for Kayser–Fleischer rings (Wilson's disease).

Congestion

Signs of CCF. Peripheral oedema. Tense tender liver. JVP ↑. With Budd–Chiari syndrome there will be acute ascites and right upper quadrant pain. In constrictive pericarditis there will be right heart failure associated with ascites. The JVP rises paradoxically with inspiration. Pulsus paradoxus. Hypotension.

Biliary tract disease

Deep jaundice. There may be a palpable mass associated with the primary malignancy. The gall bladder may be palpable with carcinoma of the head of the pancreas (Courvoisier's law). With primary biliary cirrhosis there will be clubbing, xanthomata, arthralgia, hirsutism, portal hypertension and skin pigmentation.

Storage disease

With haemochromatosis there will be signs of portal hypertension and skin pigmentation.

Malignancy

Jaundice and ascites may be present. There may be an abdominal mass representing the primary malignancy. With myeloproliferative disorders, in addition to hepatomegaly, there will be splenomegaly and lymphadenopathy.

GENERAL INVESTIGATIONS

■ FBC, ESR
   Hb ↓ malignancy, myeloproliferative disorders. WCC ↑ infection, leukaemia. Platelets ↓ leukaemia. ESR ↑ infection and malignancy.

■ U&Es
   Creatinine. Often deranged in liver failure. Renal failure may occur with amyloidosis.

- **LFTs**
  Liver enzymes deranged in hepatitis. Alkaline phosphatase grossly raised in obstruction. The pattern varies according to the cause of hepatomegaly.

- **Clotting screen**
  PT ↑ absence of clotting factors.

- **Hepatitis serology**
  Raised according to cause.

SPECIFIC INVESTIGATIONS

- **Serum iron, TIBC and serum ferritin**
  Abnormal in haemochromatosis.

- **Blood, urine, CSF culture**
  Positive in leptospirosis.

- **Antibody screen**
  Antimicrosomal antibodies raised in primary biliary cirrhosis.

- **Bone marrow aspiration**
  Myelofibrosis. Leukaemia.

- **US**
  Cirrhosis. Secondaries. Amoebic abscess. Hydatid cyst. Riedel's lobe.

- **CT**
  Pancreatic lesions. Cirrhosis. Liver cysts.

- **MRCP**
  Ductal abnormalities, e.g. stricture, stone.

- **Liver biopsy**
  Establish cause, e.g. malignancy, amyloid.

- **The liver edge is normally palpable during infancy until about the end of the third year. It is also palpable in thin adults.**

- **A normal liver can appear enlarged if displaced downwards by lung disease, e.g. COPD.**

- **Remember Riedel's lobe. It can be mistaken for pathological enlargement of the liver. It is a normal anatomical variation. Its presence should be confirmed by ultrasound scan.**

HICCUPS

Hiccups (hiccoughs) are the characteristic sounds produced by the involuntary contractions of the diaphragm terminated by sudden closure of the glottis. In the majority, it is a self-limiting condition. The most common cause of hiccups is thought to be gastric distension after rapid ingestion of food, fluid or air. The causes of intractable hiccups are listed below.

CAUSES

PHRENIC NERVE IRRITATION

- Oesophageal carcinoma
- Lung tumour
- Thoracic surgery

DIAPHRAGMATIC IRRITATION

- Lower lobe pneumonia
- Empyema
- Subphrenic abscess
- Diaphragmatic hernia
- Gastric distension

CNS CONDITIONS

- Meningitis
- Tumours
- Intracranial haemorrhage
- Brainstem stroke
- Encephalitis

OTHERS

- Uraemic
- Hysterical
- Toxic

HISTORY

The causes of hiccups predominantly originate in the respiratory, abdominal and nervous systems, therefore the history is structured similarly.

Respiratory history

The presence of cough with purulent sputum production implies respiratory tract infection. However, patients with pneumonia tend to be more unwell and may complain of rigors with high temperatures. Following pneumonia or thoracic surgery, chronic pyrexia and pleuritic chest pains with failure of resolution of symptoms of the original infection may herald the onset of an empyema. Hiccups may (rarely) complicate routine thoracic surgery. When a chronic cough is associated with haemoptysis and weight loss in a smoker, bronchial tumour is the most likely diagnosis.

Abdominal history

Symptoms of rapid progressive painless dysphagia (p. 105) may be due to oesophageal carcinoma. At birth, a diaphragmatic hernia may present with respiratory distress; adults with diaphragmatic hernias may, however, be completely asymptomatic, the hernia being detected incidentally on a chest X-ray. Unremitting pyrexia and malaise in patients after abdominal surgery, or following localised inflammatory conditions such as appendicitis and cholecystitis, may have developed an intra-abdominal abscess. The subphrenic region is the most common site of a collection of pus. This is associated with intractable hiccups and pain referred to the shoulder, scapula or neck. A pleural effusion may be an accompanying feature.

Neurological history

Pyrexia, headache, photophobia and neck stiffness are associated with meningitis. Patients with encephalitis tend to present with confusion, alterations in consciousness and seizures. The brainstem is a very anatomically complex structure, therefore symptoms of infarction or tumour may be very variable, depending on distribution of involvement of the lower cranial nerves. The presenting features may be diplopia, difficulty swallowing, dysarthria and facial sensory loss. Cortical lesions arising from infarction or haemorrhage may present with aphasia, visual field defects and hemiplegia. The principal differentiating feature between infarction and tumour is the speed of onset; in general, stroke presents suddenly and tumours progressively.

Others

Amelioration of hiccups by sleep, bizarre accompanying symptoms and inconsistencies in the history are suggestive of hysterical hiccups. Uraemia may be responsible for hiccups.

EXAMINATION

A substantial number of causes of intractable hiccups are associated with pyrexia. High swinging fevers are suggestive of collections of pus, such as empyema and subphrenic abscesses.

An abdominal examination should be performed. Areas of tenderness may suggest appendicitis or cholecystitis as a predisposing cause for a subphrenic abscess. More specifically, an abdominal abscess may point to the skin surface, or present with tenderness over the lower chest wall.

Respiratory examination may reveal tracheal deviation with a large empyema or pleural effusion from carcinoma. Areas of percussion dullness correspond to consolidation, effusion and empyema. A large diaphragmatic hernia may elevate the diaphragm sufficiently to produce clinical signs suggestive of an effusion. Localised coarse crepitations may be auscultated, corresponding to areas of consolidation by pneumonia. Vocal resonance is increased with consolidation but attenuated with effusion and empyema.

A neurological examination is performed to identify the presence of and define the anatomical territory of any deficit. Specialised tests should be performed for meningitis. This will include Kernig's sign (pain on extension of the knee from a flexed hip and knee position) and Brudzinski's sign (flexion of the neck produces flexion of the hip and knee).

GENERAL INVESTIGATIONS

In the absence of features in the history to guide specific investigations, the following general investigations should be performed.

- **FBC**
  WCC ↑ with infection, malignancy.
- **ESR**
  ↑ infection, malignancy.
- **U&Es**
  ↑ urea, ↑ creatinine with renal failure.
- **CXR**
  Peripheral shadow or cavitation, hilar mass, collapse of a lobe may suggest carcinoma. Consolidation is seen with pneumonia. Fluid with a meniscus may be due to empyema, effusion from malignancy, or as a result of a subphrenic abscess. Elevation of a hemidiaphragm may be due to phrenic nerve palsy from carcinomatous infiltration or apparent elevation due to the presence of a diaphragmatic hernia.

SPECIFIC INVESTIGATIONS

- **Upper GI endoscopy and biopsy**
  Oesophageal carcinoma.
- **Bronchoscopy and mediastinoscopy**
  Biopsy for bronchial carcinoma.
- **CT thorax**
  Biopsy for bronchial carcinoma, definition and identification of loculations with empyema.
- **US abdomen**
  Subphrenic abscess; aspiration and drainage may also be performed.

- **CT/MRI head**
  Infarction and tumour may be appreciated as low-density areas. Mass effects may be produced by tumour or bleeding causing midline shifts. Intracranial bleeding may be identified as a high-density area. Cortical swelling may be seen with encephalitis. Raised intracranial pressure can be identified and is a contraindication to lumbar puncture.

- **EEG**
  Encephalitis – periodic complex formation and slowing of the background rhythm.

- **Lumbar puncture**
  Meningitis. Encephalitis – high lymphocyte count as the majority are due to viral aetiology.

- **If hiccups are persistent, chronic, interfere with work, eating or sleep, or are associated with weight loss, full investigation is required to exclude a serious underlying disorder.**

HIRSUTISM

Hirsutism is the presence of male-pattern hair growth in women.
This is not synonymous with virilism, which, in addition to hirsutism,
is associated with the development of male secondary sexual
characteristics in women. Hypertrichosis refers to the excessive
growth of hair and may occur in either sex.

CAUSES

PHYSIOLOGICAL

- Senility
- Familial (varies with ethnicity)

PATHOLOGICAL

DRUGS

- Ciclosporin
- Antiepileptic drugs, e.g. phenytoin
- Corticosteroids
- Progestogens
- Testosterone (including anabolic steroids)
- Minoxidil

PITUITARY

- Prolactinoma
- Cushing's disease
- Acromegaly

OVARIAN

- Polycystic ovarian syndrome
- Menopause
- Androgen-producing ovarian tumour

ADRENAL

- Cushing's syndrome
- Androgen-producing adrenal tumours
- Congenital adrenal hyperplasia

OTHER

- Anorexia nervosa

HISTORY

General

The onset and duration of hirsutism are useful features in the histor
to help determine the aetiology. Onset in childhood is suggestive of

congenital adrenal hyperplasia, whereas sudden onset of hirsutism in adult females raises concerns of androgen-producing tumours of the ovaries or adrenal glands. Enquiries should be undertaken as to whether any relatives have similar problems as the aetiology may be familial. However, beware of family cancer syndromes, such as BRCA gene mutation, which is associated with familial ovarian carcinoma. Excessive androgens may result in virilisation, producing symptoms such as acne and deepening of the voice.

Menstrual history

A detailed history regarding the onset, periodicity and regularity of the menstrual cycle should be taken, as amenorrhoea is a feature of polycystic ovarian syndrome, congenital adrenal hyperplasia and prolactinomas. In addition, galactorrhoea may also be an accompanying feature of prolactinomas.

Drug history

A drug history may identify the use of progestogen-containing hormone replacement therapy or oral contraceptive pills. Hirsutism may also result as a side-effect of anabolic steroid use by body builders; phenytoin for epilepsy; minoxidil for hypertension; and ciclosporin as an immunosuppressive agent in organ transplantation.

Associated symptoms

Weight gain may result from Cushing's syndrome, but is also a common complaint with polycystic ovarian syndrome. Symptoms such as headaches, vomiting and visual field loss are suggestive of a pituitary adenoma, which can result in acromegaly, Cushing's disease or hyperprolactinaemia (prolactinoma). Additional symptoms that may accompany Cushing's syndrome are easy bruising of the skin, abdominal striae and proximal muscle weakness. Patients with acromegaly may also complain of muscle weakness, joint pains, enlarging features of the face, jaw, hands and feet, with corresponding increases in hat, glove and shoe sizes. Paraesthesia may also result as a consequence of entrapment neuropathies. Infertility may result from hyperprolactinaemia and polycystic ovarian syndrome.

EXAMINATION

An assessment should be made regarding the pattern of hair distribution. With a degree of normal variation, the distribution of hair growth with hirsutism is on the face, chin, chest and extremities. The pubic hair may adopt a male pattern, and male type frontal balding can also be present. Careful inspection for virilism may identify increased shoulder-girdle muscle mass and enlargement of the clitoris. Truncal obesity is a feature of Cushing's syndrome, and generalised obesity occurs with polycystic ovarian syndrome. This may also be accompanied by acanthosis nigricans.

Inspection is then continued to identify co-existing endocrine disease. Features of acromegaly are thick greasy skin, prominent supraorbital ridging, broad nose, prognathism, macroglossia, poor jaw occlusion, wide interdental separation, enlarged hands and feet. Features of Cushing's syndrome are moon-like facies, truncal obesity, buffalo hump, skin bruising, striae and proximal muscle weakness. Hypertension, diabetes and visual field defects (bitemporal hemianopia) are associated with both Cushing's disease and acromegaly. In addition, visual field defects may also result from a prolactinoma. Hypertension is also associated with congenital adrenal hyperplasia.

Following this, an abdominal and pelvic examination should be performed to exclude a mass, which may be suggestive of a large adrenal or ovarian tumour.

GENERAL INVESTIGATIONS

- **Urine dipstick**
  The presence of glucose may be due to diabetes, which is a feature of Cushing's syndrome and acromegaly. In addition, polycystic ovarian disease is also associated with insulin resistance.

- **U&Es**
  ↓ potassium with congenital adrenal hyperplasia.

- **Serum glucose**
  Diabetes or insulin resistance with Cushing's syndrome, acromegaly and polycystic ovarian disease.

- **Serum testosterone and DHEA**
  ↑↑ suggests an excess of androgens from a neoplastic origin and warrants detailed investigation.

SPECIFIC INVESTIGATIONS

- **24-hour free urinary cortisol**
  ↑ with Cushing's syndrome.

- **Low-dose dexamethasone suppression test**
  Failure of suppression occurs with Cushing's syndrome.

- **Oral glucose tolerance test with serial growth hormone estimations**
  Failure of suppression or increasing growth hormone concentrations occur with acromegaly.

- **IGF-1**
  ↑ with acromegaly.

- **Plasma prolactin**
  ↑ with prolactinomas.

- **Plasma 17-hydroxyprogesterone**
  ↑ with congenital adrenal hyperplasia.

- **CA 125**
  ↑ with ovarian carcinoma.

- **US abdomen and pelvis**
  Polycystic ovaries, ovarian carcinoma.

- **CT abdomen and pelvis**
  Adrenal carcinoma, ovarian carcinoma.

- **CT/MRI head**
  Pituitary tumour.

- **Rapid onset or severe hirsutism may give a clue to underlying serious pathology, e.g. androgen-producing tumours of the ovaries or adrenal glands.**

- **Pituitary tumours may present with hirsutism and associated visual field defects.**

HYPERTENSION

Hypertension is the elevation of blood pressure. An individual is classified as hypertensive when there is a sustained rise in blood pressure to more than 140/90 mmHg on three or more readings, each at least a week apart. Most patients have essential hypertension and an underlying cause is identified in less than 10%.

CAUSES

RENAL

- Renal parenchymal diseases, e.g. glomerulonephritis
- Diabetic nephropathy
- Renal artery stenosis
- Chronic pyelonephritis
- Polycystic kidney disease
- Connective tissue disease (especially systemic sclerosis)

ENDOCRINE

- Adrenal
  - Cushing's syndrome
  - Conn's syndrome
  - Phaeochromocytoma
- Acromegaly

DRUGS

- Oestrogen-containing oral contraceptives
- Glucocorticoids – corticosteroids
- Monoamine oxidase inhibitors and tyramine
- Mineralocorticoids – liquorice
- Sympathetomimetics – nebulised salbutamol

CARDIOVASCULAR

- Coarctation of the aorta

OTHER

- Pregnancy (pre-eclampsia and eclampsia)

HISTORY

Patients with uncomplicated essential hypertension are asymptomatic and are identified only in the course of routine physical examination; however, patients with secondary hypertensio may complain of symptoms from the underlying disorder.

Patients with chronic pyelonephritis may have experienced recurrent urinary tract infections, with loin pain, pyrexia and rigors, or have a history of childhood urinary tract infections or prolonged enuresis. Hypertension can also complicate glomerular disease; in particular it is associated with acute nephritic syndrome. Patients with nephritic syndrome may have experienced an acute illness with fatigue, malaise, haematuria, oliguria and oedema.

With Conn's syndrome, patients may complain of muscle weakness and fatigue due to hypokalaemia and polyuria from impaired urine-concentrating ability. Paroxysms of headache, sweating, palpitations with flushing may be experienced by patients with phaeochromocytoma. Classically these patients have attacks of hypertension; however, in the majority the hypertension is sustained.

Weight gain, hair growth, acne, abdominal striae, muscle weakness, back pain and depression may be some of the symptoms experienced by patients with Cushing's syndrome. With acromegaly, patients may complain of headaches, galactorrhoea, deepening of the voice, muscle weakness and joint pains. Hats and rings may no longer fit due to increasing size of the cranium and hands.

A complete drug history will identify offending drugs that may precipitate hypertension.

EXAMINATION

Inspection

On inspection, patients with acromegaly may have thick greasy skin, large hands, feet and tongue. Prominent supraorbital ridging with a large nose and protruding jaw accompanied by interdental separation may be noted on close inspection of the face and teeth. Confrontational testing of the visual fields may reveal bitemporal hemianopia, which may also be present with Cushing's syndrome owing to compression of the optic chiasma by a pituitary adenoma. Additional features of Cushing's disease include truncal obesity, acne, moon-like facies, bruising, striae, kyphosis and proximal muscle weakness.

Palpation and auscultation

In coarctation of the aorta, radiofemoral delay may be appreciated with simultaneous palpation of the radial and femoral arteries; bruits may be auscultated across collateral blood vessels along the axilla, chest wall and scapula. A systolic bruit may also be auscultated over the fourth left posterior intercostal space. Wide discrepancy of measured blood pressure may exist between the arm and leg.

Palpation of the abdomen may reveal bilateral ballotable masses due to enlarged polycystic kidneys, and bruits may be auscultated over stenosed renal arteries.

SECTION A

GENERAL INVESTIGATIONS

- **Urinalysis**
  Dipstick may indicate the presence of blood and protein. Urine microscopy is necessary to confirm the presence of red blood cells and also casts.

- **U&Es**
  Levels of serum potassium may be reduced with Conn's syndrome due to hyperaldosteronism. High levels of creatinine and urea are found with renal failure.

- **Blood glucose**
  Atherosclerosis, renal vascular disease and nephropathy may be associated with diabetes. All of these may contribute to hypertension. Moreover conditions such as Cushing's syndrome, acromegaly and phaeochromocytoma are associated with hyperglycaemia.

- **Serum lipids**
  Serum lipid estimation is used to screen for risk factors for atherosclerosis, and therapy may be initiated for the prevention of cerebrovascular and ischaemic heart disease.

- **ECG**
  A 12-lead ECG is recommended for all patients to provide a baseline and screen for left ventricular hypertrophy which may result as a complication of hypertension.

SPECIFIC INVESTIGATIONS

- **Autoantibodies**
  Anti-GBM and ANCA may be positive with glomerulonephritis. ANA for connective tissue diseases.

- **Plasma catecholamines**
  Elevated in phaeochromocytoma.

- **Urinary catecholamines, metanephrines and vanillylmandelic acid**
  Elevated in phaeochromocytoma.

- **24-hour urinary free cortisol**
  Excess cortisol in Cushing's syndrome.

- **Low-dose dexamethasone suppression test**
  Failure of suppression of cortisol occurs in Cushing's syndrome.

- **Oral glucose tolerance test**
  Failure of suppression of serum growth hormone occurs in acromegaly.

- **Plasma renin and aldosterone**
  Hypersecretion of aldosterone in the presence of low plasma renin levels confirms autonomous secretion in Conn's syndrome.

- **Pregnancy test**
  Hypertension occurring with pre-eclampsia and eclampsia.

- **US abdomen**
  Polycystic kidneys. Duplex Doppler can screen for renal artery stenosis.

- **Renal angiography**
  Renal artery stenosis.

- **Renal biopsy**
  Renal causes of hypertension.

- **MRA**
  This is increasingly useful in the diagnosis of renal artery stenosis and avoids the need for potentially nephrotoxic radiocontrast administration.

- **Cardiac catheterisation**
  Coarctation of the aorta.

- **Severe hypertension must be investigated and treated urgently due to the poor prognosis. Improvement in cardiovascular outcomes has been clearly shown when hypertension is adequately controlled.**

IMPOTENCE

Impotence is failure in the adult male to sustain an adequate erection for vaginal penetration. Impotence leads to psychological problems, often with marital breakdown. Psychological causes of impotence are common but the most common organic disease is diabetes mellitus. The term 'loss of libido' should be reserved for sexual dysfunction relating from a loss of sexual desire or sexual drive.

CAUSES

VASCULAR

- Diabetic vascular disease
- Aortoiliac disease (Leriche's syndrome)

NEUROLOGICAL

- Spinal lesions
- Neuropathies, e.g. diabetes
- Spina bifida
- Pelvic surgery (damage to nervi erigentes)

ENDOCRINE

- Diabetes mellitus
- Hypogonadism
- Hypothyroidism
- Cushing's syndrome
- Addison's disease

DRUGS

- Antihypertensives
- Antidepressants
- Alcohol
- Oestrogens
- Cocaine

LOCAL PAINFUL CONDITIONS

- Phimosis
- Peyronie's disease
- Short frenulum

SYSTEMIC DISEASE

- Malignancy
- Cirrhosis
- Chronic renal failure

PSYCHOGENIC

● Depression

OTHER

● Ageing

HISTORY

Is there a clear history of stress to account for the onset of impotence? Does the patient experience erections at any time, especially during the night? History of peripheral vascular disease, especially buttock claudication (Leriche's syndrome). History of neurological disease. Take a full drug history, including any recreational drugs. Check for a history of diabetes, hypothyroidism, Addison's disease or Cushing's disease. Pelvic surgery, e.g. abdominoperineal resection of the rectum with damage to the nervi erigentes. Check for any local, painful conditions of the penis. History of malignant disease. History of chronic renal failure: nausea, lethargy, nocturia, peripheral oedema, pulmonary oedema, dyspnoea, vomiting, hiccups, convulsions.

EXAMINATION

Vascular

Check all the pulses in the lower limb. Listen for bruits in the abdomen and pelvis.

Neurological

Carry out a full neurological examination.

Endocrine

There will usually be a clear history of diabetes. Complications may be apparent. Check for peripheral neuropathy. Check for hypothyroidism – weight gain, dislike of cold weather, hoarse voice, lethargy, constipation. Check for Cushing's syndrome – thin skin, cushingoid facies, abdominal striae, obesity, buffalo hump, hypertension. Check for Addison's disease – weakness, weight loss, pigmentation of palmar creases and buccal mucosa, hypotension. Examine the testes for hypogonadism. Check for development of male secondary sexual characteristics.

Local painful conditions

Examine the penis for phimosis, Peyronie's disease or short frenulum.

Systemic disease

Malignant disease may be obvious. Check for chronic renal failure: pallor of skin, peripheral oedema, pericarditis, pleural effusions, hypertension. Check for cirrhosis, liver palms, spider naevi, ascites, leuconychia, flapping tremor, testicular atrophy, Dupuytren's contracture.

GENERAL INVESTIGATIONS

History and examination suggests the diagnosis in most cases.

- **FBC, ESR**
  Hb ↓ anaemia, e.g. chronic renal failure and malignancy.
  ESR ↑ malignancy.

- **U&Es**
  Creatinine raised in chronic renal failure.

- **LFTs**
  Abnormal in cirrhosis.

- **Blood glucose**
  Diabetes mellitus.

- **TFTs**
  ↑ TSH ↓ T_4 in hypothyroidism.

- **Doppler studies**
  Peripheral vascular disease. Penile–brachial pressure index <0.6 suggests a vascular cause.

SPECIFIC INVESTIGATIONS

- **Nocturnal penile tumescence study**
  Erection versus no erection.

- **Intracorporeal injection of papaverine**
  If no abnormality of arterial inflow, this should cause an erection. If there is excessive venous leakage the penis remains flaccid.

- **MRI or CT head**
  Pituitary abnormality.

- **Arteriography**
  May show vascular lesion, especially isolated narrowings of the internal iliac arteries.

- **Serum prolactin**
  Hypoprolactinaemia.

- **Serum testosterone**
  Low in hypogonadism.

- **Serum FSH and LH**
  Low in pituitary dysfunction.

- **ACTH stimulation test**
  Addison's disease.

- **Urinary cortisol assay**
  Cushing's syndrome.

- **Plasma cortisol**
  Cushing's syndrome.

- Loss of libido may be an early manifestation of significant depressive illness. Thorough investigation for possible organic or psychogenic disease is necessary.

INTESTINAL OBSTRUCTION

Mechanical obstruction of the bowel may be simple (one-point obstruction) or closed loop (obstruction at two points enclosing a segment of bowel). If the bowel is viable the obstruction is termed non-strangulating. If the arterial blood supply is compromised, strangulating obstruction occurs with subsequent infarction of the bowel. Intestinal obstruction is a common surgical emergency.

CAUSES

SMALL BOWEL

IN THE LUMEN
- Gallstone ileus
- Food bolus (after pylorus-destroying or bypass surgery)

IN THE WALL
- Crohn's disease
- Atresia
- TB
  - (common in areas of the world where TB is endemic)
- Tumour, e.g. lymphoma, carcinoma

OUTSIDE THE WALL
- Hernia
- Adhesions
- Volvulus
- Intussusception

LARGE BOWEL

IN THE LUMEN
- Faeces

IN THE WALL
- Carcinoma
- Diverticular disease
- Crohn's disease
- Hirschsprung's disease

OUTSIDE THE WALL
- Volvulus
- Hernia
- Adhesions

ADYNAMIC OBSTRUCTION (PARALYTIC ILEUS)

- Peritonitis

- Post-operative
- Hypokalaemia
- Spinal and pelvic fractures
- Retroperitoneal haemorrhage
- Retroperitoneal malignancy
- Drugs, e.g. ganglion blockers, anticholinergics
- Immobilisation

HISTORY

Small bowel

Central abdominal colicky pain. Vomiting – food, bile, faeculent, depending upon the level of obstruction. Distension – degree depends on level of obstruction. There may be very little distension with high small bowel obstruction. It may be gross with low small bowel obstruction. Constipation. There may be a history of abdominal surgery to suggest adhesive obstruction. The patient may be aware of a hernia.

Large bowel

Central (right colon to two-thirds of the way along the transverse colon) or lower abdominal colicky pain (remainder of the colon). Constipation. Vomiting is a late feature with large bowel obstruction. Abdominal distension. There may be a previous history of change in bowel habit and bleeding PR to suggest carcinoma. A long history of constipation (years) and abdominal distension suggest Hirschsprung's disease. Development of a constant severe pain suggests infarction.

Adynamic obstruction

Carefully check the drug history. Patients on anticoagulants may have retroperitoneal haemorrhage. Precipitating cause may be obvious, e.g. recent surgery or spinal fracture. The abdominal distension may be painless but uncomfortable. Vomiting, constipation. The elderly immobilised in bed are especially vulnerable.

EXAMINATION

Small bowel

Observe for scars. Exclude obstructed incisional hernia. Check hernial orifices. It is easy to miss a small femoral hernia in an obese patient. Distended tympanitic abdomen usually non-tender. High-pitched tinkling obstructed bowel sounds. Pyrexia, tachycardia and localised tenderness suggest impending infarction. A palpable mass in the right iliac fossa may suggest Crohn's disease or caecal carcinoma (obstructing the ileocaecal valve and causing small bowel obstruction). Carry out a digital rectal examination.

SECTION A

Large bowel

Distended tympanitic abdomen, which may be very tense. Obstructed bowel sounds. Rectum may be empty on examination PR unless obstruction is due to faecal impaction. A mass may be palpable to suggest an obstructing carcinoma. A palpable, tense, tender caecum suggests closed loop obstruction with a competent ileocaecal valve. Caecal perforation may be imminent.

Adynamic obstruction

Abdominal distension. Tense tympanitic abdomen. Absent bowel sounds. Evidence of previous surgery, trauma, retroperitoneal haemorrhage and peritonitis, fractures.

GENERAL INVESTIGATIONS

- ■ **Hb, FBC**
  Hb ↓ malignancy. WCC ↑ infection, infarcted bowel.

- ■ **U&Es and creatinine**
  Dehydration. Hypokalaemia leading to paralytic ileus.

- ■ **Clotting screen**
  May be abnormal with retroperitoneal haemorrhage, especially if patient on anticoagulants.

- ■ **AXR**
  Distended loops of bowel in central abdomen. Proximal small bowel shows lines closely together crossing completely the lumen of the bowel (valvulae conniventes). These get progressively further apart until there are none seen in the terminal ileum. Gas in the biliary tree (gallstone ileus). Large bowel obstruction – distended bowel with air–fluid levels at the periphery of the abdomen. Sigmoid volvulus – distended loop of bowel, the shape of a 'coffee bean', arising out of the pelvis on the left side.

- ■ **Sigmoidoscopy**
  Tumour at rectosigmoid. Sigmoid volvulus may be decompressed by careful insertion of sigmoidoscope. Biopsy – carcinoma, absence of ganglion cells in Hirschsprung's disease.

SPECIFIC INVESTIGATIONS

- ■ **Barium enema**
  Limited barium enema may show 'apple core' lesion of carcinoma. 'Bird's beak' sign of sigmoid volvulus. Intussusception.

- ■ **Small bowel enema**
  Crohn's disease. TB of the terminal ileum. Small bowel carcinoma.

■ CT
Retroperitoneal haemorrhage. Retroperitoneal tumour.

- Tachycardia, pyrexia, localised tenderness and neutrophil leucocytosis are signs of impending infarction. Urgent surgical exploration is required.
- In large bowel obstruction a tense, tender palpable caecum is a sign of closed loop obstruction with a risk of impending caecal perforation. Urgent laparotomy is required.
- A radiological diameter of the caecum of over 10 cm is a sign of imminent rupture of the caecum. Urgent laparotomy is required.
- It can be difficult to distinguish between pseudo-obstruction (ileus or adynamic obstruction) and large bowel obstruction. Gaseous distension all the way along the large bowel, including rectum, suggests pseudo-obstruction. A sharp 'cut off' of the gas shadow in the colon suggests obstruction, e.g. in the LIF with recto-sigmoid carcinoma.

JAUNDICE

Jaundice is yellow discoloration of the tissues, noticed especially in the skin and sclera, due to accumulation of bilirubin. For jaundice to be clinically apparent, the circulating bilirubin levels should be in excess of 35 μmol/L. Jaundice may be prehepatic (due to haemolysis), hepatic (due to intrinsic liver disease) or cholestatic (due to either intrahepatic cholestasis or post-hepatic biliary tract obstruction).

CAUSES

PREHEPATIC (UNCONJUGATED HYPERBILIRUBINAEMIA)

CONGENITAL DEFECTS
- Gilbert's disease
- Crigler–Najjar syndrome

HAEMOLYSIS
Congenital red cell defects
- Hereditary spherocytosis (congenital acholuric jaundice)
- Sickle cell disease
- G6PD deficiency
- Thalassaemia

Acquired
- Malaria
  - (common in parts of the world where malaria is endemic)
- Incompatible blood transfusion
- Autoimmune
- Haemolytic disease of the newborn
- Absorbing large haematoma
- Hypersplenism

HEPATIC

ACUTE HEPATOCELLULAR DISEASE
- Viral hepatitis
  - Hepatitis A, B, C
  - EBV
  - CMV
- Drugs, e.g. paracetamol, halothane
- Other infections
  - Leptospirosis
- Toxins, e.g. carbon tetrachloride
- Autoimmune

Chronic hepatocellular disease

- Chronic viral hepatitis
- Chronic autoimmune hepatitis
- End-stage liver disease
  - Alcohol
  - Cirrhosis
  - Haemochromatosis
  - Wilson's disease

CHOLESTATIC

INTRAHEPATIC

- Drugs, e.g. chlorpromazine
- TPN
- Viral hepatitis
- Primary biliary cirrhosis
- Pregnancy

EXTRAHEPATIC (OBSTRUCTIVE)

In the lumen

- Gallstones
- Infestation
  - Clonorchiasis (liver fluke)
  - Schistosomiasis

In the wall

- Stricture, e.g. inflammatory, post-operative
- Cholangitis
- Congenital biliary atresia
- Cholangiocarcinoma
- Sclerosing cholangitis
- Choledochal cyst

Outside the wall

- Carcinoma of the head of the pancreas
- Carcinoma of the ampulla of Vater
- Malignant nodes in the porta hepatis
- Chronic pancreatitis
- Mirizzi syndrome

HISTORY

General

Fever, malaise, weight loss, dark urine, pale stools, itching.

Newborn

Biliary atresia presents as deepening jaundice within 2–3 days of birth. Liver failure develops over 3–6 months. Physiological jaundice is common and is due to immaturity of liver function. It usually settles within the first week of life.

Prehepatic

Ask about family history, racial origin, drugs, haematuria, history of anaemia. Gilbert's disease is inherited as an autosomal dominant. There is a failure of uptake of unconjugated bilirubin by the hepatocyte. Crigler–Najjar syndrome is a failure of conjugation within the hepatocyte.

Hepatocellular

Occupation. Contact with jaundice. Travel. Alcohol. Sexual activity. Drugs (tablets, injections, anaesthetic agents, drug abuse). Exposure to industrial solvents. Previous episodes of jaundice. Infection. Influenza-like symptoms. Rashes. Joint pains. Blood transfusions.

Cholestatic

Drugs, e.g. chlorpromazine. Travel abroad. Severe upper abdominal pain preceding jaundice (biliary colic followed by impaction of stone in common bile duct). Insidious onset of painless jaundice (malignancy). Dark urine, pale stools, itching.

EXAMINATION

Prehepatic (haemolytic)

Often the jaundice is not intense, with only a mild lemon tinge. Anaemia. Splenomegaly.

Hepatic

Tender liver in hepatitis. Signs of liver failure: spider naevi, palmar erythema, leuconychia, clubbing, gynaecomastia, testicular atrophy, ascites, peripheral oedema, bruising, Dupuytren's contracture, caput medusae, liver flap. Haematemesis may have occurred from bleeding oesophageal varices.

Cholestatic

Hepatomegaly – usually smooth liver with 'sharp' edge. Palpable gall bladder (Courvoisier's law – in the presence of obstructive jaundice if the gall bladder is palpable, the cause is unlikely to be due to gallstones). Epigastric mass, e.g. carcinoma of the pancreas. Other abdominal masses, e.g. carcinoma of the stomach and carcinoma of the colon with secondary deposits in the porta hepatis. Recent surgical scars. Scratch marks on abdomen from itching.

GENERAL INVESTIGATIONS

■ **FBC, ESR, blood film**
Hb ↓ malignancy, haemolysis. WCC ↑ infection, e.g. hepatitis, cholangitis. ESR ↑ infection, malignancy. Blood film – spherocytosis.

■ **Reticulocyte count**
Haemolysis.

■ **U&Es**
Deranged renal function with hepatorenal syndrome.

■ **LFTs**
See the Table below.

Urine and blood biochemistry in jaundice			
Biochemical parameter	**Prehepatic**	**Hepatic**	**Cholestatic**
Blood			
Bilirubin			
Unconjugated	↑	N/↑	N
Conjugated	N	N/↑	↑
Alkaline phosphatase	N	N/↑	↑↑
Transaminases	N	↑	N/↑
Urine			
Bilirubin	0	↑	↑
Urobilinogen	N/↑	↑	↓↓/0

N, normal; 0, no bilirubin present in urine.

■ **Clotting screen**
PT ↑.

■ **Viral antibodies**
Hepatitis A, hepatitis B, hepatitis C, CMV, EBV.

■ **US**
Gallstones. Dilated biliary tree. Level of obstruction (may not show cause of obstruction). Hepatic secondaries. Cirrhosis.

■ **ERCP**
Periampullary carcinoma. Stones in common bile duct. Tumour of common bile duct. Stricture of common bile duct. Biopsy. Brush cytology. Stenting.

■ **PTC**
Undertaken if ERCP fails.

- **MRCP**
  Bile duct anomalies. Stones.

- **CT**
  Carcinoma of the head of the pancreas – assess spread and local resectability. Liver secondaries.

- **Liver biopsy**
  Hepatocellular disease. Carcinoma.

SPECIFIC INVESTIGATIONS

- **Serum copper**
  Reduced in Wilson's disease.

- **Serum ceruloplasmin**
  Reduced in Wilson's disease.

- **Serum α_1-antitrypsin**
  α_1-Antitrypsin deficiency. Serum iron and TIBC.
  Iron raised in haemochromatosis. TIBC saturation >70%.

- **Leptospirosis complement fixation test**
  Leptospirosis.

- **Blood culture**
  Septicaemia. Leptospirosis.

- **Lumbar puncture**
  Leptospirosis.

- Painless progressive jaundice suggests carcinoma of the pancreas, especially in the presence of a palpable gall bladder (Courvoisier's law).

- Ask about foreign travel contact, drug abuse contact and sexual history in patients with sudden onset of jaundice and fever.

JAW PAIN AND SWELLINGS

Pain and/or swelling of the jaw results most commonly from dental conditions. In the upper jaw, pain may also result from infection of the paranasal sinuses. The latter condition is considered under facial swellings (p. 127).

CAUSES

TRAUMATIC

INFECTIVE

- Dental abscess
- Acute osteomyelitis
- Actinomycosis

TEMPOROMANDIBULAR JOINT

- Temporomandibular joint pain dysfunction syndrome
- Rheumatoid arthritis
- Osteoarthritis
- Dislocation

CYSTIC

- Dental cysts
- Dentigerous cysts

NEOPLASTIC

BENIGN
- Giant cell granuloma

LOCALLY INVASIVE
- Ameloblastoma

MALIGNANT
- Osteogenic sarcoma
- Burkitt's lymphoma
  - endemic in equatorial Africa
- Secondary deposits

OTHER

- Referred pain (e.g. myocardial ischaemia)
- Post-herpetic neuralgia

HISTORY

Traumatic

History of trauma, e.g. fights, road traffic accidents. Fracture of the mandible is the most common.

Infective

Dental abscess presents with a dull ache in the jaw, becoming throbbing and severe. There is often accompanying malaise and loss of appetite. Previous history of dental caries. Acute osteomyelitis of the mandible is rare. It may follow dental infection or tooth extraction. There may be a history of fractures, irradiation, leukaemia, diabetes, malnutrition, alcoholism or immunosuppression. There is a severe, throbbing deep-seated pain. The patient has difficulty opening the mouth and swallowing due to muscle oedema. Actinomycosis presents with swelling of the jaw with persistent low-grade infection.

Temporomandibular joint

Temporomandibular joint pain dysfunction syndrome results from grinding and clenching the teeth. The patient may have had a stress-related illness. Pain arises in the region of the temporomandibular joint or ear, which may be associated with a clicking noise and is aggravated by wide opening of the mouth, as with yawning and chewing. Rheumatoid arthritis of the temporomandibular joint is rare. Other signs and symptoms of rheumatoid arthritis are usually apparent. Osteoarthritis usually causes pain, swelling and limitation of jaw movement. Temporomandibular joint dislocation may be recurrent, habitual or isolated. The condyle is displaced forwards and upwards into the temporal fossa. The patient's mouth remains open and cannot be closed following yawning, tooth extraction or general anaesthesia. The condition may be unilateral or bilateral. The patient presents with an open mouth, which he or she cannot close, and pain due to muscle spasm.

Cystic

Cysts often present as asymptomatic lucencies on radiographs. Otherwise they present as painless swellings, which may reach a large size. If the cyst becomes infected the patient presents with pain, swelling and discharge. Occasionally pathological fractures occur. A dental cyst is attached to the root of a normally erupted but decayed tooth; the swelling grows slowly. Dentigerous cysts contain an unerupted tooth.

Neoplastic

The patient presents with a jaw swelling which grows steadily and often painlessly. Giant cell granuloma may erode through bone to produce a soft-tissue purplish swelling on the gum. Ameloblastomas usually occur around the age of 30–50 years and are symptomless until the swelling becomes obtrusive. Osteogenic sarcoma of the jaw is extremely rare. Initially it is painless but becomes painful as it grows. Teeth may be loosened. The patient may complain of paraesthesia due to involvement of the mental nerve. Coughing may be a symptom if lung metastases have occurred. Burkitt's tumour is associated with EBV. It is a malignant tumour of B lymphocytes. It is endemic in certain parts of Africa and New Guinea. It affects most commonly children below the age of 12 years. The child presents with a progressive painless swelling of the jaw. Secondary deposits in the jaw are uncommon but may arise from lung, breast, thyroid, prostate or kidney.

Others

With post-herpetic neuralgia there is usually a history of herpes zoster in the distribution of the trigeminal nerve. The pain tends to be distributed in a division of the trigeminal nerve. Pain may involve a large area of the face rather than just the region of the jaw. Referred pain to the jaw is common with angina. The patient usually complains of associated chest pain and radiation of the pain down the left arm.

EXAMINATION

Traumatic

Check for a normal bite. Bruising, swelling, crepitus, tenderness. Bloodstained saliva. Broken teeth. Step deformities in occlusion.

Infective

With dental abscesses there is reddening of the mucosa with a firm, hot, acutely tender, boggy swelling. The dental abscess may point on the outer side of the jaw. There may be associated dental caries and gingivitis. Cervical lymphadenopathy is usually present. With acute osteomyelitis there is usually difficulty in opening the mouth and swallowing due to muscle oedema. There is a tender, red, painful swelling overlying the mandible. In actinomycosis there may be multiple discharging sinuses, usually near the angle of the jaw, on which characteristic 'sulphur granules' may be seen discharging.

Temporomandibular joint

Diagnosis of temporomandibular joint dysfunction syndrome is usually made from the history. There is usually trismus and spasm around the joint. In rheumatoid arthritis there may be tenderness and swelling over the joint. In osteoarthritis there may be swelling over the joint and limitation of movement. In temporomandibular joint dislocation the condyles are palpable anterior to the articular eminence. The mouth is gagged open.

Cystic

Often the only abnormality on examination is a swelling in the bones. Sometimes the bone is so thin that it crackles when touched, like a broken eggshell. With dentigerous cysts the tooth remains unerupted and therefore a tooth will be missing when the teeth are counted.

Neoplastic

Often the only abnormality is a bony swelling, which grows steadily, initially without pain. With giant cell granuloma it may rarely erode through the bone to produce soft-tissue purplish swelling on the gum. Osteogenic sarcoma is initially painless but as it grows it may loosen the teeth. Check for loose teeth and paraesthesia in the distribution of the mental nerve. Examine the lung for metastases. With Burkitt's lymphoma there is progressive painless swelling. The eye may be displaced and the mouth partly occluded by the swelling. Secondary deposits often present as painful lesions within the bone. Check for a previous history of malignancy and check the lungs, breast, prostate, kidney and thyroid for the site of a primary.

Other

The diagnosis of post-herpetic neuralgia is usually made on the history, as is referred pain from myocardial ischaemia.

GENERAL INVESTIGATIONS

- **FBC, ESR**
  Hb ↓ malignancy. WCC ↑ infection, leukaemia, acute osteomyelitis.

- **LFTs**
  Alcoholism (acute osteomyelitis commoner).

- **Blood glucose**
  Diabetes (acute osteomyelitis).

- **Swab**
  C&S. Dental infection. Actinomycosis.

- **Temporomandibular joint X-rays**
  Dislocation. Osteoarthritis. Rheumatoid arthritis.

- **Skull X-rays with special views**
  Fractures, cysts, tumours.

- **CXR**
  Secondary deposits.

SPECIAL INVESTIGATIONS

■ **Blood cultures**
Osteomyelitis.

■ **ECG**
Myocardial ischaemia.

■ **EBV serology**
Burkitt's lymphoma.

■ **Biopsy**
Benign versus malignant lesions.

- Painless, progressive swelling of the jaw suggests tumour or dental cyst and requires urgent dental referral.

JOINT DISORDERS

Disorders of joints are common problems. They may be acute, as in
gout or rheumatic fever, or chronic, as in osteoarthritis. Some acute
disorders go on to become chronic, e.g. rheumatoid arthritis. The
first part of this section deals with causes of arthropathy in general;
the second part deals with disorders of specific joints. The list of
causes of arthropathies is legion and only the more common ones
will be mentioned.

CAUSES

CONGENITAL

- Achondroplasia (dwarfism)
- Ehlers–Danlos syndrome
- Marfan's syndrome
- Osteogenesis imperfecta

ACQUIRED

INFECTIVE

- Pyogenic arthritis
- Viral
- TB
  - (very common in the developing world and on the increase
    in developed countries)
- Rheumatic fever
  - (very common in developing countries)
- Endocarditis
- Brucellosis
- Typhoid
  - (very common in developing countries)

INFLAMMATORY

- Rheumatoid arthritis
- Polymyalgia rheumatica (predominantly in Caucasian
  women)
- Psoriatic arthropathy
- Henoch–Schönlein disease
- Reactive arthritis (Reiter's disease)
- Ankylosing spondylitis
- Connective tissue disease

DEGENERATIVE

- Osteoarthritis

ENTEROPATHIC
- Acute gastrointestinal infections
- Inflammatory bowel disease
- Gastrointestinal bypass surgery

ENDOCRINE
- Acromegaly

METABOLIC
- Gout
- Pseudogout
- Haemochromatosis

NEUROPATHIC
- Charcot's joints

HAEMATOLOGICAL
- Haemophilia
- Leukaemia
- Sickle cell disease

DRUGS
- Anticoagulants
- Steroids

NEOPLASTIC
- Hypertrophic pulmonary osteoarthropathy

OTHER
- Avascular necrosis of bone
- Sarcoidosis
- Behçet's disease (more common in certain Mediterranean countries)

HISTORY

Congenital

Premature osteoarthritis may occur in achondroplasia. In Ehlers–Danlos syndrome, a genetic disorder of connective tissue, patients display hypermobile joints and hyperextensible skin. They may present with joint subluxation, dislocation and swelling due to effusions. They may also present with the bleeding complications of Ehlers–Danlos syndrome. In Marfan's syndrome generalised joint laxity occurs with patients presenting with joint pain and swelling due to effusions. In osteogenesis imperfecta bony fracture is common.

Acquired
Infective

Septic arthritis usually presents as a monoarthritis with a red, swollen, painful, immobile joint. Spread has usually occurred by the haematogenous route but may occur from adjacent osteomyelitis. Organisms responsible include *Staphylococcus aureus streptococci*, gonococcus, *Brucella* and *Salmonella spp*. With TB the patient usually presents subacutely with swelling and stiffness of the joint. It is not as erythematous or warm as with acute septic arthritis. Patients on steroids or who are immunosuppressed are particularly at risk from infective arthritis. Viral arthritis may occur with rubella, mumps, hepatitis and certain enteroviruses. Rheumatic fever usually follows a streptococcal infection, e.g. scarlet fever or tonsillitis. There is a migratory polyarthritis together with carditis, erythematous skin lesions and subcutaneous nodules.

Inflammatory

Rheumatoid arthritis most often presents with swollen, painful, stiff hands and feet. Eventually characteristic hand deformities with swelling of the metacarpophalangeal joints, swan-neck and boutonnière deformities, and ulnar deviation occur. Large joints are also involved. The patient may complain of extra-articular manifestations, i.e. rheumatoid nodules, pulmonary disease and eye changes. Psoriatic arthropathy usually follows several years after the skin lesions. Reactive/Reiter's disease may present with a mono-or oligoarthritis. A history of gastrointestinal or genitourinary infection is present with associated urethritis and conjunctivitis. Ankylosing spondylitis most commonly affects young males and initially presents with morning stiffness in the lower spine. The sacroiliac joints are invariably involved. Eventually, bony ankylosis occurs with a fixed kyphotic spine. The patient may also complain of symptoms in peripheral large joints. Arthritis may occur in SLE. Other manifestations may be present, e.g. cutaneous, pulmonary or renal. Polymyalgia rheumatica occurs in elderly Caucasian women. There is aching and morning stiffness with a mild polyarthritis. Henoch–Schönlein purpura presents with a purpuric rash often over the buttocks and extensor surfaces. There may be associated nephritis and abdominal pain. Pain, swelling and stiffness in the joints, usually the ankles and knees, is transient.

Degenerative

Osteoarthritis usually occurs after the age of 50 years unless it is secondary to previous joint pathology. The patient complains of pain on movement, worse at the end of the day, together with stiffness and instability of joints. Bony swelling may be present.

Enteropathic

Check for a history of Crohn's disease or ulcerative colitis. There may also be a history of gastric bypass surgery. The spine or the peripheral joints may be affected.

Endocrine

Acromegaly will lead to arthralgia. The patient will usually complain of other symptoms, namely enlarged hands and feet (increase in shoe size) and deepening of the voice.

Metabolic

Gout usually presents with severe pain, redness and swelling in the first metatarsophalangeal joint; however, any joint may be affected. There may be a history of polycythaemia, leukaemia or medication with cytotoxic or immunosuppressive drugs. With haemochromatosis the diagnosis will usually be apparent when the patient presents. There will be cirrhosis, diabetes, cardiomyopathy and skin pigmentation.

Neuropathic

The patient usually complains of swollen joints, which are unstable but painless. There may be a history of diabetes, tabes dorsalis (syphilis), syringomyelia or leprosy.

Haematological

Bleeding into joints (haemarthrosis) occurs in haemophilia. The history will be apparent. Eventually crippling arthropathy occurs. Pain in bones and joints may occur in both childhood and adult leukaemia. In sickle cell disease, painful crises may occur in bones and joints. Avascular necrosis of bone may occur.

Drugs

Anticoagulants may cause bleeds into joints. Steroids may lead to septic arthritis or avascular necrosis of bone with subsequent secondary degenerative disease.

Neoplastic

Rarely a patient will present with direct infiltration of a joint with malignant disease. However, hypertrophic pulmonary osteoarthropathy is more common, occurring usually in association with bronchial carcinoma but it may occur in association with congenital heart disease.

Other

Avascular necrosis of bone may lead to secondary arthritis. The most common sites are the head of the femur, proximal tibia, proximal scaphoid, talus and lunate. Check for a history of steroid use. Avascular necrosis of the scaphoid will follow scaphoid fracture, and avascular necrosis of the head of the femur may follow fractures of the neck of the femur or slipped upper femoral epiphysis. Arthralgia may occur in sarcoidosis. The patient presents with fever, malaise and lymphadenopathy and erythema nodosum. Behçet's disease may present with arthritis. Usually there are eye signs, mouth ulcers and genital ulcers. CNS involvement with meningoencephalitis may occur.

EXAMINATION

Congenital

Achondroplasia is obvious. In Ehlers–Danlos syndrome there will be hypermobile joints and hyperextensible skin. There may be evidence of dislocation or subluxation of joints. In Marfan's syndrome the patient will be tall with long extremities, long fingers (arachnodactyly), high-arched palate, lens dislocation and aortic incompetence. Diagnosis of osteogenesis imperfecta will usually be obvious. There is stunted growth due to repeated fractures with deformities. The patient has blue sclerae and often hypotonia.

Acquired
Infective

With infective arthritis there is usually a red, painful, swollen, tender joint which has virtually no active or passive movement. The patient will be pyrexial. Usually a single joint is involved. With viral infections there may be signs of childhood illness, e.g. mumps (swollen salivary glands), rubella (rash), hepatitis (jaundice). With rheumatic fever there will be carditis with changing murmurs, migratory polyarthritis, subcutaneous nodules, erythema marginatum and occasionally chorea (Sydenham's).

Inflammatory

With rheumatoid arthritis there will be swelling of the metacarpophalangeal, PIP and wrist joints. Swan-neck and boutonnière deformities will be apparent, as will ulnar deviation. There may be subluxation at the wrist. Tendon ruptures may occur. Large joint involvement is common and atlantoaxial subluxation with myelopathy may develop. General signs include anaemia, nodulosis and eye signs. With psoriatic arthropathy psoriasis of the skin is usually present. With reactive/Reiter's disease there may be urethritis, conjunctivitis, keratoderma blenorrhagica, circinate balanitis, plantar fasciitis and Achilles tendonitis. With ankylosing spondylitis there may be minimal signs initially, the first sign usually being a reduced range of movement of the lumbar spine, but eventually there will be involvement of the sacroiliac joints together with a loss of the lumbar lordosis and a fixed kyphotic spine. Reduced respiratory excursion may occur. SLE may present with malaise, arthralgia, myalgia, a butterfly rash on the face, Raynaud's phenomenon, splenomegaly, pleurisy, pleural effusion, pericarditis. Polymyalgia rheumatica is associated with tender muscles, mild polyarthritis and there may be associated temporal arteritis.

Degenerative

Osteoarthritis usually involves the distal interphalangeal joints (Heberden's nodes), the metacarpophalangeal joint of the thumb, the first metatarsophalangeal joint, the cervical spine, the lumbar spine, the hips and knees. There will be joint tenderness and limitation of movement.

Enteropathic

There is normally spondyloarthritis with sacroiliitis. Large joint monoarthropathy is common although many peripheral joints may be involved.

Endocrine

With acromegaly there will be large hands and feet, a macroglossia, prognathism, arthralgia, kyphosis, deep voice and heart failure. There may be signs of the pituitary tumour, i.e. bilateral hemianopia due to local pressure on the optic chiasma.

Metabolic

There is an acutely painful, red, swollen joint with gout. The first metatarsophalangeal joint is most often involved (podagra) but any joint may be affected. There may be evidence of gouty tophi, e.g. pinna, tendons, joints. With haemochromatosis, in addition to arthropathy there may be evidence of hepatomegaly, cirrhosis, diabetes, cardiomyopathy and skin pigmentation.

Neuropathic

Deformed, painless joints with subluxation may occur. There is usually no warmth or tenderness in relation to the joint. Abnormal movement may occur. Neurological examination may reveal dorsal column signs. If the condition is due to syphilis (tabes dorsalis) there may be Argyll Robertson pupils.

Haematological

With haemophiliacs the patient will present with an acute, painful, immobile joint following a bleed. Eventually there will be deformed joints. Joints may be involved in leukaemia and acute sickle cell crises.

Drugs

Steroids may cause avascular necrosis, especially of the hips. There will be pain and limitation of movement. Osteoarthritis develops eventually. Patients on anticoagulants may have acute haemarthroses.

Neoplastic

Hypertrophic pulmonary osteoarthropathy usually occurs in association with bronchial carcinoma. The ends of long bones are affected by symmetrical but irregular widespread thickening. Clubbing usually occurs. Pain from local tumours is constant and may progress to a pathological fracture.

Other

With avascular necrosis of bone there is usually severe pain, tenderness and limitation of movement. Ultimately osteoarthritis develops. With sarcoidosis there is usually fever, lymphadenopathy, hepatosplenomegaly, erythema nodosum, eye signs, cardiac signs and CNS involvement. With Behçet's disease there will be arthritis, keratitis, uveitis, mouth ulcers, genital ulcers and occasionally CNS involvement.

GENERAL INVESTIGATIONS

- **FBC, ESR**
  Hb ↓ anaemia of chronic disease, e.g. rheumatoid arthritis, SLE. WCC ↑ infective causes, leukaemia. ESR ↑ chronic infection, rheumatoid arthritis, ankylosing spondylitis, rheumatic fever.

- **CRP**
  ↑ infective and inflammatory causes.

- **U&Es**
  Renal involvement, e.g. SLE.

- **LFTs**
  Hepatic involvement, e.g. haemochromatosis.

- **Serum uric acid**
  Gout.

- **Rheumatoid factor, anti-CCP antibodies**
  Rheumatoid arthritis.

- **PSA**
  Prostatic carcinoma.

- **Sickling test**
  Sickle cell disease.

- **Joint X-ray**
  Osteoarthritis – loss of joint space, subchondral sclerosis and cyst, osteophytes. Rheumatoid arthritis – soft-tissue thickening, juxta-articular osteopenia, loss of joint space, erosion of bone, subluxations. Avascular necrosis – avascular bone is more dense than adjacent bone. Gout – soft-tissue swelling initially then 'punched-out' lesions in juxta-articular bone. Ankylosing spondylitis – syndesmophytes, bamboo spine, obliteration of sacroiliac joints.

- **CXR**
  Bronchial carcinoma

SPECIFIC INVESTIGATIONS

- **Antistreptolysin O titre**
  Rheumatic fever.

- **Blood culture**
  Septic arthritis – *Staphylococcus aureus*, *Brucella*, *Salmonella*, streptococci.

- **Antibody screen**
  ANA positive. Anti-double-stranded DNA ↑ SLE.

- ***Brucella* serology**
  Brucellosis.

- **Viral titres**
  Viral infections.

- **Hepatitis screen**
  Hepatitis B-associated arthralgia.

- **Sickling test**
  Sickle cell disease.

- **Coagulation screen**
  Anticoagulant therapy. Haemophilia.

- **Mantoux test/ELISpot assay**
  TB.

- **Skeletal survey**
  Tumours are usually visible only when more than 50% of bone mineral is lost. Acromegaly – pituitary fossa changes, hand and skull changes.

- **Bone scan**
  Metastatic disease. Primary bone tumours. Paget's disease. Inflammatory bone lesions. Osteoarthritis. Rheumatoid arthritis. Bone fractures.

- **MRI**
  Soft-tissue injuries. Meniscal injuries. Ligamentous injuries. Early rheumatoid arthritis.

- **Joint aspirate**
  Microscopy and culture and sensitivity. Crystals in gout.

- **Synovial biopsy**
  Confirms type of arthritis in rare cases.

INDIVIDUAL JOINTS

The following section covers individual joints. It must be appreciated that the conditions covered in joint disorders (above) can involve almost any joint; however, the conditions described under the individual joints (below) will refer to those conditions that normally affect, or cause pain in, the region of the particular joint.

SHOULDER

CAUSES

CONGENITAL

- Klippel–Feil syndrome

ACQUIRED

TRAUMATIC
- Dislocation
- Fracture of the neck of the humerus
- Fracture of the clavicle
- Fracture of the scapula

DEGENERATIVE
- Supraspinatus tendinosis
- Impingement syndromes
- Rotator cuff tears
- Frozen shoulder (adhesive capsulitis)
- Osteoarthritis
  - Acromioclavicular
  - Glenohumeral

INFLAMMATORY
- Rheumatoid arthritis
- Crystal disease (gout, pseudogout)

INFECTIVE
- Septic arthritis
- Tuberculous arthritis

NEOPLASTIC
- Metastases in the upper end of the humerus/ribs/neck

REFERRED PAIN
- Cervical spondylosis
- Diaphragmatic irritation
- Pancoast's tumour

NEUROLOGICAL
- Winged scapula

HISTORY

Congenital

In Klippel–Feil syndrome, the neck is short and there are anomalies of the cervical vertebrae; the scapula is placed superiorly.

Acquired

Traumatic

With dislocation of the shoulder there is usually a history of a fall on the outstretched hand. Recurrent dislocation may occur. The patient presents in pain supporting the arm, which is abducted. Anterior dislocation is the most common but posterior dislocation is often missed and can occur after trauma such as fits or electric shocks. With dislocation of the acromioclavicular joint there is usually a history of a fall on the shoulder (common in rugby players). Fracture of the surgical neck of the humerus occurs with a fall on the shoulder. The patient presents with pain, deformity and inability to move the shoulder. Clavicular fracture is usually caused by a fall on the outstretched hand or point of the shoulder. Scapular fractures are usually high-energy injuries often due to RTAs.

Degenerative

Supraspinatus tendinosis results from degeneration, inflammation or calcification of the tendon. There may be sudden pain or there may be just a painful arc at the initiation of movement. With impingement syndromes the rotator cuff becomes compressed under the acromion, or acromioclavicular joint, resulting in pain on abducting the arm. A painful arc suggests subacromial pathology. Rotator cuff tears often occur in older patients and probably relate to degeneration of the cuff. In the younger, fit patient, the rotator cuff tear may be due to violent trauma with rupture of supraspinatus. The patient is unable to initiate abduction of the arm but passive movement is normal. Frozen shoulder (adhesive capsulitis) usually affects the middle-aged and there may be a history of minor injury. There is pain and limitation of both active and passive movement of the shoulder. The pain is often severe and disturbs sleep. It may occur in the elderly following immobilisation of the arm, e.g. following a Colles' fracture or stroke. It is more common in diabetics. Osteoarthritis of the acromioclavicular joint presents as pain associated with overhead movement and a high painful arc (>140°). Osteoarthritis of the glenohumeral joint may be idiopathic or follow avascular necrosis, or radionecrosis following radiotherapy for carcinoma of the breast. The patient complains of pain on shoulder movement and night pain.

Inflammatory

Rheumatoid arthritis is more common than osteoarthritis in the shoulder joint. There is usually a history of rheumatoid arthritis elsewhere. A history of gout or pseudogout may be evident.

Infective

The patient presents with a painful, red, swollen joint with limited movement. TB of the shoulder is extremely rare in the UK. There are systemic symptoms of malaise and fever and there is usually wasting of the muscle around the shoulder joint.

Neoplastic

Secondary deposits may occur in the upper end of the humerus, giving rise to pain. Pathological fractures may occur. Check for a history of carcinoma of the bronchus, breast, thyroid, prostate or kidney.

Referred pain

This is an extremely common cause of shoulder pain. Cervical spondylosis often results in referred pain to the upper part of the shoulder. Check for a history of neck pain with limitation of movement of the neck. Irritation of the diaphragm may refer pain to the dermatome C4 at the shoulder tip. This may be due to peritonitis below the diaphragm or pleurisy above. The symptoms of peritonitis will be obvious. A history of chest problems should be sought if Pancoast's tumour is suspected, especially if Horner's syndrome is present.

Neurological

Winged scapula may cause difficulty with shoulder movements. Check for recent surgery to the neck or axilla, e.g. axillary clearance in breast carcinoma which may damage the long thoracic nerve. Carrying heavy loads on the shoulders over a prolonged period of time may also be responsible.

EXAMINATION

Congenital

Klippel–Feil syndrome. The patient will present with a short neck and a highly placed scapula. Other congenital conditions may be present.

Acquired

Traumatic

With dislocation of the shoulder the patient supports the arm. The normal contour of the shoulder is lost. Check for axillary nerve damage (anaesthesia over the 'badge' area). With acromioclavicular dislocation there will be a palpable lump at the site of dislocation. With fracture of the surgical neck of the humerus there will be pain and tenderness, and inability to abduct the arm due to pain. Check for axillary nerve damage. With fractures of the clavicle the patient supports the weight of the arm with the other hand. The site of the break is usually palpable.

Degenerative

There will be limitation of movement. Check for a painful arc. Check for the ability to initiate abduction (supraspinatus tendon tears). With frozen shoulder and osteoarthritis there is limitation of active

nd passive movements. Check for mastectomy scars or signs of
diotherapy. With osteoarthritis of the acromioclavicular joint there
usually obvious prominence of the joint with localised tenderness
d a high painful arc.

flammatory

ith rheumatoid arthritis there are often signs elsewhere. There may
e fever, malaise and heat in the joint. Glenohumeral movements
ay cause crepitus. Features of gout may be evident such as the
resence of tophi.

fective

here will be a red, hot, swollen, tender joint. There may be a focus
f infection elsewhere in the body.

eoplastic

here may be little to find on examination or there may be a
athological fracture with pain, local tenderness and limitation of
ovement.

eferred pain

heck for movements of the cervical spine. Carry out a full
eurological examination. With referred pain from the diaphragm,
xamine the abdomen for tenderness, guarding and rigidity. Examine
e chest for signs of pneumonia, pleurisy or tumour.

eurological

heck for scars in the neck or axilla. Note the winging of the scapula
hen the patient pushes the hand against a wall with the arm
orward flexed to 90° (protraction of the scapula).

ENERAL INVESTIGATIONS

- FBC, ESR
  Hb ↓ anaemia of chronic disease, e.g. rheumatoid arthritis. WCC ↑
  infection. ESR and CRP ↑ infection/inflammatory disease.

- X-ray
  X-rays in two planes. Arthritis. Dislocation. Fracture. Secondary
  deposits.

PECIFIC INVESTIGATIONS

- Blood culture
  Septic arthritis.

- Mantoux test/ELISpot assay
  TB.

- Bone scan
  Secondary deposits.

- ■ **Aspiration**
  Gram stain. C&S. Septic arthritis. Characteristic crystals in gout and pseudogout.
- ■ **Arthroscopy**
  Cause of arthritis.
- ■ **CT/MRI**
  Painful arc syndrome. Rotator cuff tears.

ELBOW

CAUSES

TRAUMATIC

- ● Supracondylar fracture of the humerus
- ● Dislocation of the elbow
- ● Pulled elbow
- ● Fracture of the radial head
- ● Fractured olecranon
- ● Fractured epicondyle/condyle
- ● Myositis ossificans

DEGENERATIVE

- ● Osteoarthritis
- ● Osteochondritis dissecans

INFLAMMATORY

- ● Rheumatoid arthritis

NEUROLOGICAL

- ● Nerve entrapment, e.g. ulnar, posterior interosseous and median

OTHER

- ● Olecranon bursitis
- ● Tennis elbow
- ● Golfer's elbow
- ● Cubitus varus/valgus

HISTORY

Traumatic

Supracondylar fracture is chiefly a fracture of childhood. There is a history of a fall on the outstretched hand followed by pain and swelling around the elbow. This is a significant injury with several serious complications. Dislocation of the elbow may occur in children or adults. The symptoms are similar to those of supracondylar fracture. Pulled elbow occurs in children aged 2–6 years. The radial head slips out of the annular ligament. The child may have been 'swinging' with the parents holding the hands. Fractures of the olecranon may result as a fall on the point of the elbow or by sudden contraction of the triceps. Condylar and epicondylar fractures are rare and easily missed. With myositis ossificans there will be a history of a supracondylar fracture or dislocation of the elbow. A calcified haematoma forms in front of the joint. Movement of the joint, especially flexion, is affected. It may follow ill-advised physiotherapy with passive stretching of the joints after trauma or after surgery.

Degenerative

Osteoarthritis of the elbow may occur in heavy manual workers or following complicated fractures involving the joint. Osteochondritis dissecans may cause elbow pain and restrict movement because of a loose body in the joint.

Inflammatory

Rheumatoid arthritis may affect the elbow joint. There will usually be signs of rheumatoid arthritis elsewhere. If there is gross disorganisation of the joint with deformity, the ulnar nerve may be involved and there may be symptoms of ulnar nerve palsy. Gout may affect the elbow joint.

Neurological

Various nerve entrapment syndromes can occur around the elbow. Symptoms may present in the distribution of ulnar, median or posterior interosseous nerves.

Other

Olecranon bursitis results in painful or painless swelling over the olecranon. It is common in carpet layers and students (students rest their heads in their hands while studying late into the night with their elbows resting on the desk). The bursa may become infected with a red, tender, hot swelling. Tennis elbow is common between the ages of 30 and 50 years. It presents with pain on the lateral side of the elbow. It affects tennis players and anyone whose job involves extending and twisting the forearm. The pain is often worse on gripping. Golfer's elbow is similar to tennis elbow but affects the medial epicondyle. The patient complains of pain and tenderness over the medial epicondyle and also of pain on hyperextending the fingers and wrists. Cubitus valgus/varus may follow fractures around the elbow in childhood. Cubitus valgus may progressively stretch the ulnar nerve, with a slowly developing ulnar nerve palsy.

EXAMINATION

Traumatic

With supracondylar fractures there will be swelling around the elbow joint and limitation of movement. The olecranon, medial epicondyle and lateral epicondyle preserve their normal relationship with one another in an equilateral triangle. Damage to the brachial artery and median or radial nerve may occur. With posterior dislocation at the elbow, the triangular relationship referred to above is lost. Otherwise the findings are similar. It is important to check the distal circulation and to assess for median and radial nerve palsies. With a fracture of the olecranon there is swelling and tenderness directly over the olecranon. With damage to the medial epicondyle it is important to test the integrity of the ulnar nerve. With myositis ossificans a calcified mass occurs in front of the elbow joint and there will be limitation of flexion. With radial head fractures the patient will be focally tender over the radial head and there will be lack of full extension.

Degenerative

With osteoarthritis there are often few signs. There may be bony swelling of the joint with loss of movement and crepitus. With osteochondritis dissecans there may be restriction in movement, crepitus and locking of the joint due to a loose body.

Inflammatory

With rheumatoid arthritis there will often be signs elsewhere. In long-standing arthritis there will be a swollen, disrupted joint with deformity. Check the integrity of the ulnar nerve. Tophi may be present in gout.

Neurological

Examine carefully in the distribution of the median, ulnar and radial nerve.

Other

With olecranon bursitis there will be a swelling over the olecranon. This is fluid-filled and exhibits fluctuation and transilluminates. With infection it may become red and tender. With tennis elbow there is tenderness over the lateral epicondyle. Pronating the forearm while extending the elbow exacerbates the pain. With golfer's elbow there is tenderness over the medial epicondyle. With cubitus valgus/varus the deformity is usually obvious. With cubitus valgus it is important to check the integrity of the ulnar nerve.

GENERAL INVESTIGATIONS

■ **FBC, ESR**
Hb ↓ anaemia of chronic disease, e.g. rheumatoid arthritis. WCC ↑ septic arthritis. ESR and CRP ↑ in infection/inflammatory disease.

■ **Rheumatoid factor/anti-CCP antibodies**
Rheumatoid arthritis.

■ **X-ray**
Fractures around the elbow. Fracture of the radial head – anterior fat pad sign ('sail' sign). Dislocation of the elbow. Osteoarthritis. Rheumatoid arthritis. Osteochondritis dissecans with loose body. Myositis ossificans.

SPECIFIC INVESTIGATIONS

■ **US**
Olecranon bursitis (diagnosis should be obvious on clinical examination).

■ **MRI**
Will detect abnormalities of all structures, e.g. synovitis in rheumatoid arthritis ligament disruption in tennis and golfer's elbow

■ **Aspiration**
Gram stain. C&S – infection. Crystals – gout.

WRIST

CAUSES

TRAUMATIC

● Distal radial fracture, e.g. Colles', Smith's

● Scaphoid fracture

● Dislocations

● Carpal dislocations

DEGENERATIVE

● Osteoarthritis

INFLAMMATORY

● Rheumatoid arthritis

OTHER

● Ganglion

● Tenosynovitis

  ● de Quervain's

  ● Extensor tenosynovitis

● Carpal tunnel syndrome
● Avascular necrosis of the lunate (Kienböck's disease)

HISTORY

Traumatic

The patient with a Colles' fracture is usually an elderly osteoporotic woman. There is a history of a fall on the outstretched hand (extended wrist). The patient presents with pain and deformity. A Smith's fracture is the reverse of a Colles' (fall onto flexed wrist). Again there is pain and deformity. Dislocations of the carpus are rare, the most common being dislocation of the lunate. This is usually due to a fall on the dorsiflexed hand. There may be involvement of the median nerve. Fracture of the scaphoid results from a fall on the outstretched hand or a blow to the palm of the hand. The patient presents with a painful, swollen wrist.

Degenerative

Osteoarthritis of the wrist is uncommon and usually a sequel to injury, e.g. a fracture of the scaphoid. The patient complains of pain and stiffness in the wrist.

Inflammatory

The wrist is commonly affected in rheumatoid arthritis. In the early stages, there will be swelling, heat, pain and stiffness. Ultimately, ulnar deviation of the wrist and palmar subluxation occur.

Other

A ganglion is a painless lump, usually on the dorsum of the wrist. de Quervain's tenosynovitis usually occurs in the middle-aged. It involves the abductor pollicis longus and extensor pollicis brevis. The patient complains of pain on movement of the wrist and a weakness of the grip. Extensor 'tenosynovitis crepitans' follows excess activity and may affect all or only one of the extensor tendons. The patient usually complains of pain and tenderness over the dorsum of the wrist occurring with activity. With carpal tunnel syndrome there is often a history of pregnancy, rheumatoid arthritis, hypothyroidism, osteoarthritis, anterior dislocation of the lunate or an arteriovenous fistula created for dialysis. Middle-aged women are most affected with carpal tunnel syndrome. There is pain in the distribution of the median nerve in the hand, worse in bed at night. It is relieved by hanging the hand out of bed and shaking the hand. The patient often complains of clumsiness with fine movements due to median nerve involvement. With avascular necrosis of the lunate there may be a history of trauma. The patient is usually a young adult who complains of ache and stiffness.

EXAMINATION

Traumatic

With a Colles' fracture there is a classical 'dinner fork' deformity. The distal fragment is displaced backwards and radially. With Smith's fracture there is forward angulation of the distal fragment. Pain, limitation of movement and swelling occur. With dislocation there is a swollen wrist. Test the median nerve. Scaphoid fractures result in swelling around the wrist, with localised tenderness in the anatomical snuff box.

Degenerative

With osteoarthritis, the wrist may appear normal. There may be limited painful movement with crepitus.

Inflammatory

With rheumatoid arthritis there may be gross swelling with increased local heat, pain and stiffness. Ultimately, ulnar deviation occurs and there may be palmar subluxation with a significantly reduced movement.

Other

A ganglion is a well-defined cystic non-tender lump which transilluminates. With tenosynovitis there is usually localised tenderness and occasionally swelling. Often there is little else to find except for a weak grip. Look for a precipitating cause for carpal tunnel syndrome, e.g. pregnancy, hypothyroidism. The diagnosis is often made on the history. There may be wasting of the thenar eminence and sensory abnormalities in the distribution of the median nerve. Tinel's sign (percussion over the median nerve in the carpal tunnel causes paraesthesia in the median nerve distribution) and Phalen's sign (paraesthesia following prolonged wrist flexion) may be positive. With Kienböck's disease there will be localised tenderness and limited dorsiflexion.

GENERAL INVESTIGATIONS

■ **FBC, ESR**
   Hb ↓ anaemia of chronic disease, e.g. rheumatoid arthritis. WCC ↑ infection. ESR and CRP ↑ infection/inflammatory disease.

■ **Rheumatoid factor/anti-CCP antibodies**
   Rheumatoid arthritis.

■ **X-ray**
   Fractures. Dislocation. Scaphoid views for suspected scaphoid fractures. Increased density of bone in avascular necrosis. Osteoarthritis. Rheumatoid arthritis.

SPECIFIC INVESTIGATIONS

- ■ Blood culture
  Septic arthritis.
- ■ Aspiration
  Infection – Gram stain, C&S. Crystals in gout.
- ■ Nerve conduction studies
  Carpal tunnel syndrome.
- ■ Bone scan
  Fracture or avascular necrosis.
- ■ MRI
  Fracture or avascular necrosis.

HIP

CAUSES

CONGENITAL

- DDH (formerly congenital dislocation of the hip)

ACQUIRED

TRAUMATIC

- Fractured neck of femur
- Fracture of the pubic ramus
- Dislocation of the hip
- Acetabular fracture

INFECTIVE

- Acute pyogenic arthritis
- TB
  - (common in developing countries)

INFLAMMATORY

- Rheumatoid arthritis
- Reactive/Reiter's syndrome
- Ankylosing spondylitis

DEGENERATIVE

- Osteoarthritis
  - Primary
  - Secondary
- Avascular necrosis

NEOPLASTIC
- Metastases
- Leukaemia in childhood

OTHER
- Transient synovitis
- Perthes' disease
- Slipped upper femoral epiphysis
- Transient osteoporosis of the hip

HISTORY

Congenital

DDH is usually picked up on routine examination of the neonate with Ortolani's test and confirmed by US scan. If the diagnosis is missed on routine testing, the child may present with a limp and waddling gait (Trendelenburg gait). There is an increased risk of DDH if one parent has a history of the disease and it is commoner with breech delivery, primigravidas and female infants. Check for other congenital anomalies.

Acquired
Traumatic

Fracture of the neck of the femur usually occurs in an elderly female. The trauma may be minor, e.g. tripping over the carpet. The patient presents with pain in the hip especially with movement and weight-bearing is often impossible. In the young patient there is usually a history of major trauma. Dislocation of the hip, which is usually posterior, is associated with other severe injuries. It often occurs with road traffic accidents, the knee striking the dashboard. Pelvic fractures (usually pubic rami) are usually a result of a fall in the elderly. The patient feels deep-seated pain in the region of the hip. Walking is painful. Acetabular fractures usually result from direct violence, e.g. a fall on the side, or indirect, such as a fall on the feet or from impact of the knee on a car dashboard.

Infective

The infection is usually blood-borne. It may occur in children where the metaphysis is intracapsular, as in the hip. Check for a history of steroid medication or other immunosuppression. The patient presents with a hot, painful, tender joint. There is limitation of movement and weight-bearing is painful. With TB there is usually a history of contact. The patient presents with malaise, weight loss and night sweats. There is local pain and swelling with limitation of movement and local muscle atrophy.

Inflammatory

Reactive/Reiter's disease presents with a history of genitourinary or gastrointestinal infection, urethritis and conjunctivitis. There may be a history of sexual contact or dysentery. Rheumatoid arthritis usually presents with a symmetrical small joint polyarthritis; however, the hip may be involved. Ankylosing spondylitis may affect the hips. Spinal stiffness is usually the presenting symptom.

Degenerative

Osteoarthritis presents with pain and stiffness and the patient often has difficulty walking. Secondary osteoarthritis may follow a history of fractures, Perthes' disease, slipped upper femoral epiphysis, avascular necrosis, haemophilia. Avascular necrosis of the head of the femur may occur following intracapsular fractures of the neck of the femur. It may also occur in patients on steroid therapy.

Neoplastic

The upper end of the femur near the neck is a common site for metastases. Hip pain in children may be due to leukaemic infiltration.

Other

Transient synovitis gives rise to an irritable hip with a limp, pain and restriction of movement. Perthes' usually occurs with a maximum incidence around 7–8 years. There is pain in the hip and a limp. The patient is otherwise well. The pain may be referred to the knee joint. Slipped upper femoral epiphysis usually presents between 11 and 16 years. It occurs more commonly in boys. There is usually pain in the hip and a limp and it may present with referred pain to the knee. Transient osteoporosis of the hip may occur during pregnancy and is a self-limiting condition.

EXAMINATION

Congenital

Ortolani's test is carried out after birth. The hips and knees are flexed to a right angle and the thighs are abducted. There is a 'clunk' as the head of the femur slips into the joint over the acetabulum (Ortolani's test). In Barlow's test the surgeon holds the upper femur between the middle finger on the great trochanter and the thumb in the groin and levers the femoral head in and out of the acetabulum, readily demonstrating dislocation.

Acquired

Traumatic

The patient with a fractured neck of femur classically shows shortening, adduction and external rotation of the leg. If the fracture is undisplaced, limb alignment may be normal; however, movements are painful. With dislocation the patient is usually shocked with other injuries. With posterior dislocation the thigh is flexed, adducted and internally rotated. Check for sciatic nerve injury. There may be associated injury to femur or patella. With isolated fractures of the pubic ramus there may be little to find on examination, although a second fracture/joint injury is common at the back of the pelvic ring.

Infective

Acute pyogenic arthritis presents with a hot, tender, painful swollen hip. All movements are painful. There is spasm in the surrounding muscles. The patient usually has a high fever. TB presents with local tenderness, swelling and effusion. There is muscle wasting and spasm. There is usually a constitutional upset with malaise and fever.

Inflammatory

With reactive/Reiter's disease there is usually associated urethritis and conjunctivitis. With rheumatoid arthritis other joints are usually involved and the patient may describe constitutional symptoms. The hip is often held in flexion and movements are painful. Ankylosing spondylitis usually presents with a stiff spine with a limited range of movement, although the hips may also be stiff.

Degenerative

Osteoarthritis usually presents with a limp. The leg lies externally rotated and appears shortened because of fixed adduction. There is usually a degree of fixed flexion. Restriction in movement occurs: abduction, extension and internal rotation loss occurring early and being most restricted. There is apparent shortening. Avascular necrosis results in distortion of joint shape with stiffness, limitation of movement and ultimately secondary osteoarthritis.

Neoplastic

Check for localised pain over the hip joint. Check for any tumour of breast, bronchus, thyroid, prostate or kidney. In children with leukaemic infiltration there may be other signs, e.g. spontaneous bruising, lymphadenopathy, splenomegaly.

Other

Transient synovitis presents with a limp. There is no systemic upset. There is limitation of movement at the joint. Perthes' disease presents with a limp and a decreased range of joint movement. With slipped upper femoral epiphysis the leg lies in external rotation and passive internal rotation is diminished. Limitation of movement due to pain is usually present in transient osteoporosis of the hip.

GENERAL INVESTIGATIONS

■ **FBC, ESR**
Hb ↓ anaemia of chronic disease, e.g. rheumatoid arthritis. WCC ↑ infection. ESR and CRP ↑ in infection/inflammatory disease.

■ **Hip X-ray**
AP and lateral. Fractures, osteoarthritis, rheumatoid arthritis, dislocation, Perthes' disease, slipped upper femoral epiphysis, TB, avascular necrosis, transient osteoporosis.

SPECIFIC INVESTIGATIONS

■ **Blood culture**
Septic arthritis.

■ **Aspiration**
Infection – Gram stain, C&S. Crystals in gout.

■ **US**
Developmental dysplasia of the hip.

■ **Bone scan**
Avascular necrosis. Occult fracture.

■ **MRI**
Fractures, osteoarthritis, rheumatoid arthritis, dislocation, Perthes' disease, slipped upper femoral epiphysis, TB, avascular necrosis, transient osteoporosis.

KNEE

CAUSES

TRAUMATIC

BONES
● Patellar fractures
● Supracondylar fractures of the femur
● Tibial fractures involving the joint

LIGAMENTS
● Medial and lateral collateral ligament damage
● Cruciate ligament damage
● Rupture of quadriceps tendon
● Rupture of the patellar tendon

MENISCI
● Meniscal tears

INFECTIVE
● Pyogenic arthritis

INFLAMMATORY

- Rheumatoid arthritis
- Reactive/Reiter's syndrome
- Ankylosing spondylitis

DEGENERATIVE

- Osteoarthritis

METABOLIC

- Gout
- Pseudogout

NEUROPATHIC

- Charcot's joint

NEOPLASTIC

- Osteogenic sarcoma

OTHER

- Bursitis
  - Pre-patellar bursitis (housemaid's knee)
  - Infra-patellar bursitis (clergyman's knee)
  - Semi-membranosus bursitis
- Baker's cyst
- Disorders of alignment
  - Genu varum (bow legs)
  - Genu valgum (knock knee)
- Patellofemoral instability
- Referred pain from the hip/back
- Osteochondritis dissecans
- Osgood–Schlatter's disease (osteochondritis of the tibial tuberosity)
- Chondromalacia patellae

HISTORY

Traumatic

With fractures around the knee joint there will usually be an obvious history of trauma. Fractures of the patella may arise because of violent contraction of quadriceps or because of direct blows to the patella. With ligamentous tears there is often a history of damage during sport, e.g. footballers. The patient will present with a painful, swollen knee joint. Posterior cruciate ligament injury is usually due to a force drawing the tibia backwards on the femur with the knee flexed, e.g. in a car accident when the upper tibia strikes the dashboard. Meniscal tears often occur in sportsmen when the knee is twisted while it is flexed. The patient presents with a swollen knee with pain and tenderness on the side on which the meniscus is torn. The knee may be 'locked', i.e. lacks the last 10–15° of extension. Very rapid swelling indicates bleeding into the joint, and hence fracture or cruciate damage or peripheral meniscal detachment.

Infective

Usually blood-borne. More common in children. May occur in adults on steroids or who are immunosuppressed. The patient presents with a hot, painful, tender joint with malaise and fever. The patient is reluctant to move the joint.

Inflammatory

In rheumatoid arthritis the patient complains of pain, swelling and stiffness together with constitutional upset. Symptoms of rheumatoid arthritis may be present elsewhere. Reactive/Reiter's syndrome may present with swelling and discomfort in the knee. There is often a history of urethritis, conjunctivitis or dysentery. Ankylosing spondylitis may present with knee joint involvement. Usually the patient also complains of stiffness of the spine.

Degenerative

Osteoarthritis is common in the knee. The patient may be overweight and elderly. There is pain on movement, stiffness and deformity. There may be a history of previous joint pathology, e.g. septic arthritis, meniscal tear, meniscal surgery or osteochondritis dissecans.

Metabolic

Gout may present with pain and swelling of the knee. Pseudogout (pyrophosphate deposition disease) may also present in the knee joint. The condition is associated with chondrocalcinosis, i.e. there is calcification visible in hyaline and fibrocartilage.

Neuropathic

The patient presents with a painless joint, which is grossly deformed and hypermobile. There may be a history of diabetes, syphilis or leprosy.

Neoplastic

The lower end of the femur and the upper end of the tibia are common sites of osteogenic sarcoma. The patient is usually male and under the age of 30 years. There is pain, swelling and deformity around the knee. The patient may also complain of cough due to lung metastases.

Other
Bursitis

Bursitis presents with swelling, either in front of or behind the knee. The swelling may be painless. Patients who work on their knees leaning forwards, e.g. carpet fitters, may get prepatellar bursitis (housemaid's knee). Infrapatellar bursitis occurs in those who sit back on their heels (e.g. vicars praying, hence the name clergyman's knee). A semi-membranosus bursa presents behind the knee on the medial side. A bursa may become infected, in which case the patient will present with a tender, red, hot swelling.

Baker's cyst

Baker's cyst presents in the midline of the popliteal fossa. The patient will notice a lump and reduced flexion of the knee. There may also be pain associated with concurrent osteoarthritis of the joint.

Disorders of alignment

With genu varum the patient presents with bow legs. In children, this is usually associated with a disorder of growth, often with a bony injury to the area of epiphyses. In adults, there may be a history of rickets, Paget's disease, rheumatoid or osteoarthritis. In genu valgum (knock knee), the patient is often a child who has flat feet. In adults, there may be a history of rheumatoid arthritis.

Patellofemoral instability

Dislocation of the patella may occur. In the acute form there may be a history of a blow to one side of the knee. Recurrent dislocation of the patella affects adolescent girls. It is usually associated with flattening of the lateral condyle, a high-riding patella (patella alta) or genu valgum.

Referred pain

It is very common for pain to be referred from the hip or the back to the knee. Always enquire about hip and back symptoms.

Osteochondritis dissecans

This occurs most commonly in the second decade of life. A segment of bone undergoes avascular necrosis, separates and forms a loose body in the joint. The patient complains of pain, swelling and intermittent 'locking' of the joint.

Osgood–Schlatter's disease

The patient is usually a boy aged between 10 and 14 years. There is a history of physical activity, e.g. football. Pain and swelling occur, accurately located to the area of the tibial tuberosity.

Chondromalacia patellae

The patient presents with ill-localised pain in front of the knee. It is most common in females in the 15–35 years age group. There may be a history of injury. There is usually some swelling, and pain occurs especially when climbing stairs. The knee tends to give way.

EXAMINATION

Traumatic

Fractures will usually be obvious. There will be pain, tenderness, deformity and crepitus. With supracondylar fractures it is important to check the distal circulation. With ligamentous injuries, test for joint stability, effusion and tenderness over the affected ligament. Testing for active straight-leg raising will exclude injury to the extensor mechanism (rupture of quadriceps, rupture of patellar tendon, patellar fracture). Valgus and varus strain testing may be necessary to diagnose ligamentous injury. Test for anterior and posterior drawer signs and carry out Lachman's test. With meniscal injuries there is tenderness, swelling and effusion in the acute phase. The joint may be locked, i.e. loss of the last 10–15° of extension. In the chronic phase there will be wasted quadriceps, effusion, tenderness over the meniscus in the joint line. McMurray's test will be positive with medial meniscus injury, although it is rarely carried out these days.

In acute knee injuries little examination can be performed at the time due to pain and re-assessment at 10 days is appropriate.

Infective

The patient will be febrile with a hot, red, tender, painful, swollen joint. There will be spasm in the surrounding muscles and no active or passive movement will be possible (occasionally, movements are possible in diabetics and patients on steroids and immunosuppressive drugs).

Inflammatory

With rheumatoid arthritis there will be fever, pain and swelling with decreased range of movement and synovial thickening. There will often be signs of rheumatoid arthritis in other joints. With reactive/Reiter's syndrome there will be swelling and reduced movements. Urethritis and conjunctivitis may be apparent. Ankylosing spondylitis may affect the knee joints, in which case there will be swelling and stiffness. There is usually reduced movement of the spine.

Degenerative

With osteoarthritis there will be swelling due to osteophytes, and possibly thickened synovium or effusion. There will be wasting of quadriceps, reduced mobility of the joint and gait is invariably disturbed. Alignment may be distorted if only one side of the joint is affected.

Metabolic

With gout the joint is red, hot and swollen and there is limitation of movement. A similar appearance occurs in pseudogout.

Neuropathic

The joint will be grossly swollen and deformed. There will be abnormal mobility which is painless. Test for abnormality of dorsal column sensation (joint position sense).

Other

Bursitis – soft, fluctuant swelling in front of the patella (prepatellar bursitis) or below the patella (infrapatellar bursitis). Semi-membranosus bursitis presents as a cystic swelling on the medial aspect of the popliteal fossa. If the bursa becomes infected then the swelling becomes hot, red and tender. With osteochondritis dissecans there will be joint swelling due to effusion, and intermittent locking of the joint. Genu valgum and genu varum will be apparent on examination. Patellofemoral instability may result from acute or chronic dislocation. With acute dislocation the patella is visibly displaced laterally with the knee flexed. There will be localised tenderness and swelling. With chronic dislocation the knee locks in semiflexion. Spontaneous reduction often occurs. The patella may feel too high or too small. With Osgood–Schlatter's disease there is tenderness and swelling over the tibial tuberosity. With chondromalacia patellae there is slight swelling and pain when the patella is rocked against the femur. Always remember to examine the hip joint and spine as pain may be referred. Baker's cyst is a soft, diffuse swelling in the popliteal fossa. Pain occurs if the cyst ruptures and can mimic a DVT.

GENERAL INVESTIGATIONS

- ■ **FBC, ESR**
  Hb ↓ anaemia of chronic disease, e.g. rheumatoid arthritis. WCC ↑ infection, e.g. pyogenic arthritis. ESR and CRP ↑ infection/inflammatory disease.

- ■ **Rheumatoid factor/anti-CCP antibodies**
  Rheumatoid arthritis.

- ■ **Serum uric acid**
  Gout.

- ■ **Knee X-ray (AP, lateral, tunnel and skyline views)**
  Fractures. Osteoarthritis. Rheumatoid arthritis. Loose bodies. Osteogenic sarcoma. X-ray stressing the joints may be necessary to diagnose ligamentous injuries.

- ■ **CXR**
  Secondary deposits in osteogenic sarcoma.

SPECIFIC INVESTIGATIONS

- ◀ **Blood culture**
  Pyogenic arthritis.

- ■ **Joint aspiration**
  Gram stain and culture and sensitivity – infection. Microscopy shows crystals in gout and pseudogout.
- ■ **Isotope scan**
  Tumour. Infections.
- ■ **MRI**
  All pathology but especially good for meniscal and other cartilage injuries. Ligamentous injuries, e.g. cruciates. Avascular necrosis. Synovitis.
- ■ **Arthroscopy**
  Loose bodies. Effusion. Meniscal injuries.
- ■ **Synovial biopsy**
  Confirmation of diagnosis.

ANKLE

CAUSES

TRAUMATIC

- Sprains (lateral ligaments)
- Fractures around the ankle
- Rupture of the Achilles tendon

INFECTIVE

- Pyogenic arthritis
- TB

INFLAMMATORY

- Rheumatoid arthritis

DEGENERATIVE

- Osteoarthritis

OTHERS

- Tenosynovitis
- Footballer's ankle
- Tarsal tunnel syndrome
- Osteochondritis of the talus

HISTORY

Traumatic

History of recent injury. Sprains usually affect the lateral ligament. With fractures there will be swelling, deformity, bruising and crepitu around the ankle. With tibiofibular diastasis there may be a high fibular fracture. Rupture of the Achilles tendon often occurs during sport (occasionally in bed!), particularly in middle-aged men. Patients feel as though they have been kicked in the back of the heel.

Infective

Pyogenic arthritis will result in a red, hot, tender joint. Tuberculous arthritis is rare. There will be pain on walking. There is usually a history of TB elsewhere.

Inflammatory

Rheumatoid arthritis is the commonest cause of chronic pain and swelling at the ankle joint. There will invariably be other symptoms of rheumatoid arthritis. Fever and malaise may also be present.

Degenerative

Primary osteoarthritis of the ankle is rare. Osteoarthritis is often a sequel to an imperfectly reduced fracture, or avascular necrosis of the talus. Symptoms are often mild.

Others

Tenosynovitis may occur in the tendons behind either the lateral or medial malleolus. Pain is present on either side of the ankle, particularly during inversion or eversion. Footballer's ankle, as the name implies, occurs in those who play football. The patient presents with poorly localised pain in front of the ankle. Osteochondritis of the talus is rare. It occurs in teenagers and young men. There is often severe pain in the ankle. In tarsal tunnel syndrome the tibial nerve may be compressed as it passes beneath the flexor retinaculum, giving rise to paraesthesia and a burning pain in the medial aspect of the sole of the foot and toes.

EXAMINATION

Traumatic

In fractures there will be deformity, a palpable swelling, tenderness and crepitus. With ruptures of the Achilles tendon there is usually an obvious gap in the Achilles tendon, and a weakness of plantar flexion of the foot against resistance. Apply the Thomson squeeze test. Normally when the calf is squeezed the foot plantar flexes. This does not occur with rupture of the Achilles tendon.

Infective

In pyogenic arthritis there will be a hot, tender, swollen, painful ankle. With TB the ankle will be swollen, with wasting of calf muscles.

Inflammatory

Rheumatoid arthritis seldom affects the ankle only. It presents with a swollen, tender ankle but there will be signs of arthritis elsewhere.

Degenerative

In osteoarthritis there is swelling, with a decreased range of movements of the ankle with crepitus.

Others

With tenosynovitis there is a puffy swelling and tenderness along the tendons. There may be pain on forced eversion (peroneus longus) and inversion (tibialis posterior). With footballer's ankle there is tearing of the anterior capsule of the joint with subsequent calcification. Examination often reveals restriction in dorsiflexion. With osteochondritis of the talus there is ankle swelling and tenderness. Loose bodies may present in the joint.

GENERAL INVESTIGATIONS

- **FBC, ESR**
  Hb ↓ anaemia of chronic disease, e.g. rheumatoid arthritis. WCC ↑ infection, e.g. pyogenic arthritis. ESR and CRP ↑ infection/inflammatory disease.

- **Ankle X-ray**
  Fractures. Stress X-rays may be required to delineate the type of fracture. Always include the upper fibula in the X-ray, as in diastasis of the joint there may be a fracture of the upper part of the shaft of the fibula. Rheumatoid arthritis. Osteoarthritis. Osteochondritis of the talus. Calcification of the anterior part of the capsule in footballer's ankle.

SPECIFIC INVESTIGATIONS

- **Blood culture**
  Pyogenic arthritis.

- **Joint aspiration**
  Gram stain and C&S in infection. Crystals in the fluid in gout.

- **Bone scan**
  Infections. Acute arthritis.

- **MRI**
  Osteochondritis of the talus. Fractures. Synovitis. Avascular necrosis. Tenosynovitis.

- Septic arthritis is an emergency. Immediate assessment and management is required in order to avert long-term joint damage.

- New onset inflammatory arthritis dictates rapid referral to a specialist, as early intensive intervention has been shown to markedly improve prognosis.

KIDNEY SWELLINGS

Kidney swellings are not uncommon. They may present silently or may be associated with haematuria, urinary tract infections and pyrexia.

CAUSES

CONGENITAL
- Polycystic kidney

ACQUIRED

INFECTIVE
- Perinephric abscess
- TB
  - (common where TB is endemic)

OBSTRUCTIVE
- Hydronephrosis
- Pyonephrosis

DEGENERATIVE
- Solitary cyst

NEOPLASTIC
- Hypernephroma
- Nephroblastoma

HISTORY

Congenital

There will often be a family history with adult polycystic kidney disease; however, it does not usually present until the third or fourth decade, when the patient may present with an abdominal mass, haematuria, loin pain (infection or bleeding into a cyst) or chronic renal failure. Hypertension may be a presenting symptom. Rarely, hydronephrosis may present at birth. Hydronephrosis in infants may be a cause of failure to thrive.

Acquired

There may be a history of TB. The patient may present with haematuria, dysuria or pyuria. With perinephric abscess there may be a history of diabetes. Nephroblastoma presents with an abdominal mass, pain, haematuria, pyrexia and weight loss within the first 3 years of life.

EXAMINATION

A mass may be palpated in either the right or the left loin. This moves with respiration and is palpable bimanually and ballotable.

Generally, a kidney swelling is dull to percussion, but there may be a strip of resonance across the swelling due to the gas-filled overlying transverse colon. A solitary cyst may be large, tense and smooth. Polycystic kidneys may be very large and extend down to the groin. They are smooth and embossed with many cysts. They may be tender if the cysts are infected or tense following bleeding. Hydronephrotic kidneys may be very large, smooth and tense. Perinephric abscesses may be associated with redness, swelling and oedema in the loin. Occasionally they may point in the loin, but this is rare nowadays. Hypernephromas are usually firm, irregular, nodular, and may be fixed. A nephroblastoma presents with a large mass in the loin and abdomen.

GENERAL INVESTIGATIONS

- **FBC, ESR**
  Hb ↑ (hypernephroma may be associated with polycythaemia). Hb ↓ blood loss due to haematuria. WCC ↑ pyonephrosis, perinephric abscess. ESR ↑ hypernephroma, nephroblastoma, TB, infection.
- **U&Es**
  Urea and creatinine raised if bilateral disease.
- **Blood glucose**
  Perinephric abscess in diabetes.
- **KUB**
  Hydronephrosis due to renal or ureteric stones. Renal outline.
- **CXR**
  Metastases – hypernephroma (cannonball metastases), nephroblastoma. TB.
- **Urinalysis**
  Blood, pus cells, organisms, EMSUs for TB.
- **US**
  Cystic versus solid. Biopsy.

SPECIFIC INVESTIGATIONS

- **IVU**
  Absent function. Hydronephrosis. Distortion of calyces (hypernephroma).
- **CT**
  Solid versus cystic. Spread of tumour. Biopsy.
- **Cystoscopy**
  Bladder tumour obstructing ureters. TB. Bladder outlet obstruction.
- **Antegrade pyelography**
  Site of obstruction.

- **Retrograde pyelography**
  Site of obstruction.

- **Angiography**
  Tumour circulation (rarely used).

- **MRI**
  Renal parenchymal lesions. Vascular lesions.

- Painless frank haematuria in association with an abdominal mass is an ominous sign and indicates malignancy.

- Always take a full family history. If polycystic kidney is a possible diagnosis, others in the family may be affected or there may be a past history of deaths in the family from chronic renal failure.

LEG PAIN

This section deals with causes of pain arising from local lesions within the leg, or referred into the leg. Pain in the leg is a common complaint and the majority of cases are of vascular or orthopaedic origin. Joint problems are dealt with in the section on joint disorders (p. 250).

CAUSES

TRAUMATIC

- Fractures
- Dislocations
- Crush injuries

INFLAMMATORY

- Rheumatoid arthritis
- Reiter's disease
- Ankylosing spondylitis

INFECTIVE

- Cellulitis
- Septic arthritis
- Myositis
- Osteomyelitis

DEGENERATIVE

- Osteoarthritis
- Meniscal lesions
- Baker's cyst

VASCULAR

- Intermittent claudication
- Deep venous thrombosis
- Acute arterial occlusion

NEUROLOGICAL

- Sciatica
- Peripheral neuropathy
- Neurogenic claudication

METABOLIC

- Gout

NEOPLASTIC
- Osteogenic sarcoma
- Secondary deposits

OTHER
- Cramp
- Polymyalgia rheumatica
- Strenuous exercise

HISTORY

Traumatic

Obvious history of trauma.

Inflammatory

History of joint swelling, stiffness, limitation of movement. Pain on walking. There may be an obvious history of rheumatoid arthritis with signs elsewhere, e.g. the hands. Reiter's disease – conjunctivitis, urethritis. Ankylosing spondylitis – stiffness of the spine, especially in the morning; hip and knee involvement.

Infective

Cellulitis may arise from puncture wounds, e.g. insect bites, or in a lymphoedematous leg. The patient presents with pain, redness, tenderness, malaise and fever. Myositis may occur in association with collagen diseases, e.g. scleroderma, dermatomyositis. Osteomyelitis is rare but more common in childhood. History of immunosuppression or diabetes. Recent history of infection elsewhere. Pain aggravated by movement. Swelling and redness of the affected area. Septic arthritis presents with a red, hot, tender, painful joint. More common in children. In adults, enquire about a history of steroid therapy or diabetes.

Degenerative

Osteoarthritis presents with pain, stiffness and deformity. The pain is often worse on starting walking and then improves. Baker's cyst presents with a lump behind the knee. The patient may complain of pain and swelling of the calf if the cyst ruptures. With meniscal lesions, there is usually a history of twisting the knee, e.g. playing football. The knee may lock.

Vascular

Deep venous thrombosis presents with painful swelling of the leg. There may be a history of the contraceptive pill, prolonged immobilisation, recent surgery, malignancy. Acute arterial occlusion results in sudden onset of severe pain in the affected limb. The patient is unable to move the leg and complains that the leg feels cold.

With intermittent claudication there is a pain on walking, relieved by rest. It may affect the calf, thigh or buttock. Rest pain in the foot may occur with advanced arterial disease. The pain is often worse in bed at night and the patient obtains relief by hanging the foot out of bed.

Neurological

Pain down the back of the leg (sciatica) often made worse by coughing, movement or straining. The patient may also complain of backache with painful spasm in the back muscles. There are restricted movements of the spine. Neurogenic claudication results from central spinal canal stenosis. Symptoms improve with flexion as this increases the diameter of the canal. Therefore, patients find it easier to cycle than walk and easier to walk upstairs than downstairs. With neurogenic claudication, the claudication distance becomes progressively shorter with each bout of pain during one walk but not with vascular claudication. It also takes the pain of neurogenic claudication longer to settle than the pain of vascular claudication. The two forms of claudication may co-exist, making diagnosis difficult.

Metabolic

Gout presents as acute severe pain with redness and swelling of a joint. There may be a history of previous episodes. History of trauma, surgery, infection, diuretics, polycythaemia, leukaemia, cytotoxic therapy or immunosuppressive therapy.

Neoplastic

Osteogenic sarcoma usually presents in men between 20 and 40 years old. There is usually swelling around the knee, the commonest sites of the tumour being the lower femur or upper tibia. The patient often complains of bone pain, swelling or cough due to lung secondaries. Pain or pathological fractures may be due to secondary deposits. These may occur from the breast, lung, thyroid, prostate or kidney. Check for symptoms related to these or previous surgery for malignancy.

Other

Polymyalgia rheumatica usually occurs in elderly women. There is aching, morning stiffness in proximal muscles and often associated arthritis. Cramp is painful muscle spasm. The patient often complains of severe pain in the legs, especially at night or after exercise. It may occur with salt depletion, myopathy or muscle ischaemia. It is common in chronic renal failure.

EXAMINATION

Traumatic

Pain, loss of function, tenderness, deformity, crepitus, abnormal mobility. Check for associated nerve and vascular injuries.

Inflammatory

Pain in joints, swelling, tenderness, loss of movement, fixed deformities, disturbances of gait. Signs of rheumatoid arthritis elsewhere. Reiter's disease – conjunctivitis, urethritis. Ankylosing spondylitis – stiffness of the spine, reduced thoracic excursion, fixed kyphotic spine, hyperextended neck.

Infective

In acute cellulitis there is redness and tenderness over the affected area. Inguinal lymphadenopathy may be present. With acute osteomyelitis there is tenderness and heat over the site of infection. With myositis there is tenderness and wasting of the muscles. There may be other signs of collagen diseases, e.g. polyarteritis nodosa, SLE, scleroderma or dermatomyositis. In septic arthritis there is a hot, tender, painful, swollen joint and all movements are painful. Surrounding muscle spasm is present.

Degenerative

In osteoarthritis there is deformity, synovial thickening, bony enlargement due to osteophytes, effusion, loss of movement and fixed deformities. Baker's cyst presents as a swelling in the popliteal fossa. If it has ruptured there is pain and swelling of the calf. Meniscal lesions present with swelling of the knee and tenderness over the joint line in the early phase. Later there may be a continued effusion with wasted quadriceps and a positive McMurray sign.

Vascular

Deep vein thrombosis presents with pain, tenderness, swelling and heat, usually over the calf. There is ankle oedema. Homans' sign is positive. With iliofemoral thrombosis there may be phlegmasia alba dolens (white leg) or phlegmasia cerulea dolens (painful blue leg). Acute ischaemia presents with the five Ps: pain, pallor, pulselessness, paraesthesia and paralysis. Check for atrial fibrillation. With intermittent claudication, examine for absent pulses. Buerger's test.

Neoplastic

There is usually a hot, tender swelling around the knee joint in either the lower femur or upper tibia. Examine the chest for lung metastases. With secondary deposits, check the lung, breast, thyroid, prostate and kidney.

Neurological

Lordosis, limited straight leg raising, restricted back movements. Reduced reflexes in the lower limb. Areas of absent sensation.

Metabolic

With gout there will be a tender, red, swollen joint with limitation of movement. Check for gouty tophi elsewhere.

Other

Polymyalgia rheumatica presents with tenderness over muscles and arthritis. Occasionally there is associated giant cell arteritis.

Examine the temporal artery for tenderness. With cramp there may be signs of chronic renal failure.

GENERAL INVESTIGATIONS

- **FBC, ESR**
  Hb ↓ anaemia of chronic disease, e.g. rheumatoid arthritis, collagen disease. WCC ↑ infection, e.g. osteomyelitis, septic arthritis. ESR ↑ inflammation, e.g. rheumatoid arthritis, malignancy, polymyalgia rheumatica.

- **CRP**
  ↑ infection/inflammatory disease.

- **U&Es**
  Chronic renal failure. Renal involvement in collagen disease.

- **LFTs**
  Alkaline phosphatase ↑ in liver secondaries.

- **Rheumatoid factor**
  Rheumatoid arthritis.

- **Blood glucose**
  Diabetes – neuropathy, peripheral vascular disease.

- **Serum uric acid**
  Gout.

- **Local X-rays**
  Fractures. Osteoarthritis. Rheumatoid arthritis. Chronic osteomyelitis. Tumours.

- **Lumbosacral spine X-ray**
  Disc lesions. Osteophytes. Narrowing of joint spaces. Lordosis.

- **CXR**
  Secondary deposits in osteogenic sarcoma.

SPECIFIC INVESTIGATIONS

- **CT**
  Local lesion. Spine, e.g. disc lesion, tumour, neurogenic claudication – narrowing of canal.

- **MRI**
  Spine, disc lesion, tumour.

- **Duplex Doppler**
  DVT. Arterial disease.

- **Arteriography**
  Vascular disease.

- **Venography**
  DVT.

- **Nerve conduction studies**
  Nerve lesions, peripheral neuropathy.

- Always carefully examine the pulses. Vascular disease in the lower limbs is a common condition.

- Acute ischaemia presents with the five Ps. Treatment is urgent.

- Homans' sign is not reliable in DVT. It is positive in most painful conditions of the calf.

- Vague swelling and thickening around the knee joint in 20–40 year olds may be due to osteogenic sarcoma. Refer for X-ray.

LEG SWELLINGS

Swelling of the lower limb may be unilateral or bilateral. Bilateral swellings are usually due to medical conditions such as cardiac, renal or hepatic failure. Unilateral swellings are commonly due to trauma, venous disease or lymphatic disease.

CAUSES

LOCAL

ACUTE SWELLING

- Trauma
- DVT
- Cellulitis
- Rheumatoid arthritis
- Allergy

CHRONIC SWELLING

- Venous
  - Varicose veins
  - Obstruction to venous return, e.g. pregnancy, pelvic tumours, IVC, obstruction, post-phlebitic limb
- Dependency
- Lymphoedema
- Congenital malformations, e.g. arteriovenous fistulae
- Paralysis (failure of muscle pump)

GENERAL

- Congestive cardiac failure
- Hypoproteinaemia, e.g. liver failure, nephrotic syndrome, malnutrition
- Renal failure
- Fluid overload
- Myxoedema

HISTORY

Pain will be associated with trauma, DVT, infection or complications of varicose veins. Other causes of swelling of the lower limb may be painless, although the limb may be uncomfortable if the oedema becomes tense. Evidence of the following should be sought in the past medical history: trauma to the limb, recent pregnancy (DVT), abdominal or pelvic malignancy, previous surgery or radiotherapy to lymph nodes, thyroid disease, congestive cardiac failure, renal failure, liver failure, malnutrition, poliomyelitis in childhood, nerve lesions. With primary lymphoedema the leg may have been swollen since birth or oedema may have developed at puberty (lymphoedema praecox) or in the third decade (lymphoedema tarda).

EXAMINATION

The presence of fracture, contusion or haematoma should be obvious. With cellulitis the limb will be red, swollen, hot and tender. A puncture wound may be visible. DVT may be suspected if the limb is tender and swollen, particularly the calf with a positive Homans' sign, i.e. pain in the calf on dorsiflexion of the foot. Tenderness may be present over the femoral vein with femoral vein thrombosis. The limb may be pale and swollen to the groin (phlegmasia alba dolens) or tense and purplish and extremely painful (phlegmasia cerulea dolens) with iliofemoral thrombosis. Bilateral swelling with dilated collateral veins on the abdominal wall suggests IVC thrombosis. Swelling and tenderness over the joints may suggest rheumatoid arthritis. Lymphoedema pits in the early stages but in the later stage it becomes non-pitting, when the skin and subcutaneous tissue become thick and eventually hyperkeratotic and warty. Previous scars in the groin, a mass of malignant nodes or signs of previous radiotherapy will suggest lymphoedema as a possible cause.

In the presence of an arteriovenous fistula there will be dilated veins which do not collapse on elevation of the limb. The limb will be warmer than the opposite limb; palpation will reveal a thrill and auscultation will reveal a continuous machinery bruit.

Localised swelling of the limb may be due to a tumour. There may also be associated distal swelling due to venous or lymphatic obstruction.

Swelling due to neurological damage, e.g. nerve lesions or poliomyelitis, will result in wasting, which should be apparent. Examination of the abdomen may reveal hepatomegaly or an abdominal mass, which could obstruct the venous outflow. It is appropriate to carry out a rectal examination for a pelvic tumour, which may be causing back pressure on the venous and lymphatic system or may have resulted in a 'frozen' pelvis.

GENERAL INVESTIGATIONS

- **FBC, ESR**
  A large haematoma associated with trauma or fracture may result in a low Hb. WCC ↑ will suggest infection. Haematoma may be associated with a reduced platelet count.

- **Urinalysis**
  Proteinuria may suggest a renal cause.

- **U&Es and creatinine**
  Raised urea and creatinine will be associated with renal failure

- **LFTs**
  May indicate impaired liver function with associated hypoalbuminaemia.
- **Blood glucose**
  Cellulitis or other infections of the leg may be associated with diabetes.
- **CXR**
  Findings suggestive of cardiac failure are cardiomegaly, pulmonary oedema and pleural effusions. Pulmonary oedema may be associated with fluid overload associated with renal failure. Secondary deposits may be seen in association with sarcoma of the limb.
- **Limb X-ray**
  May show fracture, tumour or gas in the tissues associated with gas gangrene.

SPECIFIC INVESTIGATIONS

- **Clotting screen**
  There may be abnormal clotting associated with coagulopathy, resulting in spontaneous haematoma.
- **TFTs**
  Myxoedema
- **US**
  Haematoma or soft-tissue sarcoma.
- **CT**
  Haematoma or tumour.
- **MRI**
  Soft-tissue sarcoma.
- **US or CT pelvis**
  May show an abdominal or pelvic mass causing extrinsic pressure on the veins.
- **Duplex Doppler**
  Will show DVT or arteriovenous fistula.
- **Venography**
  Will confirm DVT.
- **Arteriography**
  Will confirm the presence of an arteriovenous fistula.
- **Lymphangiography**
  May demonstrate the cause of lymphoedema, e.g. hypoplasia or obstruction.
- **Lymph node biopsy**
  Infection or tumour.

- Patients with unexplained DVT may have underlying malignancy. Take a full systematic history.

- In the young patient with unilateral oedema of slow onset, always consider lymphoedema. Lymphoedema does not pit.

LEG ULCERS

An ulcer is a discontinuity of an epithelial surface. Leg ulcers are common and the site of an ulcer on the leg may provide a clue to its aetiology.

CAUSES

INFECTIVE

- Syphilis
- TB
  - (common where TB is endemic)

NEOPLASTIC

- Squamous cell carcinoma
- Malignant melanoma
- Basal cell carcinoma

VASCULAR

- Venous stasis ulcers
- Arterial (ischaemic) ulcers
- Arteriovenous fistulae

NEUROPATHIC

- Diabetes
- Leprosy
- Tabes dorsalis (syphilis)

AUTOIMMUNE/VASCULITIC

- Rheumatoid arthritis
- SLE

HAEMATOLOGICAL

- Sickle cell anaemia
- Polycythaemia rubra vera
- Thrombotic thrombocytopenic purpura

OTHER

- Dermatitis artefacta (self-inflicted)
- Pyoderma gangrenosum

HISTORY

A history of trauma may be apparent. In self-inflicted injury it may not. Pain suggests trauma, ischaemia or infection. Lack of pain suggests a neuropathic cause, e.g. diabetes mellitus or tabes dorsalis. A history of varicose veins or DVT suggests a venous stasis ulcer. A prior history of intermittent claudication suggests ischaemic ulcers, as does a history of atrial fibrillation or subacute bacterial endocarditis (embolic). The presence of a long-standing venous ulcer with recent change in the shape of the ulcer suggests development of a squamous cell carcinoma (Marjolin's ulcer).

A history of rheumatoid arthritis or collagen disease may suggest a vasculitic lesion. A pigmented ulcerating lesion arising at the site of a previous mole or *de novo* may suggest a malignant melanoma, especially if there is a history of prolonged exposure to the sun or sunburn. A history of any haematological conditions should be sought. Pyoderma gangrenosum may occur in association with Crohn's disease or ulcerative colitis.

EXAMINATION

Site

The site of an ulcer may give a clue to the aetiology. Venous stasis ulcers usually occur on the medial aspect of the lower third of the leg, usually over the medial malleolus. Arterial ulcers occur over the metatarsal heads, tips of the toes, lateral aspect of the head of the fifth metatarsal, around the heel, in between the toes, and on the tips of the toes. Diabetic ischaemic ulcers occur at the same sites. Diabetic neuropathic ulcers usually occur at pressure points, e.g. under the heel, under the heads of the first and fifth metatarsals and under the toes. They are often associated with callosities.

Edge

Classically, five types are described. A sloping edge suggests a healing ulcer, e.g. venous stasis ulcer. A punched-out edge suggests an ischaemic ulcer or a syphilitic gummatous ulcer (rare). An undermined edge suggests a tuberculous ulcer (rare). A rolled edge is characteristic of a rodent ulcer, while an everted edge is suggestive of a malignant ulcer, e.g. squamous cell carcinoma.

Base

This may contain slough or granulation tissue. Ischaemic ulcers may contain no granulation tissue but have black necrotic tissue, or tendon or bone visible in the base. Syphilitic ulcers have a classical appearance of slough in the base which resembles a wash leather.

Surrounding tissues

Is the surrounding skin pink and healthy with normal innervation? Are there black satellite lesions associated with malignant melanoma?

Examine the regional lymph nodes for sites of secondary infection or metastases. Examine for varicose veins, changes following DVT, or the absence of pulses and the presence of bruits. Examine the whole patient, e.g. signs of rheumatoid arthritis.

Remember that, although the initial lesion may have been caused by trauma, other abnormalities may be present to prevent healing, e.g. poor circulation, malnutrition or steroid therapy. Ulcers over the shin in elderly women with thin skin may have been due to minor trauma. However, the fact that the skin here is poorly supported on the periosteum of the underlying bone means that they may be extremely slow to heal. Ulcers occurring in inflammatory bowel disease may be due to pyoderma gangrenosum. The ulcers may be multiple and may have started as pustules.

GENERAL INVESTIGATIONS

- **FBC, ESR**
  Hb ↓ suggests haematological disease. WCC ↑ infection. ESR ↑ collagen diseases (vasculitis), syphilis, TB.
- **U&Es**
  Renal involvement may suggest autoimmune disease.
- **Blood glucose**
  Diabetes mellitus.
- **Swab of ulcer**
  C&S.

SPECIFIC INVESTIGATIONS

- **Rheumatoid factor**
  Rheumatoid arthritis.
- **Antibody screen**
  e.g. ANCA (SLE).
- **VDRL**
  Syphilis.
- **Doppler studies**
  Venous disease. Arterial disease.
- **Biopsy**
  Incision biopsy for possible squamous cell carcinoma or diagnosis of the cause of an obscure ulcer. Excision biopsy is required for suspected malignant melanoma.
- **Venography**
  Assess varicose veins. Deep venous patency.
- **Arteriography**
  Assess arterial tree.

- Always carefully describe the ulcer in the notes, especially the edge. Rolled everted edges suggest malignancy.
- Deep ulcers punched out with tendon or periosteum in the base suggest an arterial aetiology.
- Painful ulcers usually have an arterial aetiology.
- Neoplastic change may occur in an existing benign ulcer (Marjolin's ulcer). This is rare.

LIP LESIONS

Lip lesions are common. They may be extremely painful and interfere with speech and feeding. They may be socially embarrassing for the patient. They may also prevent appropriate contact with a partner, leading to emotional problems. In the elderly, carcinoma is a common cause of a lump on the lip, especially in those with outdoor occupations.

CAUSES

CONGENITAL
- Cleft lip (hare lip)

ACQUIRED

FLAT LESIONS
- Junctional naevus
- Peutz–Jeghers syndrome
- Telangiectasia (hereditary haemorrhagic telangiectasia)

RAISED LESIONS
- Mucous retention cysts
- Warts
- Pyogenic granuloma
- Squamous cell carcinoma
- Malignant melanoma
- Syphilitic chancre
- Vascular malformations

EROSIONS
- Herpes simplex
- Impetigo
- Pemphigus

SWELLING
- Trauma, e.g. burns, bites, assault
- Angioneurotic oedema
- Drug reactions
- Crohn's disease

CHEILITIS
- Infection, e.g. candidiasis
- Contact dermatitis, e.g. lipstick, pen-sucking
- Lip-licking (especially in children)

HISTORY

Congenital

Cleft lip occurs due to failure of fusion of the nasal and maxillary processes which form the upper lip and the maxilla. The only abnormality may be a slight indentation in the outer part of the middle third of the upper lip. However, it may extend to the anterior nares. It may be associated with a cleft palate. The condition may be unilateral or bilateral. Abnormal phonation occurs.

Acquired

Flat lesions

Junctional naevi develop at or before puberty. Ensure that there has been no change in a junctional naevus to suggest development of malignant melanoma. In Peutz–Jeghers syndrome pigmentation will be on the gums as well as the lips. There will usually be a family history (autosomal dominant). These pigmented lip lesions do not become malignant. There may be associated history of bowel problems, e.g. bleeding or intussusception. In hereditary telangiectasia, the patient may also have noticed lesions in the mouth and on the skin, especially the fingertips.

Raised lesions

Mucous retention cysts may occur at any age. The patient complains of a lump on the inner aspect of the lip which interferes with eating. With warts, pyogenic granuloma and squamous cell carcinoma, the patient's only complaint is usually of a lump on the lip. With carcinoma, there may be a history of leucoplakia, betel-nut chewing or pipe smoking. Classically it used to relate to clay-pipe smoking. There may also be a history of exposure to sunlight, and carcinoma is common in outdoor workers, e.g. sailors, farmers, fisherman and fair-skinned people in sunny climates. Ulcerating and bleeding of the lesion may be a presenting complaint. Syphilitic lesions are now extremely rare. A primary chancre may present on the lip. They are highly contagious. A gummatous lesion on the lip is extremely rare. Malignant melanoma may present as a black, ulcerating or raised lesion at the site of a junctional naevus.

Erosions

The commonest are herpes simplex lesions. Small painful ulcers, which itch, may present on the lips. They are common in immunocompromised patients. Impetigo is common around the mouth and face of children but may affect any age. Pemphigus is a blistering disorder which affects the mucosa and skin.

Swelling

Swelling of the lips may be due to a variety of causes. Trauma is probably the most common, usually following assault, but may arise as a result of burns (hot fluids), sun rays or angioneurotic oedema, which is rare and may affect the tongue and other parts of the body. Drug reactions may cause oedema when associated with urticaria. They usually affect the whole face rather than just the lips. Crohn's disease may also cause swelling of the lips. Other symptoms and signs of Crohn's disease, e.g. diarrhoea, abdominal pain or perianal sepsis, may be present.

Cheilitis

This usually refers to inflammation of the lips and may occur at the angles of the mouth, i.e. angular cheilitis or angular stomatitis. Contact dermatitis may be apparent from either lipstick or pen-sucking. A history of lip-licking should be sought, especially in children. *Candida* may cause cheilitis in the immunocompromised, infants, those with dentures, and those with iron-deficiency anaemia.

EXAMINATION

Congenital

Cleft lip is obvious at birth. Cleft palate is discovered on routine inspection soon after birth or may be discovered when difficulties occur with feeding. Beware missing a submucous cleft in which the palate initially appears intact. Late presentation may occur with speech and hearing difficulties.

Acquired

Flat lesions

Junctional naevi are flat, pigmented lesions. The lesions of Peutz–Jeghers syndrome are also flat lesions but, in addition to occurring on the lips, occur also on the gums. In hereditary telangiectasia, telangiectasia may also be present in the mouth, on the palate and on the skin, especially the fingertips.

Raised lesions

Mucous retention cysts tend to occur on the inner aspects of the lips. They are generally pale pink with a grey glairy appearance when the cyst contents show through the stretched overlying mucosa. They are usually smooth, well localised and rarely get bigger than 2 cm in diameter. A warty lesion is usually obvious, with a rough hyperkeratotic surface. Warts may be pedunculated. A pyogenic granuloma is a firm, small, cherry-red nodule consisting of hyperplastic granulation tissue. A squamous cell carcinoma is usually a hard ulcerated lesion with a raised everted edge. The regional lymph nodes may be palpable due to metastases. Malignant melanoma may arise *de novo* or in a pre-existing junctional naevus. The lesion is usually raised, pigmented, occasionally friable and bleeds easily. There may be satellite nodules and regional nodes may be palpable due to metastases. Syphilitic lesions are rare nowadays. A chancre associated with primary syphilis may occur on the lips. The initial lesion is elevated, flat, hard and painless. Eventually, however, ulceration may occur, to give a slightly painful ulcer which crusts over. The regional lymph nodes become enlarged and tender, usually 7–10 days after the appearance of the chancre.

Erosions

Herpetic lesions begin as a patch of painful, itchy erythema. Vesicles form subsequently, which dry up and crust over after 4–5 days, the crust eventually separating, leaving tiny scars. Impetigo causes golden-coloured crusts, usually on the faces of children. In pemphigus, blisters erode quickly and become painful erosions on the mucous membrane and skin.

Swellings and cheilitis

These are usually diagnosed from the history. They usually cause reddening and inflammation of the lips.

GENERAL INVESTIGATIONS

- **FBC, ESR**
  Hb ↓ iron-deficiency anaemia (associated with cheilitis). WCC ↑ infection. WCC ↓ immunosuppression. ESR ↑ Crohn's disease, syphilis, malignancy.

- **Swab**
  C&S. Dark-ground illumination of fluid from syphilitic chancre (spirochaetes visible).

SPECIFIC INVESTIGATIONS

- **VDRL**
  Syphilis.

- **Biopsy**
  Benign versus malignant. Pyogenic granuloma. Squamous cell carcinoma. Malignant melanoma (excision biopsy). Crohn's disease.

- **FNAC**
  May be diagnostic when lymph node enlargement is associated with lip lesion.

- **Gastroscopy**
  Peutz–Jeghers Syndrome. Mucosal lesions.

- **Colonoscopy**
  Peutz–Jeghers Syndrome. Mucosal lesions.

- Ulcers on the lips in the elderly are likely to be malignant. Biopsy is indicated.
- Recurrent herpetic lesions suggest an immunosuppressed state. Further investigation is necessary.

LYMPHADENOPATHY

Lymphadenopathy is a common presenting condition. It may be localised or generalised. The causes are multiple but a careful history and clinical examination will often simplify the diagnosis. Lymphadenopathy, especially cervical, is extremely common in children who are otherwise healthy. Painful tender nodes are usually associated with infection. Firm or hard, painless nodes are commonly the seat of malignancy. Only the commoner causes, which the student would be expected to know, are described in this section.

CAUSES

PRIMARY INFECTION

VIRAL
- Infectious mononucleosis
- HIV
- CMV
- Rubella
- Measles

BACTERIAL
- TB
  - (common in some parts of the world where TB is endemic)
- Syphilis
- Brucellosis
- Cat scratch disease
- Septicaemia

PROTOZOAL
- Toxoplasmosis

PARASITIC
- Filariasis
  - (common in tropical regions of Asia, Africa)

SECONDARY INFECTION

- e.g. tonsillitis with cervical lymphadenitis, abscess with regional lymphadenitis

PRIMARY MALIGNANCY

- Acute lymphoblastic leukaemia
- Chronic lymphatic leukaemia
- Hodgkin's disease

- Non-Hodgkin's lymphoma
- Myeloproliferative disorders

SECONDARY MALIGNANCY

- Metastases from local malignancy
- Metastases from distant malignancy

OTHERS

- Sarcoidosis
- SLE
- Rheumatoid arthritis

HISTORY

Infection

Local infections will be usually obvious, e.g. dental abscess with cervical lymphadenopathy. With generalised lymphadenopathy there may be a history of malaise, lethargy and fever. Check for exposure to TB, which may be a cause of lymphadenopathy in the immunocompromised patient. Check for visits abroad. Check if there are animals in the household, e.g. cats (cat scratch fever) or dogs (toxoplasmosis). In the case of cat scratch fever the scratches are often healed before the patient presents. Note any history of local trauma.

Primary malignancy

There will normally be a history of malaise, fever or night sweats. The patient may have noticed lumps at several sites. Spontaneous bruising and bleeding associated with thrombocytopenia may also be present.

Secondary malignancy

The primary may be obvious or may be very small and have not been noticed by the patient (e.g. a malignant melanoma in an inaccessible site). There may be a history of malignancy that has been treated several years previously with metastases presenting late (e.g. axillary lymphadenopathy or cervical lymphadenopathy occurring several years after an apparently curative operation for carcinoma of the breast). Occasionally the lymph node swelling is distant from the primary, e.g. cervical lymphadenopathy (left supraclavicular fossa) from testicular cancer; Virchow's node in gastric cancer.

Other conditions

Sarcoidosis causes bilateral hilar lymphadenopathy but may present with lymphadenopathy at other sites. Check for a history of SLE or rheumatoid arthritis.

EXAMINATION

Examine the enlarged lymph nodes. Are they painful and tender, suggesting infection, or are they firm and painless, suggesting malignancy? Check the sites draining to these nodes for a site of infection or primary malignancy. Check for linear scratches suggestive of cat scratch disease. Examine for bruising. Examine all other sites of potential lymphadenopathy: cervical, axillary, inguinal, popliteal and epitrochlear nodes. Check for splenomegaly and hepatomegaly. Carry out a full general examination.

GENERAL INVESTIGATIONS

- **FBC, ESR**
  Hb ↓ blood dyscrasias. Platelets ↓ dyscrasias. WCC ↑ infection, leukaemia. ESR ↑ tumour, infection. Blood film. Leukaemia.

- **LFTs**
  Malignant infiltration of the liver.

- **Clotting screen**
  Blood dyscrasias.

- **Viral titres**
  Viral infections, e.g. EBV, HIV.

- **CXR**
  Hilar glands in sarcoidosis. TB. Secondary deposits.

- **Mantoux test**
  TB.

- **Swab**
  Local infection. C&S.

SPECIFIC INVESTIGATIONS

- **Antibody screen**
  SLE, rheumatoid arthritis.

- **Blood film**
  Filiariasis.

- **Blood cultures**
  Septicaemia.

- **VDRL**
  Syphilis.

- **Kveim test**
  Sarcoidosis.

- **Toxoplasma screen**
  Toxoplasmosis.

- **PCR**
  Filiariasis
- **OGD**
  Virchow's node with gastrointestinal malignancy.
- **CT**
  Nodal distribution. Staging of Hodgkin's disease.
- **FNAC of lymph node**
  Malignancy versus other conditions.
- **Biopsy**
  Lymph node, e.g. Hodgkin's disease, secondary deposit. Biopsy of local lesion, e.g. infective versus malignant.

- **An enlarged left supraclavicular lymph node in a patient with weight loss suggests gastrointestinal malignancy.**
- **Persistent generalised lymphadenopathy with night sweats suggests lymphoma or AIDS.**
- **Persistent cervical lymphadenopathy in the older patient suggests malignancy and, in the absence of an obvious cause, an ENT assessment is required.**
- **A solitary left supraclavicular node in a young male should prompt examination of the testes.**

MELAENA

Melaena is the passage of altered blood PR. A melaena stool is black and tarry and has a characteristic smell. The blood is degraded by hydrochloric acid and intestinal enzymes high in the gastrointestinal tract. Melaena is unlikely to occur if bleeding comes from lower than the jejunum, although occasionally melaena may result from a bleeding Meckel's diverticulum.

CAUSES

SWALLOWED BLOOD

- Epistaxis
- Haemoptysis

OESOPHAGUS

- Reflux oesophagitis
- Oesophageal varices
- Oesophageal carcinoma

STOMACH

- Peptic ulceration
- Acute gastric erosions
- Mallory–Weiss syndrome
- Carcinoma
- Leiomyoma (gastro-intestinal stromal tumour – GIST)
- Hereditary haemorrhagic telangiectasia
- Vascular malformations

DUODENUM

- Peptic ulceration
- Duodenal diverticulae
- Aortoduodenal fistulae
- Invasive pancreatic tumours
- Haemobilia

SMALL INTESTINE

- Leiomyoma (gastro-intestinal stromal tumour – GIST)
- Meckel's diverticulum

BLEEDING DISORDERS

- Liver disease-associated

- Thrombocytopenia
- Haemophilia

DRUGS

- Anticoagulants
- Aspirin
- NSAIDs
- Steroids

OTHERS

- Uraemia
- Connective tissue disorders

OTHER CAUSES OF DARK STOOLS

- Iron therapy
- Bismuth preparations
- Liquorice
- Charcoal biscuits
- Red wine (large quantities)

HISTORY

Swallowed blood

Check for a recent history of epistaxis or haemoptysis.

Oesophagus

There may be a history of excess alcohol consumption or a history of other liver disease to suggest oesophageal varices. Check for retrosternal burning pain and heartburn, which would suggest oesophagitis. Check for a history of dysphagia. The bleeding associated with varices is often torrential. That associated with oesophagitis is minor.

Stomach

History of epigastric pain to suggest peptic ulceration. There may be a history of steroid or NSAID medication. Mallory–Weiss syndrome usually occurs in the younger patient who has had a large meal with much alcohol and has a forceful vomit. The first vomit contains food, the second contains blood. Acute gastric erosions may occur with stressful illnesses, e.g. major surgery, acute pancreatitis, burns (Curling's ulcer), head injuries (Cushing's ulcer). It is unusual to get a large bleed with a carcinoma. Anaemia is a common presentation, and there may be 'coffee ground' vomit. Leiomyoma causes a moderate haematemesis.

There is usually no preceding history. There will also be no preceding history with vascular malformations. Hereditary haemorrhagic telangiectasia is rare. The patient may present with a history of the condition, or it may be apparent from the telangiectasia around the lips and oral cavity.

Duodenum

Melaena tends to be a more common symptom than haematemesis with duodenal lesions. There may be a history of chronic duodenal ulceration, although often presentation may be acute with little background history. Bleeding from invasive pancreatic tumours is rare. The patient will present with malaise, lethargy, weight loss and vomiting. Haemobilia is rare. Aortoduodenal fistula is rare and usually follows repair of an aneurysm with subsequent infection of the graft. There is massive haematemesis and malaise.

Small intestine

Leiomyomas are rare but may bleed, resulting in melaena. Bleeding from a Meckel's diverticulum, if it occurs fast enough, usually causes dark-red bleeding rather than characteristic melaena.

Other causes of dark stools

Take a full dietary and drug history.

EXAMINATION

Depending upon the severity of the bleed, there may be shock. The patient will be cold, clammy, with peripheral vasoconstriction; there will be a tachycardia and hypotension.

Swallowed blood

Check for blood around the nose. Examine the chest for a possible cause of haemoptysis.

Oesophagus

There may be little to find on examination except clinical signs of anaemia and weight loss unless the cause is oesophageal varices, in which case there may be jaundice, abdominal distension due to ascites, spider naevi, liver palms, clubbing, gynaecomastia, testicular atrophy, caput medusae, splenomegaly or hepatomegaly.

Stomach

There may be little to find on examination. There may be an epigastric mass with a carcinoma, or a palpable left supraclavicular node (Virchow's nodes). There may be epigastric tenderness. With hereditary haemorrhagic telangiectasia there may be telangiectasia on the lips and mucous membrane of the mouth.

Duodenum

Again, there may be little to find on examination other than epigastric tenderness. In the rare case where duodenal bleeding comes from an invasive pancreatic carcinoma, there may be a palpable mass in the region of the pancreas.

Small intestine

Often there is little to find. Leiomyomas may be palpable.

Bleeding disorders

There may be sites of bruising or bleeding from other orifices.

GENERAL INVESTIGATIONS

- **FBC, ESR**
  Hb ↓ anaemia due to chronic bleeding, e.g. from carcinoma. ESR ↑ connective tissue disease.

- **U&Es**
  Urea and creatinine will be raised in uraemia. Urea may be raised due to absorption of blood from the bowel.

- **LFTs**
  Liver failure, oesophageal varices, haemobilia.

- **Clotting screen**
  Liver disease. Bleeding diatheses. Anticoagulants.

SPECIFIC INVESTIGATIONS

- **OGD**
  Will demonstrate most lesions, e.g. varices, oesophagitis, peptic ulcer, gastric erosions, Mallory–Weiss tear, carcinoma and rarer causes of bleeding. Biopsy may be carried out where necessary.

- **Angiography**
  Vascular malformations. Also may diagnose rarer distal duodenal causes, e.g. aortoduodenal fistulae.

- **Technetium scan**
  Meckel's diverticulum containing gastric mucosa.

- **Labelled red cell scan**
  Rare small bowel causes of bleeding.

- **Small bowel enema**
  Leiomyoma. Meckel's diverticulum

- Melaena is altered blood PR. It is black and tarry and has a characteristic smell. Take care to distinguish it from rectal bleeding, which is either bright red or dark red and free from odour.

- Melaena is unlikely to occur if bleeding comes from lower down than the jejunum, although occasionally melaena may result from a bleeding Meckel's diverticulum.

MOUTH ULCERS

Ulceration in the mouth is common. It is important to be able to distinguish between simple benign ulcers, e.g. traumatic or aphthous, and those that are malignant. Tongue lesions are dealt with on p. 446.

CAUSES

- Traumatic
- Aphthous

INFLAMMATORY

- Crohn's disease

INFECTIVE

BACTERIAL
- Acute ulcerative gingivitis (Vincent's angina)
- Syphilis

VIRAL
- Herpes simplex

FUNGAL
- Candidiasis

NEOPLASTIC

- Squamous cell carcinoma
- Haematological disorders
- Agranulocytosis

SKIN DISEASE-ASSOCIATED

- Lichen planus
- Pemphigus
- Pemphigoid
- Bullous erythema multiforme

CONNECTIVE TISSUE DISEASE

- SLE

OTHER

- Behçet's syndrome
- Reiter's disease

HISTORY

Traumatic

Diagnosis usually obvious, such as ill-fitting dentures or sharp teeth and ulcers heal when precipitating cause is removed.

Aphthous

Patient presents with small, painful ulcers, usually inside the cheeks or lips. They heal in about 1 week but others may occur while the initial ulcers are healing. A number of patients will have a history of gastrointestinal disease, e.g. coeliac disease or Crohn's disease. They may also arise in patients with debilitating disease.

Inflammatory

Chronic granulomatous disease (Crohn's) may affect the oral cavity. The patient may complain of painful ulcers, swelling of the lips or gum swelling.

Infective

Vincent's angina (acute ulcerative stomatitis) presents with swollen gums with small ulcers, which may spread to the buccal mucosa. The patient will complain of bleeding gums, together with constitutional upset with fever and malaise. Syphilis is now rarely seen but chancres, snail-track ulcers and gummas may occur within the mouth. *Candida* is not uncommon in the oral cavity. There may be a history of debilitating disease, diabetes or immunosuppressive therapy. Herpes simplex presents as painful vesicles, which ulcerate. The patient may be immunocompromised. Herpes zoster may occur on the palate in the distribution of the maxillary division of the trigeminal nerve. There will be severe pain and ulceration.

Neoplastic

Squamous cell carcinomas occur as ulcers with hard edges, which bleed. They tend to occur in the older patient. There may be a history of leucoplakia or the six Ss: syphilis, smoking, sharp tooth, spirits, spices, sepsis.

Haematological disorders

Agranulocytosis may be due to drugs or marrow infiltration. Take a careful drug history. The ulceration may be due to bacterial infection consequent on the low WCC. Leukaemia may also present with mouth ulcers.

Skin disease-associated

These include lichen planus, pemphigus pemphigoid and bullous erythema multiforme. The reader is referred to a textbook of dermatology for the characteristics of these conditions.

Connective tissue disease

Oral ulceration may be associated with SLE. The patient may present with other features of this disease, e.g. skin lesions, joint pains or renal failure.

Other

Although Behçet's disease may present with mouth ulcers, the patient may also complain of arthritis, eye disease, scrotal or labial ulcers. With Reiter's disease the patient will complain also of urethritis, conjunctivitis and arthritis. There will usually be a history of sexual contact.

EXAMINATION

Traumatic

There will be ulceration related to ill-fitting dentures or sharp teeth. Observe for healing when the precipitating cause has been removed.

Aphthous

Small, white, circular, deep, painful ulcers with surrounding erythema. There may be signs and symptoms of gastrointestinal disease or other debilitating disease, or they may occur in otherwise healthy patients.

Inflammatory

With Crohn's disease, there may be lip swelling, nodular thickening of the buccal mucosa, diffuse granular gingival swelling or painful linea oral ulcers.

Infective

Vincent's angina presents with red, swollen, bleeding gums covered with yellowish ulcers. The ulcers may also be seen on the buccal mucosa and occasionally on the tonsils. There is usually tender lymphadenopathy. With syphilis there may be a chancre, snail-track ulcers or gummas. Herpes simplex presents with small 2-mm vesicles which ulcerate and coalesce and produce erosions with surrounding erythema. Herpes zoster shows small ulcers surrounded with erythema in the distribution of the maxillary nerve on the palate. There will usually be skin lesions in the distribution of the nerve. Candidiasis appears as red patches on the buccal mucosa, which are covered with white patches of desquamated epithelium mixed with fungus.

Neoplastic

There will be an ulcer with hard, everted edges which bleeds on touching. Cervical lymphadenopathy may be present.

Haematological disorders

These present with bleeding gums and ulceration.

Skin disease-associated

The reader is referred to a textbook of dermatology for the characteristic features of these.

Connective tissue disorders

Oral ulceration may occur with SLE. Other features may be present on examination, e.g. skin, joint or renal disease.

Other

Behçet's disease presents with painful ulcers. Other features may be apparent on examination, e.g. arthritis, keratitis, iritis, scrotal or labial ulcers. With Reiter's syndrome there will be urethritis, conjunctivitis and balanitis, as well as mouth ulcers.

GENERAL INVESTIGATIONS

- **FBC, ESR**
  Hb ↓ malignancy, debilitating disease. WCC ↑ infection, leukaemia. ESR ↑ malignancy, connective tissue disease, chronic infection, e.g. syphilis.

- **U&Es**
  Renal disease – SLE.

- **Swab**
  C&S. Infections – *Borrelia vincentii* (Vincent's angina), candidiasis.

- **Antibody screen**
  SLE – ANA positive. Anti-double-stranded DNA ↑.

- **VDRL**
  Syphilis.

- **Viral antibodies**
  Herpes simplex. Herpes zoster.

- **Biopsy**
  Squamous cell carcinoma. Crohn's disease.

- A solitary persistent and often painless ulcer which feels hard to the touch is likely to be malignant. Urgent referral is required.

- Enquire about change in bowel habit. Mouth ulcers may be associated with inflammatory bowel disease.

- Mouth ulcers may be associated with vitamin and iron deficiency. Check for associated glossitis and angular cheilitis.

- Medication, e.g. carbimazole, may be associated with agranulocytosis. Oral ulceration may be the first sign.

MUSCLE WEAKNESS AND WASTING

Muscle weakness and wasting may be caused by a variety of conditions both systemic and those confined to muscles. Subjective weakness is common and may not indicate significant illness.

CAUSES

LOCALISED

- Peripheral nerve lesions
  - Peripheral nerve compression
  - Motor neuropathy
  - Peripheral nerve transection
- Disuse atrophy
- Anterior horn cell lesions
  - Previous poliomyelitis
    - (common in developing countries)

GENERALISED

NUTRITIONAL DEFICIENCY
- Vitamin D deficiency

SYSTEMIC DISEASE
- Malignancy
- Cardiac and/or respiratory cachexia
- Thyrotoxicosis
- Sarcoidosis
- Guillain–Barré syndrome
- Cushing's disease
- Addison's disease

MUSCLE AND MOTOR END PLATE DISORDERS
- Myasthenia gravis
- Muscular dystrophies
- Motor neurone disease
- Myotonic dystrophy
- Polymyositis/Dermatomyositis/Inclusion body myositis

DRUGS AND TOXINS
- Alcohol
- Statins
- Steroids
- Ciclosporin

HISTORY

Onset

Muscle weakness and wasting in childhood is often due to congenital disease such as inherited muscular dystrophies (e.g. Duchenne's muscular dystrophy), a diagnosis further supported by a positive family history of a first-degree relative with similar problems. With myotonic dystrophy, first symptoms occur around the age of 15–30 years, while with motor neurone disease the peak age of onset is in the 50s.

Site

The distribution of muscle wasting may characterise the disease. Atrophy may be confined to the motor supply of a single nerve, such as the thenar eminence with the median nerve affected by carpal tunnel syndrome. It may also occur with a group of muscles such as the leg with polio. And finally the distribution may be generalised in conditions such as motor neurone disease. Distal weakness ascending to involve proximal muscles is characteristic of Guillain–Barré syndrome.

Precipitating factors

Precipitating factors such as trauma may result in transection of a peripheral nerve such as the ulnar nerve, commonly at the wrist.

Past medical history

The presence of carcinoma or chronic cardiorespiratory disease may give rise to peripheral muscle wasting from cachexia. Previous infection with polio is significant because, in a minority of affected individuals, degeneration of anterior horn cells with subsequent paralysis and muscle wasting occurs (post-polio syndrome). Disuse atrophy can be localised or generalised. Conditions that result in immobility such as a long-bone fracture will cause disuse atrophy of the surrounding muscles; this is commonly seen upon removal of plaster casts. Localised disuse atrophy may also result from joint pains such as quadriceps wasting with painful knee disorders. Prolonged immobility will result in generalised muscle wasting. Conditions such as diabetes and renal failure are associated with neuropathy. Poor diet and lack of sun exposure may lead to vitamin D deficiency.

Associated symptoms

Most of the causes are associated with weakness of the affected muscles. Diplopia, ptosis and fatiguability are associated features suggestive of myasthenia gravis. Motor neurone disease may present with progressive weakness and wasting of the hand or leg accompanied with dysarthria and dysphasia. Cushing's disease may be associated with weight gain, hair growth, acne, abdominal striae, muscle weakness, back pain and depression.

EXAMINATION

Inspection will identify the areas of muscle wasting. Central obesity with limb wasting occurs with Cushing's disease. Generalised uniform muscle wasting should lead to a careful examination of the organ systems for malignancy and organ failure. Muscle tenderness may occur with polymyositis.

Characteristic features of myotonic dystrophy are frontal balding, ptosis, temporal and facial muscle wasting. Cataracts may be seen with inspection of the eyes. Ptosis may also be a feature of myasthenia gravis; this is accompanied by diplopia, facial weakness and a weak nasal voice. Muscle wasting with fasciculations occurs with motor neurone disease, no sensory loss is experienced and mixed upper and lower motor neurone signs may be present.

Assessment of tone, reflexes and pattern of weakness will determine whether it is an upper or lower motor neurone lesion. Delayed relaxation of muscle contraction occurs with myotonic dystrophy and proximal muscle weakness occurs with Cushing's disease. With localised muscle wasting, examination of each muscle will allow you to determine whether the lesion arises from a single nerve or a nerve root. Weakness, areflexia and sensory loss is seen with Guillain–Barré syndrome.

The joint surrounded by wasted muscles should be examined for deformity or pain that may restrict movement. Measurements of circumference can be obtained to assess asymmetrical muscle wasting of the limbs.

Proximal muscle weakness may be more evident than distal weakness in many of the conditions listed. Specific assessment for this, such as rising from a low chair or from a squatting position, is required.

GENERAL INVESTIGATIONS

- **FBC**
  Anaemia with nutritional disorders and chronic disease.
- **ESR and CRP**
  ↑ with malignancy, polymyositis.
- **U&Es**
  ↑ urea and ↑ creatinine with renal failure.
- **Glucose**
  ↑ with diabetes.
- **LFTs**
  ↓ Albumin with malnutrition.
- **Creatine phosphokinase**
  ↑ with myopathies.
- **TFTs**
  ↓ TSH ↑ T_4 with thyrotoxicosis.

- **Vitamin D**
  Low in osteomalacia.

- **EMG**
  Allows assessment for denervation of muscle, myopathies and myotonic dystrophy, motor neurone disease.

- **Nerve conduction studies**
  Radiculopathies, peripheral neuropathy, peripheral nerve compression, motor neurone disease.

SPECIFIC INVESTIGATIONS

- **Tensilon test**
  Injection of edrophonium reverses symptoms of myasthenia gravis.

- **MRI**
  May reveal areas of abnormal muscle in myositis.

- **Lumbar puncture**
  Elevated protein in Guillain–Barré syndrome.

- **Muscle biopsy**
  Diagnosis of muscle dystrophies and the various myositides.

- **A patient presenting with rapid onset muscle weakness requires an urgent full assessment, as respiratory muscle involvement may lead to respiratory failure.**

NAIL ABNORMALITIES

Nail abnormalities are common and can give invaluable clues to underlying systemic illness. Clubbing is dealt with in a separate section (p. 62).

CAUSES

CONGENITAL

- Epidermolysis bullosa

ACQUIRED

INFECTIONS

- Fungal infection (onychomycosis)
- Chronic paronychia

TRAUMATIC

- Nail biting
- Nail bed trauma

SYSTEMIC ILLNESS

- Severe systemic illness (Beau's lines)
- Iron deficiency anaemia (koilonychia)
- Chronic liver disease (leuconychia)
- Diabetes mellitus (leuconychia)
- Psoriatic arthritis
- Plummer–Vinson syndrome (koilonychia)

DERMATOLOGICAL

- Psoriasis
- Eczema

OTHER

- Onychogryphosis
- Raynaud's syndrome
- Autoimmune disease
- Yellow nail syndrome

HISTORY

Congenital

A history of severe skin disease from birth will be apparent with epidermolysis bullosa.

Acquired

Infections

A history of discoloration of the nail will be present with chronic fungal infections. Chronic paronychia leads to pain, swelling and tenderness in the area of the nailfold.

Traumatic

A history of severe or recurrent damage to the nail may be present. Enquiry as to whether the patient is a nail-biter is important.

Systemic illness

The patient must be asked about severe illness of any description as this may have led to trophic nail changes with transverse ridges (Beau's lines), which may occur up to 3 months following the insult. Symptoms of joint pain, stiffness and swelling will be present with psoriatic arthritis. In iron deficiency anaemia patients often describe lethargy, shortness of breath and/or chest pain on minimal exertion. Frank blood loss (haematemesis, melaena) will usually be volunteered by the patient; however, history of dyspepsia or vague upper abdominal pain may be a clue to occult blood loss. Plummer–Vinson syndrome occurs in middle-aged women. It is an iron deficiency anaemia associated with koilonychia, a smooth tongue and dysphagia. A history for the possible causes of chronic liver disease should be sought such as alcohol abuse or hepatitis. Symptoms of polyuria, polydipsia and lethargy suggest diabetes mellitus.

Dermatological

The scaly rash of psoriasis is classically found on the knees, elbows and scalp; however, lesions may be described in the external meatus, umbilicus, glans penis and natal cleft. An eczematous rash may be present diffusely and is often itchy.

Other

Onychogryphosis is a 'ram's horn' deformity of the nail. It usually affects the great toenail. The nail thickens and curls over as it grows. Common in the elderly, it may follow trauma to the nail in the younger patient. The nail is greatly deformed and difficult to cut. In autoimmune disease the patient may describe hair loss in alopecia areata and sclerodactyly in systemic sclerosis. In classic Raynaud's phenomenon the fingers turn white, blue, then red upon exposure to cold environments. In yellow nail syndrome, the nails are typically slow growing with yellow discoloration. It is associated with lymphoedema, pleural effusions and in some cases bronchiectasis and chronic sinusitis.

EXAMINATION

Congenital

Severe skin disease will be apparent with epidermolysis bullosa.

Acquired

Infections

A discolored, thick and possibly malformed nail will be seen with chronic fungal infections. A swollen, red, tender nailfold will be present with chronic paronychia.

Traumatic

A malformed nail will be seen. Severe nail-biters will have nails bitten back to the nailbed.

Systemic illness

Swollen deformed joints may be seen with psoriatic arthritis. Check for associated psoriatic plaques. If the patient suffered from severe systemic illness this may have resolved; however, trophic nail changes may be seen following this. In iron deficiency anaemia pallor, angular cheilitis and spoon-shaped nails (koilonychia) may be present. Features of chronic liver disease might be present along with leuconychia. Leuconychia may also be seen with diabetes.

Dermatological

Scaly, silvery plaques of psoriasis will be seen, which may be localised or diffuse. Eczema may also be present either as localised or diffuse lesions.

Other

A grossly deformed, usually great, toenail will be seen with onychogryphosis. The nail thickens and curls over as it grows. Distal finger atrophic changes may be seen following long-standing Raynaud's phenomenon. In yellow nail syndrome the nails are typically slow growing with yellow discoloration. Lymphoedema usually affects the lower limb. Examine the chest for signs of bronchiectasis and pleural effusions. Abdominal examination may reveal ascites.

GENERAL INVESTIGATIONS

The diagnosis of most nail abnormalities is made on clinical examination alone.

- **FBC**
  ↓ Hb, ↓ MCV, ↓ MCHC.
- **Blood film**
  Microcytic RBCs in iron deficiency.
- **Serum iron and TIBC**
  ↓ serum iron, ↑ TIBC with iron deficiency.
- **Serum ferritin**
  ↓ iron deficiency anaemia.

- **Blood glucose**
  Diabetes.
- **LFTs**
  Cirrhosis.
- **Urinalysis**
  Diabetes.

SPECIFIC INVESTIGATIONS

- **Nail clippings**
  Fungal infections.
- **Skin biopsy**
  Psoriasis, eczema.
- **Hand X-rays**
  Psoriatic arthritis.
- **CXR**
  Chest abnormalities with yellow nail syndrome,
  e.g. bronchiectasis, pleural effusion.
- **ANA**
  Systemic sclerosis.

- Always examine the nails. It may be necessary to ask female patients to remove nail varnish.
- It may be difficult to differentiate between psoriatic nail dystrophy and fungal infections. Always confirm the diagnosis with nail clippings before starting a patient on a lengthy course of anti-fungal treatment.

NASAL DISCHARGE

Nasal discharges are common. The most frequent causes are the common cold and allergic rhinitis. Persistent bloodstained nasal discharge is a serious symptom requiring urgent investigation.

CAUSES

CONGENITAL
- Choanal atresia

ACQUIRED

INFECTIVE
- Common cold (coryza)
- Chronic rhinitis
- Sinusitis
- Adenoiditis (large adenoids)
- Viral infections
- Chronic infection
- Fungal infections
- Syphilis
- AIDS
  - (common in certain developing countries)

ALLERGIC
- Allergic rhinitis

INFLAMMATORY
- Nasal polyps
- Non-eosinophilic vasomotor rhinitis
- Eosinophilic vasomotor rhinitis

NEOPLASTIC
- Carcinoma
  - Nasopharynx
    - (common in South-East Asia)
  - Sinuses
- Lymphoma (malignant granuloma)

GRANULOMATOUS DISEASE
- Wegener's granulomatosis
- Churg–Strauss syndrome

TRAUMATIC
- Foreign body

- Fracture of the anterior fossa
- Irritant gases, e.g. chlorine, tobacco smoke

DEGENERATIVE
- Senile rhinorrhoea

HISTORY

Congenital

Choanal atresia is rare. Check for other congenital abnormalities. Bilateral choanal atresia is a life-threatening condition in newborn infants. Unilateral atresia may not be picked up until 5–10 years of age, when it becomes apparent that one nostril is blocked and there is a thick mucus discharge.

Acquired
Infective

The patient will often have a common cold. There is a mucoid nasal discharge, which settles rapidly once the cold has settled. With chronic rhinitis there may be a chronic purulent discharge. This is often thick and mucoid. There may be a history of immunological deficiency or cystic fibrosis. With sinusitis there may be pain or discomfort over the maxillary sinuses or a headache with pain over the frontal sinuses. With large adenoids there may be a complaint of mouth breathing, recurrent pharyngeal infections, snoring and recurrent ear infections. Fungal infections of the nose are rare, occurring in immunosuppressed patients. *Candida albicans* and *Aspergillus* spp are the most common organisms. Chronic infective lesions include syphilis. Secondary syphilis can affect the nose and cause a catarrhal rhinitis. Usually other lesions of syphilis will be present. AIDS may be associated with a watery nasal discharge. Check for HIV risk factors. Other symptoms of AIDS may be present.

Allergic

Allergic rhinitis   There may be a history of infantile eczema, allergic asthma or nasal or conjunctival allergy. It may be seasonal with allergy to pollen or perennial with exposure to animal dander (cats) or house-dust mites. The patient complains of watery rhinorrhoea, sneezing attacks, nasal obstruction, and conjunctival irritation and lacrimation. There is usually a family history.

Inflammatory

Vasomotor rhinitis   Eosinophilic vasomotor rhinitis presents with a watery nasal discharge and sneezing. No type I allergic reaction is involved in this condition. The condition is associated with nasal polyps and aspirin sensitivity and asthma.

Nasal polyps These occur in non-allergic eosinophilic vasomotor rhinitis. The patient will complain of nasal obstruction and discharge.

Non-eosinophilic vasomotor rhinitis The patient presents with watery nasal discharge, nasal obstruction and sneezing attacks. This condition may be associated with: (1) certain antihypertensive drugs, particularly ganglion blockers and vasodilators; (2) hormonal disturbances; (3) congestive cardiac failure; (4) anxiety states; (5) occupational irritants, e.g. ammonia, smoke.

Neoplastic

Nasopharyngeal carcinoma Nasopharyngeal carcinoma is rare in Europe but is common in South-East Asia. The patient presents with nasal obstruction and bloodstained discharge. Unilateral otitis media may occur from eustachian tube blockage. Nerve palsies may occur due to invasion of the base of the skull. The patient may complain only of a swelling in the neck due to lymphadenopathy; lymphatic spread occurring at an early stage. With this disease, unilateral deafness, cervical lymphadenopathy and cranial nerve palsies are often diagnostic.

Carcinoma of the maxillary sinus This is often diagnosed late. Early presenting symptoms include bloodstained nasal discharge and unilateral nasal obstruction. Later, swelling of the cheek occurs, with ulceration of the palate. Epiphora may occur due to invasion of the nasolacrimal duct. Erosion into the orbit results in proptosis and diplopia. Pain may be referred to the ear.

Malignant granuloma Malignant granuloma (now thought to be lymphomatous) presents with slowly progressive ulceration starting in the region of the nose. The chronic inflammatory reaction causes a nasal discharge.

Granulomatous disease

Wegener's granulomatosis and Churg–Strauss syndrome affect the nose and are associated with disease of the kidneys, lungs and respiratory tract. The patient may present with either lung manifestations or renal failure.

Traumatic

The commonest trauma causing a nasal discharge is a foreign body. The patient is usually a child aged between 1 and 5 years, or rarely a psychiatrically disturbed adult. The child is usually miserable with a smelly, bloodstained nasal discharge. In adults, rhinolith may occur. This results in unilateral obstruction and discharge. There is usually a large concretion blocking the nose, which may have a foreign body at the centre, with calcium and magnesium laid down around it. Following fracture of the anterior fossa, sustained during head injury, the patient may complain of a clear nasal discharge (CSF rhinorrhoea) or a bloodstained nasal discharge. Irritant gases, e.g. chlorine, which may be industrial or in excess in swimming pools, may cause irritation of the nasal mucosa, with discharge.

Degenerative

Senile rhinorrhoea occurs in the elderly. It is thought to be due to failure of vasomotor control.

EXAMINATION

Choanal atresia

Pass a probe or catheter into the nasal cavity. It will not pass. Posterior rhinoscopy under general anaesthetic will confirm the diagnosis.

Infective

With a common cold there will be oedematous nasal mucosa with clear mucus in the nose. With chronic rhinitis there will be thick mucus or a purulent nasal discharge. With enlarged adenoids, mirror examination will reveal the diagnosis.

Allergic

Allergic rhinitis reveals an oedematous nasal mucosa with clear mucus in the nose.

Inflammatory

The appearance of eosinophilic vasomotor rhinitis is similar to that of allergic rhinitis except that nasal polyps may be seen. Nasal polyps are usually pink and smooth or a yellowish-grey and pedunculated. With non-eosinophilic vasomotor rhinitis excessive secretions will be noted on examination, with engorgement of the inferior turbinates. Often the signs are not as severe as the symptoms would suggest.

Neoplastic

Examination should include visualisation of the post-nasal space, under general anaesthetic if necessary. A full examination of the cranial nerves must be made. With carcinoma of the maxillary sinus there may be swelling of the cheek with ulceration of the palate. Epiphora may occur due to invasion of the nasolacrimal duct. Check for proptosis and diplopia due to invasion into the orbit. Examine the neck for cervical nodes. With malignant granuloma there is slowly progressive ulceration of the face, starting in the region of the nose.

Granulomatous disease

With Wegener's granulomatosis or Churg–Strauss syndrome, necrotic mucosal ulceration occurs. There may be co-existing otitis media, ulceration of the mouth or involvement of the trachea or larynx. There may be lung involvement, eye involvement and renal disease.

Traumatic

Examination with a nasal speculum will usually reveal the foreign body. With CSF rhinorrhoea it may be difficult to distinguish bleeding from blood mixed with CSF. Place a drop of the bloodstained discharge on a clean white gauze. If CSF is present, there will be a spreading yellowish ring around the central stain of blood (halo sign). With irritant gases, there will be redness and oedema of the nasal mucosa. There will almost certainly be eye irritation and a skin reaction accompanying it.

Degenerative

With senile rhinorrhoea, there are usually no physical signs apart from the nasal drip.

GENERAL INVESTIGATIONS

- **FBC, ESR and CRP**
  Hb ↓ malignancy, granulomatous disease. WCC ↑ infection, e.g. adenoiditis. ESR and CRP ↑ infection, malignancy, granulomatous disease.
- **Swab**
  Culture and sensitivity. Bacterial versus fungal.
- **Skull X-ray**
  Anterior cranial fossa fracture involving ethmoid bone – CSF rhinorrhoea. Carcinoma of the maxillary antrum.

SPECIFIC INVESTIGATIONS

- **Biopsy**
  Carcinoma. Wegener's granulomatosis. Malignant granuloma. Chronic inflammation.
- **RAST**
  Measures allergen-specific Ig.
- **CT and MRI**
  Carcinoma and granulomatous disease: diagnosis and assessment of extent of disease.

- **Persistent bloodstained nasal discharge is a serious sign and further investigation is required to exclude malignancy.**

NECK LUMPS

A lump in the neck is a common problem in surgical practice.
It is necessary to be able to distinguish the different causes, which
may vary from a simple benign swelling to part of a generalised
malignant condition.

CAUSES

SUPERFICIAL

- Sebaceous cyst
- Lipoma
- Abscess
- Dermoid cyst
- Lymph nodes

DEEP

ANTERIOR TRIANGLE

Move on swallowing

- Thyroid
- Thyroglossal cyst

Do not move on swallowing

- Salivary glands
- Branchial cyst
- Carotid body tumour
- Carotid aneurysm
- Sternomastoid 'tumour'

POSTERIOR TRIANGLE

- Cervical rib
- Subclavian artery aneurysm
- Pharyngeal pouch
- Cystic hygroma

HISTORY

Symptoms

The diagnosis of superficial swellings of the neck should be obvious.
A sebaceous cyst will usually have grown slowly and may have been
painful and red if infected. Lipomas tend to grow slowly. An abscess
will be obvious from pain and tenderness. Lymphadenopathy may be
associated with a recent pyrexial illness, local lesions in the head and

neck, generalised infection or generalised malignancy. Swelling during mastication suggests a salivary gland origin. Blackouts or dizziness may suggest a carotid body tumour. A lump in the lower part of the posterior triangle, increasing in size after eating and gurgling when full, suggests a pharyngeal pouch. The patient may experience bouts of coughing or choking when lying down as the pouch empties itself and aspiration occurs. Neurological or vascular symptoms in the upper limb may be associated with a cervical rib. Sternomastoid tumours are rare and occur in the neonate. Cystic hygromas are rare and occur in infancy.

Past medical history

A history of HIV infection, TB and malignancy is relevant. Breech or forceps delivery may be relevant to the development of a sternomastoid tumour.

EXAMINATION

Decide whether the swelling is superficial or deep. Decide whether it is likely to be due to lymphadenopathy. If the swelling is deep, decide whether it is in the anterior triangle of the neck or the posterior triangle. If it is in the anterior triangle, decide whether it moves on swallowing (thyroid-associated) or not.

Sebaceous cyst

This is usually obvious, being in the skin and having a punctum.

Lipoma

May occur anywhere in the neck but often occurs in the midline posteriorly. Lipomas are soft and lobulated and not fixed to the skin.

Dermoid cyst

These may be congenital or acquired. The congenital ones are most common in the head and neck and occur where skin dermatomes fuse. They are not unlike sebaceous cysts on examination but lack a punctum. Acquired implantation dermoids usually occur in relation to scars.

Abscess

The diagnosis will usually be obvious. There will be a tender, red, inflamed swelling. They may occur in relation to lymph nodes or salivary glands.

Lymphadenopathy

Depending upon the cause of the condition, lymph nodes will be enlarged and tender; non-tender and firm or rubbery; or small, hard and matted together. A check should be made for enlarged lymph nodes elsewhere in the body and for hepatosplenomegaly. Generalised lymphadenopathy and splenomegaly will occur with blood dyscrasias.

Thyroid

Thyroid swellings move on swallowing. Associated lymphadenopathy will suggest malignancy. The thyroid status of the patient should be checked on clinical examination.

Thyroglossal cyst

This is a painless cystic swelling in the midline of the neck that moves on swallowing. It also moves on protrusion of the tongue. It is commonly attached to the body of the hyoid bone. Occasionally it may become infected, with pain, tenderness and increased swelling.

Salivary gland

Swelling of the submandibular salivary gland is most frequently due to obstruction of the submandibular duct. Swelling will be noted on mastication. A stone may be palpated in the submandibular duct in the floor of the mouth. Swelling of the parotid gland may be due to duct obstruction, although tumour is more common with this gland. Malignant tumours of the parotid gland may be associated with facial nerve palsy.

Branchial cyst

A branchial cyst feels soft and putty-like and abuts from the anterior border of sternocleidomastoid at the junction between its upper and middle thirds.

Carotid body tumour

This feels firm and is located at the bifurcation of the common carotid artery.

Carotid aneurysm

These are extremely rare. False ones may follow surgery or trauma to the neck. A tortuous carotid artery may be mistaken for a carotid aneurysm.

Sternomastoid 'tumour'

This appears only in babies and is a result of birth trauma. There is a swelling in the middle third of the sternomastoid. The head becomes turned to the opposite side and tilted towards the shoulder on the side of the lesion.

Cervical rib

A bony, hard swelling may be palpable in the posterior triangle of the neck.

Subclavian artery aneurysm

Obvious as a pulsatile, expansile swelling in the lower part of the posterior triangle. Often associated with a cervical rib.

Pharyngeal pouch

Presents behind the lower border of sternomastoid in the posterior triangle. It may fill after a meal and empty after lying down. Signs of aspiration pneumonitis may be present.

Cystic hygromas

This is a collection of dilated lymphatics which presents in infancy. It is soft, lobulated, fluctuant, compressible and brilliantly transilluminable.

GENERAL INVESTIGATIONS

- **FBC, ESR**
  Hb ↓ malignancy. WCC ↑ infection and leukaemia. ESR ↑ infection and malignancy.

- **CXR**
  May show TB or primary or secondary tumour. Tracheal deviation may be associated with thyroid swellings. A cervical rib may be seen. Count the ribs. If there are 13 it is likely that there is a cervical rib.

- **US**
  This may be helpful in almost any lump in the neck. It will also distinguish between solid and cystic swellings, e.g. in the thyroid.

SPECIFIC INVESTIGATIONS

A detailed history and examination may suggest the aetiology of the swelling. Further confirmatory investigations may be required for specific cases.

- **Paul–Bunnell test**
  For glandular fever.

- **Toxoplasma screen**
  Toxoplasmosis.

- **Mantoux test**
  For TB.

- **Viral titres**
  For any viral infection that may cause cervical lymphadenopathy.

- **HIV screen**
  AIDS.

- **TFTs**
  If clinical examination reveals a swelling to be a goitre.

- **FNAC**
  Especially useful for swellings of lymph nodes, thyroid or salivary glands.

- **CT**
  Helpful with the diagnosis of almost any mass but particularly helpful with confirming the diagnosis of carotid body tumours.

- **Duplex Doppler**
  For suspected carotid artery aneurysm or subclavian artery aneurysm.

- **Floor of mouth X-ray**
  Will identify a calculus in the submandibular duct.

- **Sialography**
  Contrast study of salivary duct to locate possible cause and site of obstruction, e.g. stone or stricture.

- **Barium swallow**
  To confirm the presence of a pharyngeal pouch. Never perform an endoscopy if a pouch is suspected, as perforation of the pouch may result.

- **OGD**
  To check for a primary oesophageal or gastric carcinoma causing cervical lymphadenopathy.

- **Bronchoscopy**
  Check for carcinoma of the lung associated with cervical gland metastases.

- **If cervical lymphadenopathy is thought to be due to malignancy, the patient should be referred for an urgent ENT opinion.**

- **Dysphagia in association with a neck swelling is likely to represent serious underlying pathology.**

NECK PAIN

Neck pain is a common problem. The majority of cases are due to poor posture or cervical spondylosis. If there has been a history of trauma, extreme care must be exercised in examination of the neck and any X-rays must be strictly supervised.

CAUSES

CONGENITAL

- Torticollis
- Klippel–Feil syndrome

ACQUIRED

TRAUMATIC
- Fractures
- Dislocations
- Whiplash injury

INFLAMMATORY
- Traumatic
- Rheumatoid arthritis

INFECTIVE
- TB
  - (common where TB is endemic)

DEGENERATIVE
- Cervical spondylosis
- Cervical disc lesion

NEOPLASTIC
- Secondary deposits

OTHER
- Postural
- Exposure to cold
- Meningitis
- Subarachnoid haemorrhage

HISTORY

Congenital

Torticollis may be congenital and present at birth due to sternomastoid 'tumour'. This is a rare condition often associated with breech delivery. Klippel–Feil syndrome is rare and is characterised by developmental abnormalities of the cervical vertebrae and a high-riding scapula.

Acquired
Traumatic

History of trauma may be evident and it is important to screen for any neurological sequelae, e.g. arm pain or weakness or bladder symptoms. Whiplash injuries are common. These occur in road traffic accidents where the car is struck from behind. The neck extends with sudden acceleration and flexes forward with sudden deceleration.

Inflammatory

Rheumatoid arthritis frequently affects the neck, particularly the atlantoaxial joints, which may undergo subluxation. There will usually be a history of rheumatoid arthritis elsewhere. The patient complains of pain in the neck, difficulty in walking and there may be progressive bladder involvement.

Infective

TB of the cervical spine is rare in the UK. There is usually a history of TB elsewhere.

Degenerative

Cervical spondylosis is the commonest condition involving the neck. The patient complains of neck pain and stiffness with radiation of pain into the occiput, shoulder or arms. There may be complaints of weakness of grip and wasting of the hand. Acute cervical disc lesions may cause acute neck pain, with referred pain to the arm with weakness. Central disc protrusion may cause bladder problems or even paraplegia.

Neoplastic

Primary tumours of the cervical vertebrae are extremely rare. Secondary deposits may occur from breast, bronchus, lung, prostate or kidney. The patient may have had surgery for carcinoma of one of these organs. If not, check for a history suggesting a lesion. The patient will present with pain and collapse of a vertebra, perhaps with neurological symptoms.

Other

Postural neck pain is common and relates to changes in neck posture, the patient often complaining of sleeping in an 'awkward' position. The pain is usually across the neck and shoulders. The patient may also complain of exposure to cold, e.g. 'sitting in a draught'. Meningitis may cause a stiff neck with pain, as does subarachnoid haemorrhage. The diagnosis of these will usually be obvious from the history. The headache radiates into the neck and causes neck stiffness.

EXAMINATION

Congenital

Torticollis – the head is pulled down to the affected side and often rotated to the opposite side. Klippel–Feil syndrome presents with a short neck and a high-riding scapula.

Acquired
Traumatic

Treat the patient as for spinal injury, with stabilisation of the neck. Carry out a full neurological examination. Any X-ray examination should be strictly supervised by an experienced orthopaedic surgeon. With whiplash injuries there is usually only ligamentous and soft-tissue damage. Localised tenderness may be present. Check for pain and paraesthesia in the arms and hands.

Inflammatory

Rheumatoid arthritis will be apparent elsewhere, e.g. hand deformities, ulnar deviation. Carry out a full neurological examination.

Infective

With TB the patient will be generally unwell with spasm in the neck muscles. There may be evidence of paravertebral abscess. Carry out a full neurological examination.

Degenerative

There will be reduced neck movements. Carry out a full neurological examination. There will often be weakness of grip, muscle wasting and reduced reflexes. Acute disc lesions result in pain and spasm of the neck muscles. There may be weakness of the arm and reduced reflexes. Carry out a full neurological examination.

Neoplastic

Examine the possible sites of primary tumours, e.g. breast, bronchus, prostate, thyroid, kidney. Carry out a full neurological examination.

Other

With postural neck pain or cold exposure there is usually little to find on examination. There may be some localised muscular tenderness. With meningitis the patient is usually ill, with photophobia, headache, stiff neck and a positive Kernig's sign. Subarachnoid haemorrhage is usually diagnosed from the history.

GENERAL INVESTIGATIONS

- FBC, ESR
  Hb ↓ anaemia of chronic disease, e.g. rheumatoid arthritis. WCC infection. ESR ↑ rheumatoid arthritis, TB, malignancy.

- **Rheumatoid factor**
  Rheumatoid arthritis.

- **X-ray**
  Fractures (supervised X-rays), cervical spondylosis – narrowing of joint spaces, osteophytes. Rheumatoid arthritis – atlantoaxial subluxation. Secondary deposits. Congenital anomalies.

SPECIFIC INVESTIGATIONS

- **CT**
  Disc lesion. TB. Subarachnoid haemorrhage.

- **MRI**
  Disc lesions – cord compression.

- **Bone scan**
  Secondary deposits. Acute arthritis.

- **Lumbar puncture**
  Meningitis. Subarachnoid haemorrhage.

- If there has been a history of trauma, extreme care must be exercised in examination of the neck and any X-rays must be strictly supervised.

- Neck pain and stiffness may be early signs of meningitis. Check carefully for petechiae.

NIPPLE DISCHARGE

This is a common problem. It is embarrassing for the patient as discharge may leak through and stain the clothing. Bloodstained nipple discharge may be due to an underlying carcinoma.

CAUSES

SEROUS
- Early pregnancy
- Fibroadenosis

MILKY
- Late pregnancy
- Lactation
- Lactorrhoea of the newborn (witch's milk)
- Puberty
- Prolactinoma (tumour of the anterior pituitary gland)

COLOURED

YELLOW, BROWN, GREEN
- Fibroadenosis

THICK AND CREAMY
- Duct ectasia

PURULENT
- Retroareolar abscess
- Breast abscess
- TB

BLOODSTAINED
- Intraduct carcinoma
- Intraduct papilloma
- Paget's disease of the nipple

HISTORY

Pregnancy or lactation will be apparent. Discharge may occur from the nipples of newborn babies of either sex (witch's milk). It is due to the passage of female hormones across the placenta. Discharge, either serous or milky, may occur at puberty. Cyclical mastalgia with a coloured discharge, especially greenish, suggests fibroadenosis. A patient in the fifth decade with a history of retroareolar pain and a thick creamy discharge may have duct

ectasia. A bloodstained discharge must be taken seriously
and fully investigated. The patient may describe this as frank,
red blood or altered blood, which may be darkish brown. It
is important to know whether it has come from one duct or
several. Does the patient have an underlying lump? Profuse milky
discharge associated with amenorrhoea will suggest the possibility
of prolactinoma of the anterior pituitary gland.

EXAMINATION

Is the discharge obvious? It may have stained the clothes and the
colour of it may be apparent. Is it associated with a painful and
lumpy breast to suggest fibroadenosis? Is it possible to express
the discharge by manual pressure? Occasionally it is possible, by
manual pressure on specific areas of the breast, to express blood
from one particular duct. Is there an underlying discrete lump
suggestive of a carcinoma? Is there retroareolar tenderness,
lumpiness and nipple retraction suggestive of duct ectasia? Are
there any signs of infection or abscess? Has the nipple been
destroyed, as in Paget's disease? If prolactinoma is suspected
(galactorrhoea, amenorrhoea, infertility), the visual fields should
be checked, as a macroadenoma of the anterior pituitary gland
may impinge on the optic chiasma.

GENERAL INVESTIGATIONS

- **FBC, ESR**
  WCC ↑ in infection. ESR ↑ in tumour and TB.
- **Swab**
  C&S. Infection, abscess, TB.
- **FNAC**
  Carcinoma.
- **Dipstick testing**
  Blood versus other fluid.

SPECIFIC INVESTIGATIONS

- **Mammography**
  Carcinoma, duct ectasia.
- **Microdochectomy**
  If bleeding is localised to an individual duct, this is an
  appropriate surgical investigation. It may demonstrate intraduct
  papilloma or intraduct carcinoma.
- **CT head**
  Prolactinoma of the pituitary gland.

- A bloodstained nipple discharge is serious. An underlying carcinoma is the most likely diagnosis. Referral to a breast surgeon for full assessment is required.

- Always remember pregnancy in the patient with bilateral serous discharge.

- If the discharge is bilateral and not bloodstained, serious breast disease is unlikely.

- Destruction of the nipple suggests Paget's disease.

- Nipple discharge in a male is always abnormal. Full investigation is required.

OEDEMA

Oedema is the accumulation of excessive fluid in the subcutaneous tissue. When oedema results from lymphatic stasis, the term lymphoedema is used.

CAUSES

GENERALISED

INCREASED PLASMA HYDROSTATIC PRESSURE
- Congestive cardiac failure
- Vasodilatory drugs – nifedipine

DECREASED PLASMA ONCOTIC PRESSURE
- Liver disease
- Renal disease, e.g. nephrotic syndrome
- Malnutrition/malabsorption
  - (very common in the developing world)

IMPAIRMENT OF LYMPHATIC DRAINAGE*
- Congenital deficiency of lymphatics

INCREASED CAPILLARY PERMEABILITY
- Angio-oedema – anaphylaxis

LOCALISED

INCREASED PLASMA HYDROSTATIC PRESSURE
- Venous obstruction

IMPAIRMENT OF LYMPHATIC DRAINAGE*
Congenital
- Milroy's disease
- Lymphoedema praecox
- Lymphoedema tarda

Acquired
- Malignant infiltration
- Infection, e.g. elephantiasis
  - (common in Africa)
- Radiation
- Surgical damage

INCREASED CAPILLARY PERMEABILITY
- Local infection
- Trauma

Indicates the causes of lymphoedema.

- Burns
- Animal bites/stings

HISTORY

Site and distribution

Enquiries should be made regarding the site of oedema, as localised and demarcated sites of oedema are usually due to trauma or infection. Oedema may be confined to both lower limbs, for example with IVC obstruction and pregnancy, or affect only a single limb, such as the leg with unilateral DVT, or arm following axillary lymph node clearance.

Precipitating factors

Precipitating factors such as trauma and infection may be obvious from the history, and should be excluded. Angio-oedema may be precipitated by a known allergen. Lymphoedema may result as a complication of infection with filarial nematodes while travelling in endemic areas such as Africa, Asia and Australia. Lymphoedema may also be congenital, occurring shortly after birth (Milroy's disease) or at puberty (lymphoedema praecox) or in the third decade (lymphoedema tarda).

Past medical and drug history

Interruption to lymphatic drainage may result as a complication of irradiation or surgery, especially in the region of the axilla and groin. Obstruction of lymphatic flow can also result from direct involvement of the lymph nodes by lymphoma, or secondary to metastatic lymphatic infiltration from tumours. A detailed drug history will identify any offending drug.

Associated symptoms

If there is no obvious precipitating factor in the history, then specific enquiries should be undertaken for each system. Symptoms suggestive of malignancy, in particular, should be sought.
In addition, it is important to exclude the following conditions.

Cardiac failure

Lethargy, dyspnoea, orthopnoea, paroxysmal nocturnal dyspnoea, cough, ankle oedema and abdominal distension from ascites may be some symptoms experienced by patients with cardiac failure.

Liver disease

Symptoms of jaundice, pruritus, ankle oedema, abdominal distension, haematemesis and confusion (encephalopathy) should be sought to determine the presence of liver disease.

Renal disease – nephrotic syndrome

Severe generalised oedema is the prominent feature with nephrotic syndrome. Patients may also complain of frothy urine due to proteinuria.

Malabsorption

Weight loss, diarrhoea and steatorrhoea may be some of the features associated with malabsorption.

Venous thrombosis

Unilateral leg swelling and pain are the main symptoms of DVT. Occasionally with iliofemoral vein thrombosis, the entire leg may appear blue (phlegmasia cerulea dolens) or white (phlegmasia alba dolens). Bilateral leg oedema with the onset of dilated superficial collateral veins on the trunk and abdomen is suggestive of IVC obstruction.

EXAMINATION

Inspection

Assessment of the distribution of oedema may narrow the differential diagnosis. Generalised causes tend to present with dependent oedema, with fluid accumulating in the ankles in ambulant patients and the sacrum in recumbent patients.

Cardiovascular system

With cardiac failure, palpation of the pulse may reveal tachycardia with pulsus alternans. The measured blood pressure may be low due to systolic failure. The JVP is elevated and a third heart sound with bilateral coarse pulmonary crepitations may be auscultated. Hepatomegaly due to liver congestion and ascites may also be present.

Abdominal examination

Generalised wasting from malabsorption or malignancy may be appreciated on inspection. Clubbing, palmar erythema, Dupuytren's contracture, jaundice, spider naevi and gynaecomastia are signs of liver disease. Dilated collateral veins on the abdomen may be due to portal hypertension or IVC obstruction; therefore, determine the direction of blood flow. Below the umbilicus the direction of blood flow is inferior with portal hypertension, and superior with IVC obstruction. Organomegaly due to carcinoma may be present and predispose to venous thrombosis. Pelvic malignancy may also result in venous outflow obstruction.

Legs

The legs are examined for the presence of tenderness and swelling. Circumferences of both the thighs and calves are compared. Marked painful erythematous unilateral swelling may be indicative of a DVT.

SECTION A

GENERAL INVESTIGATIONS

- **Urinalysis**
  Heavy proteinuria with nephrotic syndrome.
- **FBC**
  WCC ↑ infection and DVT. Hb ↓ malabsorption.
- **U&Es**
  Urea and creatinine ↑ with renal failure.
- **LFTs**
  Abnormal in liver disease.
- **Serum albumin**
  ↓ with nephrotic syndrome, liver disease, malabsorption and malnutrition.

SPECIFIC INVESTIGATIONS

- **24-hour urine collection**
  >3.5 g of protein with nephrotic syndrome.
- **Renal biopsy**
  To determine the cause of nephrotic syndrome in adults.
- **Echocardiography**
  Ventricular dilatation and impaired function with cardiac failure.
- **Liver biopsy**
  Liver cirrhosis.
- **Faecal fat estimation**
  ↑ malabsorption.
- **Duplex Doppler deep veins of the leg**
  DVT of the leg.
- **Venography**
  Below-knee DVT, IVC obstruction.
- **Lymphangiography**
  Lymphatic obstruction of any cause.
- **Pelvic ultrasound or CT**
  Pelvic tumours.

- **Sudden onset of oedema in the lower limb is highly suggestive of deep venous thrombosis. Urgent investigation and treatment is required to prevent pulmonary embolism.**

OLIGURIA

Oliguria is the passage of less than 400 mL of urine in 24 hours. Anuria is failure to pass any urine.

CAUSES

RENAL CIRCULATORY INSUFFICIENCY

- Dehydration, e.g. vomiting, diarrhoea
- Shock, e.g. haemorrhage and burns

RENAL CAUSES

- Nephrotoxins
- Acute tubular necrosis
- Acute cortical necrosis
- Acute glomerulonephritis
- Acute interstitial nephritis
- Vascular lesions

POST-RENAL (OBSTRUCTIVE)

- Prostatic hypertrophy
- Calculi
- Pelvic tumours
- Retroperitoneal fibrosis

OTHERS

- Mismatched transfusion (haemoglobinuria)
- Crush injuries (myoglobinuria)

ANURIA

- Blocked catheter
- Ureteric damage (bilateral)
- Stone in solitary functioning kidney

HISTORY

Renal circulatory insufficiency

There will usually be a recent history of a condition which causes renal hypoperfusion. This may include haemorrhage, burns or dehydration, e.g. from vomiting, diarrhoea or acute pancreatitis.

Renal causes

In the absence of adequate resuscitation, shock will proceed to cause damage to the tubules, resulting in acute tubular necrosis.

SECTION A

Acute cortical necrosis may arise as a result of antepartum haemorrhage, eclampsia or septic abortion. It may also follow insults similar to those that cause acute tubular necrosis. Vascular lesions may also lead to acute renal failure; these include renal vein thrombosis, renal artery stenosis and intravascular coagulation occurring in haemolytic uraemic syndrome. Other forms of acute renal failure usually present with swelling of the eyelids, ascites and peripheral oedema. Later there may be vomiting, confusion, bruising, gastrointestinal bleeding and eventually fitting and coma. Volume overload may result in pulmonary oedema. With acute interstitial nephritis, there may be a history of drug ingestion, e.g. antibiotics, NSAIDs or diuretics, or there may be a history of infection. Nephrotoxins may cause acute renal failure and among the drugs implicated are the aminoglycosides, amphotericin and radiographic contrast media. Organic solvents, particularly carbon tetrachloride used in carpet cleaning, may be responsible. Paraquat, snake bites and mushrooms may also cause acute renal failure.

Post-renal

Often the patient will present with complete anuria. This may occur if there is ureteric damage following surgery or a stone impacted in the ureter of a solitary functioning kidney. The patient may have a history of calculous disease or may have recently suffered an attack of ureteric colic. There may be a history of pelvic tumour or symptoms of prostatic hypertrophy, e.g. difficulty in starting and a poor stream. Retroperitoneal fibrosis often develops insidiously.

Others

Oliguria may follow a mismatched transfusion, due to haemoglobinuria, or crush injuries, due to myoglobinuria. The history will usually be obvious.

Anuria

Before diagnosing anuria, make sure that the patient does not have a palpable bladder (if he or she is not catheterised) and is not therefore in acute retention, or, if the patient is catheterised, that the catheter is not blocked. As indicated above, anuria is more likely to be a symptom of an obstructive lesion rather than one of renal hypoperfusion or an intrinsic renal lesion.

EXAMINATION

General

If the patient has a catheter *in situ*, make sure that it is not blocked. If the patient does not have a catheter *in situ*, palpate the lower abdomen for a distended bladder associated with acute retention.

Palpate the abdomen to exclude swelling of the kidneys and perform a rectal examination to exclude prostatic hypertrophy.

Specific

All causes of oliguria are likely to have some common features on examination. The patient will be dyspnoeic due to pulmonary oedema and will either have sacral oedema (if confined to bed) or ankle oedema (if ambulant). There may be confusion, drowsiness, fitting or coma. Hypertension and arrhythmias may be present. The patient will be nauseated, may be vomiting, have hiccups, and there may be evidence of gastrointestinal haemorrhage. Spontaneous bruising may occur eventually.

GENERAL INVESTIGATIONS

■ **FBC, ESR**
Hb ↓ anaemia, renal failure, haemorrhage. WCC ↑ infection. ESR ↑ some causes of glomerulonephritis.

■ **U&Es**
Urea ↑, creatinine ↑ in renal and post-renal causes. These may rise in renal hypoperfusion if not adequately treated.

■ **ECG**
Arrhythmias. Associated with electrolyte imbalance, e.g. hyperkalaemia.

■ **CXR**
Pulmonary oedema. Cardiomegaly.

■ **ABGs**
Metabolic acidosis.

■ **MSU**
Red cells, casts and protein in intrinsic renal disease. Hb positive but no red blood cells suggests myoglobinuria or haemoglobinuria.

■ **Urine electrolytes**
See Table on p. 350.

■ **Urine osmolality**
See Table on p. 350.

Distinction between physiological oliguria and acute renal failure		
Urine	Physiological oliguria	Acute renal failure
Specific gravity	>1020	<1010
Osmolality (mmol/kg)	>500	<350
Sodium (mmol/l)	<15	>40
Urine/serum creatinine	>40	<20
Fractional sodium excretion[a]	<1	>2
Renal failure index[b]	<1	>2

[a] Fractional sodium excretion = (urine sodium × plasma creatinine/plasma sodium × urine creatinine) × 100.

[b] Renal failure index = (urine sodium × plasma creatinine)/urine creatinine.

SPECIFIC INVESTIGATIONS

■ **US**
Obstructive lesion.

■ **Cystoscopy and ureteric catheterisation with retrograde pyelography**
Cause of obstruction, possible relief of obstruction.

■ **Antegrade pyelography**
Cause of obstruction. Relief of obstruction.

■ **DMSA scan**
Renal function. Infarction. Absent outline of kidney.

- The commonest cause of oliguria is hypovolaemia. Always check that the patient is adequately filled. CVP monitoring may be required.

- Always check for catheter blockage before diagnosing oliguria/anuria.

PALPITATIONS

Palpitation is an awareness of the heartbeat; although benign in the vast majority, palpitations are occasionally a manifestation of a life-threatening disorder.

CAUSES

SINUS TACHYCARDIA

- Anxiety/emotional stress
- Caffeine
- Nicotine
- Alcohol

CARDIAC ARRHYTHMIA

- Premature ventricular contractions (ventricular ectopic beats)*
- Premature atrial contractions (atrial ectopic beats)*
- Atrial fibrillation*
- Supraventricular tachycardia
- Ventricular tachycardia

HISTORY

A variety of symptoms is used to describe palpitations and this includes 'fluttering', 'pounding' and 'skipping a beat'. Symptoms may also be experienced in the neck. Important aspects are the frequency, regularity of palpitation (e.g. fast and irregular) and precipitating factors. Asking the patient to tap the rate and rhythm of the palpitation (on a table for example) can be very informative. Arrhythmias associated with irregular palpitations are listed above.

Knowledge of precipitating factors is important. Palpitations can be a normal manifestation of anxiety or panic reactions. However, it is vitally important that an organic cause is excluded as it is common for anxiety disorders to co-exist in a patient with supraventricular tachycardia. Exercise is associated with excess catecholamines and also a precipitator of arrhythmia (supraventricular tachycardia, atrial fibrillation and ventricular tachycardia usually originating from the right ventricle). Excessive caffeine, smoking and alcohol intake are is also thought to be precipitators of arrhythmia.

A history of any underlying heart disorder is important, as arrhythmia is associated with ischaemic heart disease (ventricular arrhythmia), hypertensive heart disease (atrial fibrillation), heart failure (ventricular arrhythmia), heart valve disease.

* Indicates causes that tend to present as irregular palpitations.

SECTION A

Early age of onset of arrhythmia (childhood or teenage years) suggests the presence of a congenital abnormality such as a bypass tract that can lead to supraventricular tachycardia. The reader should consult a cardiology textbook for further details.

Additional features

Dizziness or syncope (p. 427) is usually associated with serious arrhythmia such as ventricular tachycardia and occasionally supraventricular tachycardia.

EXAMINATION

Examination during an episode of palpitation is very informative as assessment of the rhythm and rate of the pulse can be determined. Auscultation of the rate at the cardiac apex is more accurate as not all beats are conducted to the pulse (e.g. in atrial fibrillation).

It is important to measure the blood pressure and screen for any evidence of underlying structural heart disease, especially mitral valve prolapse (systolic murmur and a systolic click), as this condition is associated with supraventricular tachycardia and atrial fibrillation.

INITIAL INVESTIGATIONS

12-lead ECG

All patients should have a resting ECG. It is very unlikely that any arrhythmia can be picked up during this investigation; however, conditions that predispose to arrhythmia may be diagnosed. The presence of an accessory pathway (and hence predisposition to supraventricular arrhythmia) is indicated by a short PR interval (less than 0.12 seconds).

Also, the presence of left ventricular hypertrophy can indicate underlying structural heart disease (hypertensive heart disease, hypertrophic obstructive cardiomyopathy). Ischaemic heart disease can be suggested by Q waves, or ST segment/T wave abnormalities.

Occasionally, atrial or ventricular premature contractions (ectopic beats) may be evident.

FURTHER INVESTIGATIONS

Further investigations are best reserved for those who are at high risk of arrhythmia: patients with evidence of underlying structural heart disease, family history of arrhythmia, regular palpitations (especially during sleep) and dizziness or syncope associated with palpitations.

Ambulatory ECG monitoring

Continuous ambulatory ECG monitoring is an excellent method to detect and identify arrhythmia. Upon further investigation, ventricular and atrial premature contractions (ectopic beats) are the most commonly identified arrhythmia. Sinus rhythm is the usual remaining finding. A serious arrhythmia is detected in approximately 7%. The reader is advised to consult ECG textbooks for a detailed discussion of the numerous configurations of each arrhythmia.

- **Although palpitations are benign in the vast majority of cases, they can occasionally be a manifestation of life-threatening disorders.**
- **Sudden onset of tachycardia in childhood or teenage years associated with breathlessness, dizziness and chest pain suggests supraventricular tachycardia. Suspect a congenital anomaly.**

PENILE LESIONS

Penile lesions are common. They interfere with sexual intercourse. The majority of surgical conditions of the penis relate to problems with the foreskin and glans and the need for circumcision. Carcinoma of the penis and Peyronie's disease are rare.

CAUSES

FORESKIN AND GLANS

- Phimosis
- Paraphimosis
- Balanoposthitis
- Balanitis xerotica obliterans
- Herpes genitalis
- Condylomata (warts)
- Trauma (bite)
- Carcinoma
- Erythroplasia of Queyrat
- Chancre (syphilis)

SHAFT OF THE PENIS

- Peyronie's disease
- Priapism

URETHRA

- Epispadias
- Hypospadias

HISTORY

Foreskin and glans

Phimosis

In most cases phimosis is congenital. The foreskin has been tight since birth and the patient complains that it will not retract over the glans. In children, this may cause ballooning of the foreskin during micturition, with resulting balanoposthitis. In adults, the complaint is that it interferes with sexual intercourse.

Paraphimosis

This is a result of a patient having a phimosis. The foreskin is pulled back over the glans while washing and then is not returned. It may also occur during sexual intercourse. In hospital practice it may occur while the patient is being catheterised and the foreskin is not returned to its correct place following this procedure. The foreskin forms a tight constriction around the glans, interfering with venous return and causing swelling of the glans and foreskin. The patient presents with considerable pain and a swollen glans penis.

Balanoposthitis

This is inflammation of the glans and foreskin. The patient complains of an attack of inflammation of the foreskin and glans. It may be associated with poor hygiene but in children it is often associated with phimosis and collection of urine under the foreskin. In diabetics it is often due to *candida*.

Balanitis xerotica obliterans

The patient will complain of thickening and tightening of the foreskin, and the inability to retract it.

Herpes genitalis

The patient will complain of painful vesicles on the foreskin or glans penis. There will usually be a history of sexual contact.

Condylomata (warts)

The patient may present with warts on the glans and contiguous surface of the prepuce. They are usually of venereal origin.

Trauma

There may be a history of trauma, often of an unusual nature. Love bites may be responsible.

Carcinoma

This usually presents in old age. It is virtually unknown in those who are circumcised. Most patients present with a lump or an ulcer which may be painful. In uncircumcised patients who cannot retract the foreskin there may be a bloodstained purulent discharge from under the foreskin.

Erythroplasia of Queyrat

The patient will present having noticed a dark, velvety, red, flat patch on the skin of the glans.

Syphilitic chancre

A chancre presents as a painless, hard ulcer on the penis.

Shaft

Peyronie's disease

The patient may have noticed a subcutaneous lump along the penis. He may complain that when he has an erection the penis appears bent.

Priapism

The patient will present with a persistent painful erection. This is unassociated with sexual desire. There may be a history of leukaemia, sickle cell disease, disseminated pelvic malignancy, or the patient may be on haemodialysis. Priapism may also result from alprostadil overdose for erectile dysfunction.

Urethra

Epispadias

This is rare. The patient, a baby or child, usually presents with the urethra opening on the dorsal surface of the glans penis.

Hypospadias

This is more common than epispadias, the patient presenting with the urethral opening on the ventral or undersurface of the penis. In both epispadias and hypospadias, the patient will complain of a problem with micturition.

EXAMINATION

Foreskin and glans

Phimosis

The foreskin is tight and has a pinhole orifice. It will be impossible to retract it over the glans penis. There may be associated balanoposthitis.

Paraphimosis

The diagnosis is usually obvious. The glans penis is swollen and oedematous and there is a deep groove just proximal to the corona glandis, where there is a tight constricting ring of skin. The patient is obviously in pain.

Balanoposthitis

There is inflammation of the glans (balanitis) and often associated inflammation of the foreskin (posthitis). There may be a discharge from under the foreskin. In the case of candidiasis there are itchy red patches on the glans. There may be evidence of poor personal hygiene.

Balanitis xerotica obliterans

The foreskin is thickened, with loss of elasticity and fibrosis. It is usually not possible to retract it over the glans.

Herpes genitalis

Initially there will be itchy vesicles but these develop into shallow, painful erosions. There may be associated painful inguinal lymphadenopathy.

Condylomata (warts)

There will be a bunch of warts, usually around the junction between the foreskin and the glans and extending onto the glans.

Trauma

Appearance will depend upon the type of trauma. Teeth marks may be apparent.

Carcinoma

The lesion is usually at the junction of the foreskin and glans. There will be a lump or ulcer. If there is an ulcer it will have raised everted edges and a necrotic base. It feels hard. The inguinal lymph nodes may be affected, either by metastases or by secondary infection. In patients in whom the foreskin cannot be retracted, it may be necessary to carry out circumcision to make the diagnosis.

Erythroplasia of Queyrat

There is a dark-red, flat, velvety, indurated patch on the glans penis. It is a premalignant condition and represents carcinoma *in situ*.

Syphilitic chancre

There will be a painless, hard ulcer with a sloping edge. The inguinal nodes will be enlarged, rubbery, discrete and non-tender.

Shaft

Peyronie's disease

There are plaques of fibrosis in the corpora cavernosa. These may be felt as hard lumps along the corpora cavernosa. The patient will volunteer the information that the penis becomes bent on erection.

Priapism

The diagnosis will be obvious, there being a painful erection.

Urethra

The diagnosis of epispadias and hypospadias will be obvious. In hypospadias the opening of the urethra may be anywhere along the line of the urethra, from a few millimetres from the tip of the penis to the perineum. In epispadias, which is rare, the urethral opening is on the dorsal surface of the glans penis.

GENERAL INVESTIGATIONS

- **FBC, ESR**
  WCC ↑ infection, leukaemia (associated with priapism). ESR ↑ malignancy.

- **Swab**
  C&S. Microscopy. Balanitis – bacterial or fungal.

- **Blood glucose**
  Diabetes – *candida* balanitis.

SPECIFIC INVESTIGATIONS

- ■ Sickle cell test
  Sickle cell disease with priapism.
- ■ VDRL
  Syphilitic chancre.
- ■ Electron microscopy
  Identification of herpes virus in vesicular fluid.
- ■ PCR
  For rapid diagnosis of herpes.
- ■ Biopsy
  Erythroplasia of Queyrat. Carcinoma. Condylomata.
- ■ Circumcision
  Diagnostic if tight phimosis prevents retraction of foreskin to inspect glans for carcinoma.

- • Always take a full sexual history. Enquire about foreign travel and sexual encounters. If STD is suspected, refer to a GUM clinic.
- • A persistent solitary ulcer needs thorough investigation as malignancy is likely.
- • Recurrent candidal balanitis may reflect underlying diabetes. Check the blood sugar.

POLYURIA

The volume of urine produced per day varies in each individual and is affected by the amount of fluid intake, physiological requirements and insensible losses. Polyuria is arbitrarily defined as urine output of more than 3 litres in 24 hours.

CAUSES

DIURETICS

THERAPEUTIC
- Frusemide
- Bendrofluazide
- Amiloride

OSMOTIC
- Hyperglycaemia
- Hypercalcaemia
- Mannitol
- Urea

DIABETES INSIPIDUS

CRANIAL
- Head injuries
- Neurosurgery
- Brain tumours (especially of pituitary)
- Idiopathic deficiency of ADH production
- Inherited (dominant or recessive)
- Pituitary granulomas, e.g. sarcoidosis, TB
  - (commoner where TB is endemic)
- Opiates

NEPHROGENIC
- Drugs
  - Lithium
  - Demeclocycline
- Hypokalaemia
- Chronic tubulointerstitial nephritis
- Recovering acute tubular necrosis
- Recovering obstructive uropathy
- Chronic hypercalcaemia
- Inherited (X-linked)

EXCESSIVE FLUID INTAKE

- Drug-induced thirst – anticholinergics
- Psychogenic
- Hypothalamic disease

HISTORY

General

Polyuria is often accompanied by polydipsia, and, as with all water-losing states, severe thirst is often a side-effect. Frequency of micturition (frequent passing of small amounts of urine) should be differentiated from polyuria (frequent passing of large amounts of urine). Diabetes insipidus may be hereditary and other family members may be affected.

Drug history

A detailed drug history is invaluable, as a significant number of drugs precipitate polyuria by various mechanisms. Therapeutic diuretics are used in a range of disorders, such as hypertension and cardiac failure. Opiates inhibit ADH secretion and may produce cranial diabetes insipidus, whereas drugs such as lithium and demeclocycline may produce nephrogenic diabetes insipidus. A side-effect of anticholinergics is dryness of the mouth; patients may therefore ingest excessive quantities of water, causing polyuria. Nephrotoxic drugs, such as aminoglycosides, ciclosporin, NSAIDs and ACE inhibitors, may precipitate acute tubular necrosis, which can result in severe polyuria in the recovery phase.

Past medical history

Hyperglycaemia causes an osmotic diuresis, therefore polyuria and polydipsia are common presenting features of diabetes mellitus. Malignancy and hyperparathyroidism are common causes of chronic hypercalcaemia, which can cause polyuria by an intrinsic osmotic effect or by precipitation of nephrogenic diabetes insipidus. Cranial diabetes insipidus can result from severe, blunt, head injuries, craniopharyngiomas, pineal gland tumours or as a transient post-operative complication following neurosurgery. Renal ischaemia from conditions such as sepsis and haemorrhage predisposes to acute tubular necrosis. Chronic tubulointerstitial nephritis can result from reflux nephropathy, polycystic kidney disease, gout and multiple myeloma.

GENERAL INVESTIGATIONS

- **Urine dipstick**
  +++ glucose with diabetes mellitus.

- **24-hour urine collection**
  >3 litres confirms polyuria, and helps differentiate from urinary frequency.

- **U&Es**
  Plasma urea and creatinine levels ↑ renal failure. Sodium ↑ with uncompensated polyuria (inadequate water intake). Sodium ↓ with urea/creatinine ↓ indicates polydipsia as the primary cause. Potassium ↓ may cause nephrogenic diabetes insipidus.

- **Urine and plasma osmolality**
  Urine osmolality low and plasma osmolality normal in pituitary and nephrogenic diabetes insipidus. Urine osmolality low and plasma osmolality normal to low in compulsive water drinking.

- **Serum calcium**
  ↑ calcium causes osmotic diuresis and chronic tubulointerstitial nephritis.

- **Serum glucose**
  ↑ diabetes.

The above tests may be all that is required to differentiate between osmotic diuresis, excess fluid intake and diabetes insipidus. If the differentiation between primary polydipsia and diabetes insipidus cannot be made confidently then proceed with the following two tests. The reader is advised to consult a reference source regarding the precautions and safety measures to be observed in the water deprivation and DDAVP tests.

- **Water deprivation test**
  Do not perform this test in volume-depleted patients nor in the presence of hypernatraemia.
  After overnight water restriction the plasma osmolality is measured.
  Plasma osmolality ↓: primary polydipsia.
  Plasma osmolality ↑: stop test and measure urine osmolality.
  Urine osmolality ↑: no diabetes insipidus.
  Urine osmolality ↓ in three consecutive samples: diabetes insipidus.

- **DDAVP test**
  Arginine vasopressin is then administered.
  Urine osmolality ↑: cranial diabetes insipidus.
  No urine osmolality ↑: nephrogenic diabetes insipidus.

SPECIFIC INVESTIGATIONS

- **CT/MRI head**
  Tumours, hypothalamic disease.

- **Renal biopsy**
  Acute tubular necrosis, chronic tubulointerstitial nephritis.

- Polyuria accompanied by polydipsia is often the first presentation of both type 1 and type 2 diabetes mellitus. Urgent investigation is required.

- Diabetes mellitus is not the only cause of polyuria accompanied by thirst. If urinalysis is negative for sugar, diabetes insipidus or hypercalcaemia are possible diagnoses.

POPLITEAL SWELLINGS

Popliteal swellings are not uncommon. The majority are easily diagnosed on clinical examination alone.

CAUSES

SUPERFICIAL

- Sebaceous cyst
- Lipoma
- Varix of the short saphenous vein

DEEP

- Lipoma
- Lymphadenopathy
- Semi-membranosus bursa
- Baker's cyst
- Popliteal artery aneurysm

BONY

- Exostoses
- Osteogenic sarcoma

HISTORY

Superficial

Sebaceous cyst

A sebaceous cyst will present as a firm swelling in the skin. It may be tender if it becomes inflamed and there may be a discharge from it.

Lipoma

This presents as a soft lobulated swelling in the subcutaneous tissue.

Varix of the short saphenous vein

This presents as a soft swelling behind the knee, usually associated with varicose veins of the short saphenous system.

Deep

Lipoma

Deeper lipomas are difficult to feel because of the tough overlying fascia. They do not always feel soft and lobulated, as superficial ones do.

Lymphadenopathy

There may be several palpable lumps within the popliteal fossa. The patient will usually draw attention to a lesion distally, either on the

SECTION A

leg or on the foot, usually on the lateral margin of the foot or the back of the leg. Other groups of nodes may be enlarged.

Semi-membranosus bursa

The patient complains of a swelling behind the knee that interferes with knee movement, particularly flexion.

Baker's cyst

A Baker's cyst is a pulsion diverticulum of the knee joint caused by chronic disease within the joint. The patient will usually give a history of a painful knee joint and may have osteoarthritis or rheumatoid arthritis. Occasionally the cyst ruptures and the patient complains of severe pain in the calf, which has to be carefully distinguished from venous thrombosis.

Popliteal artery aneurysm

These often get quite large before they are noticed. The patient may be aware of a pulsatile swelling behind the knee but often notices it when crossing the legs, the upper of the crossed limbs moving with each pulse.

Bony

Exostoses

Exostoses may grow in the region of the epiphyseal cartilage of the femur. There is a well-defined bony swelling in the popliteal fossa.

Osteogenic sarcoma

This may affect either the lower end of the femur or the upper end of the tibia. There is a rather diffuse swelling around the knee joint. Pain may be a presenting symptom. There may also be general malaise and weight loss. Occasionally pulmonary metastases have occurred at presentation, and there may be cough and haemoptysis.

EXAMINATION

Superficial

Sebaceous cyst

There will be a small, well-defined swelling in the skin with a punctum. If it is infected, the surrounding skin will be red and there may be discharge.

Lipoma

There will be a soft, lobulated swelling in the popliteal fossa.

Varix of the short saphenous vein

This is not uncommon. There will be a soft, compressible dilatation at the termination of the short saphenous vein. There may be an expansile cough impulse. A fluid thrill will be palpable when the short saphenous vein lower down the leg is tapped.

Deep

Lipoma

A deep lipoma in the fat of the popliteal fossa may be difficult to define accurately. It does not always have the soft, lobulated appearance of a more superficial lipoma.

Lymphadenopathy

There may be a number of discrete glands palpable or they may be firm and matted together. Check for a lesion distally on the leg or foot, e.g. malignant melanoma. Check for lymphadenopathy elsewhere.

Semi-membranosus bursa

The swelling lies above the level of the knee joint line, slightly to the medial side of the popliteal fossa. It tends to be firm in consistency and transilluminates.

Baker's cyst

Baker's cysts occur more often in elderly patients with long-standing arthritis or in younger patients with rheumatoid arthritis. The lump is below the level of the knee joint and deep to gastrocnemius. It may transilluminate. Pressure over the lump may reduce it into the knee joint. Examination of the knee joint reveals changes consistent with arthritis, i.e. limited movements, crepitus and occasionally an effusion.

Popliteal artery aneurysm

An expansile, pulsatile mass will be palpable in the popliteal fossa. They are often bilateral. Check the distal circulation. Popliteal aneurysms may thrombose with distal ischaemia, or may throw off small emboli causing ischaemic toes or ischaemic ulcers on the tips of the toes. Palpate the abdomen: there is an association between popliteal aneurysms and abdominal aortic aneurysms.

Bony

Exostoses

A bony mass may be felt in the popliteal fossa.

Osteogenic sarcoma

The overlying skin may be reddened, with dilated subcutaneous veins. There may be tenderness. The swelling is usually smooth until it spreads into the surrounding tissues, when it becomes irregular. The swelling feels firm but is not usually bony hard.

GENERAL INVESTIGATIONS

■ **FBC, ESR**
Hb ↓ lymphadenopathy, e.g. part of generalised lymphadenopathy associated with reticulosis. WCC ↑ reticulosis. ESR ↑ reticulosis, osteogenic sarcoma with secondaries.

■ **US**
Lipoma. Semi-membranosus bursa. Baker's cyst. Popliteal artery aneurysm.

■ **Knee X-ray**
Exostoses. Osteoarthritis (Baker's cyst). Rheumatoid arthritis (Baker's cyst). Osteogenic sarcoma – bone destruction, grows out of cortex, elevating periosteum with reposition of subperiosteal bone (Codman's triangle), radiating spicules of bone ('sunray' spicules).

■ **CXR**
Secondary deposits from osteogenic sarcoma. Hilar lymph nodes with generalised lymphadenopathy.

SPECIFIC INVESTIGATIONS

■ **Duplex Doppler**
Varix of short saphenous vein. Popliteal artery aneurysm.

■ **CT**
Shows invasion of osteogenic sarcoma. Lung secondaries.

■ **MRI**
Baker's cyst. Bone tumour.

■ **Arteriography**
Popliteal aneurysm. Distal circulation.

- There is an association between popliteal artery aneurysms and abdominal aortic aneurysms. Always examine the abdomen.

- If the lump is thought to be a gland, always examine the sole of the foot, between the toes and under the toenails to exclude a primary lesion, e.g. melanoma.

- Vague generalised swelling around the knee in a young patient may suggest an osteogenic sarcoma.

PRURITUS

Pruritus is itching of the skin. There are a vast number of dermatological causes of pruritus which are usually visible on inspection. The following are causes of generalised pruritus in the absence of dermatological disease.

CAUSES

- Obstructive jaundice
- Chronic renal failure

HAEMATOLOGICAL DISEASE

- Iron deficiency
- Polycythaemia

INTERNAL MALIGNANCY

- Bronchial carcinoma
- Hodgkin's disease

ENDOCRINE DISEASE

- Hyperthyroidism
- Hypothyroidism
- Diabetes mellitus

DRUGS

- Oral contraceptive pill (cholestasis)
- Opiates (histamine release)
- Alcohol and drug withdrawal

HISTORY

When approaching a patient with generalised pruritus, enquiries are made regarding the site and duration of symptoms. Occasionally the onset of pruritus will correlate with the initiation of drug treatment, allowing you to exclude the offending medication. It may also occur as a side-effect of alcohol or drug withdrawal. Pruritus after a hot bath classically occurs with polycythaemia. Iron deficiency, even in the absence of anaemia, can cause pruritus; therefore symptoms of blood loss in each system should be carefully elicited.

Haemoptysis, chronic cough and weight loss in smokers may be due to underlying bronchial carcinoma, which is an important subgroup of internal malignancies that present with pruritus. The presence of localised lymphadenopathy, fever, night sweats and weight loss should lead to the consideration of Hodgkin's disease. Patients with obstructive jaundice (p. 240) may present with pruritus (due to the accumulation of bile salts), even while the jaundice is not clinically apparent. With complete obstruction, patients may notice pale stools and dark urine.

Lethargy, anorexia, nocturia, oliguria, polyuria, haematuria, frothy urine from proteinuria, skin fragility, oedema and bone pains are some of the multisystemic features suggestive of chronic renal disease. Interestingly, pruritus seldom occurs with acute renal failure.

As pruritus may be due to thyroid disease, clinical assessment of the thyroid status is an important aspect of the history. Features of hyperthyroidism are tremor, heat intolerance, palpitations, increased appetite with weight loss, anxiety and diarrhoea. Features of hypothyroidism are cold intolerance, mental slowing, weight gain, constipation and menorrhagia.

EXAMINATION

Inspection

Wide, staring eyes with lid lag and tremor may be present with thyrotoxicosis. Pallor of the conjunctivae may be evident in severe anaemia, whereas, with polycythaemia, conjunctival insufflation and facial plethora occur. The sclera should also be examined for the presence of jaundice. Sallow skin with easy bruising and uraemic frost may be seen with chronic renal failure. Spoon-shaped nails of iron deficiency may be accompanied by angular cheilitis. Clubbing may be due to bronchial carcinoma.

GENERAL EXAMINATION

Asymmetrical, non-tender, localised lymphadenopathy in the absence of infection is suggestive of Hodgkin's disease. The thyroid gland is palpated for abnormalities, such as enlargement, nodularity and asymmetry. A respiratory examination is performed; features of bronchial carcinoma include monophonic inspiratory wheeze (partial endoluminal bronchial obstruction), lobar collapse of the lung, pleural effusion, and Horner's syndrome with apical lung tumours. Chest wall tenderness may also occur as a result of tumour infiltration. Splenomegaly may occur with Hodgkin's disease and polycythaemia rubra vera.

GENERAL INVESTIGATIONS

- **Urine dipstick**
  Protein and blood with renal disease.

- **FBC and blood film**
  Microcytic hypochromic anaemia with iron deficiency, normochromic normocytic anaemia with Hodgkin's, ↑ Hb with polycythaemia.

- **U&Es**
  Urea and creatinine ↑ renal failure.
- **Glucose**
  ↑ with diabetes mellitus.
- **LFTs**
  Bilirubin ↑, alkaline phosphatase ↑ with obstructive jaundice.
- **TFTs**
  TSH ↓ and T_4 ↑ thyrotoxicosis; TSH ↑ and T_4 ↓ hypothyroidism.
- **CXR**
  Bronchial carcinoma, hilar lymphadenopathy with Hodgkin's disease.

SPECIFIC INVESTIGATIONS

- **Excisional biopsy of lymph node**
  Hodgkin's disease – Reed–Sternberg cells.
- **US abdomen**
  Dilated bile ducts with obstructive jaundice, the site and cause of obstruction may be visualised. The size of the kidneys may be decreased with chronic renal disease, and multiple cysts visible with polycystic kidney disease.
- **Serum iron, serum ferritin, protoporphyrin**
  Serum iron ↓, serum ferritin ↓, free erythrocyte protoporphyrin ↑ iron deficiency.
- **CT chest and abdomen**
  Hilar lymphadenopathy in lymphoma. Chest lesion in bronchial carcinoma.

- Persistent pruritus may be the presenting symptom of lymphoma or other malignancy. Always examine the abdomen and lymph nodes.

SECTION A

PRURITUS ANI

Pruritus ani is itching around the anal canal. It is a common symptom and in approximately half the cases no cause can be found.

CAUSES

ANAL DISCHARGE
- Haemorrhoids
- Fistula-in-ano
- Skin tags
- Warts
- Carcinoma
- Polyps
- Gonococcal proctitis

FAECAL SOILING
- Incontinence
- Poor hygiene
- Diarrhoea

SKIN DISEASE
- Candidiasis
- Tinea cruris
- Lichen sclerosus
- Contact dermatitis
- Scabies
- Psoriasis
- Eczema

PARASITES
- Threadworms

PSYCHOGENIC
- Anxiety

HISTORY

Anal discharge

Any cause within the anus or lower rectum that produces moisture and sogginess of the anal skin may cause pruritus ani. Patients may volunteer the information that they have haemorrhoids or perianal warts. They may have noticed an anal discharge, which soils the underwear. Check for a history of anal sexual exposure.

Faecal soiling

The patient may complain of incontinence. This may be associated with poor hygiene. Chronic diarrhoea may be responsible. There may be an underlying cause for the chronic diarrhoea, e.g. colitis or Crohn's disease. Excessive sweating in hot weather may be associated with pruritus ani.

Skin diseases

If the patient is diabetic or immunosuppressed, candidiasis may be responsible. Recent oral antibiotic therapy may result in candidiasis. Check whether the patient has an itchy rash anywhere else. This may be particularly so with scabies or eczema. Contact dermatitis may result from the use of deodorants or a change in washing powder for the underwear. Psoriasis is usually not itchy but sometimes considerable itching occurs, especially if the area becomes infected. Lichen sclerosus is uncommon, occurring chiefly in women, when it may involve both the vulva and the perineum. In men, this may be associated with balanitis xerotica obliterans, so enquire if there is any abnormality of the foreskin.

Parasites

Threadworms usually occur in children. The parents may have noticed them.

Psychogenic

Idiopathic pruritus may occur in people with anxiety states. An itch–scratch cycle may occur, which is difficult to break.

EXAMINATION

Anal discharge

Inspection of the anus may show skin tags, the external opening of a fistula-in-ano, perianal warts or haemorrhoids. Digital rectal examination may reveal a carcinoma of the anal canal or fibrous anal polyps. Proctoscopy and sigmoidoscopy will confirm any associated anal or rectal lesion. Take a swab if purulent discharge.

Faecal soiling

Soiling of the underwear may be apparent. General poor hygiene may be apparent also in the patient. Carry out a digital rectal examination to check for sphincteric tone.

Skin diseases

Candidiasis may occur in those on long-term antibiotics, diabetics and the immunosuppressed. Tinea cruris is more common in men.

The infection often involves the groin and perineum in addition to the perianal areas. The patient may also have co-existing tinea pedis. With lichen sclerosus there are well-defined plaques of superficial atrophy of the epidermis with a whitish colour. In the male, check the penis for balanitis xerotica obliterans. With contact dermatitis there may be changes in the skin in other areas apart from the perianal area. With scabies there are usually lesions on other parts of the body. Burrows 5–10 mm deep appear as long ridges, which may be 'S' shaped. Isolation of the organism with a pin and examination under the microscope will confirm the diagnosis. With psoriasis there will usually be lesions on other areas of the body, and this will also be so with eczema.

Parasites

Threadworms may be visible around the anus.

Psychogenic

There may be an obvious history of psychiatric illness or the patient may appear anxious or depressed.

GENERAL INVESTIGATIONS

- **FBC, ESR**
  These are usually normal.
- **Urinalysis**
  Positive for sugar – diabetic.
- **Blood glucose**
  Diabetic.
- **Stool culture**
  Ova, parasites and cysts, cause of diarrhoea.
- **Anal swab**
  Gram stain – Gram-negative intracellular diplococci in gonorrhoea.
- **Skin scrapings**
  For mycotic infection, microscopy and culture.
- **Nocturnal 'Sellotape swab'**
  Threadworms.
- **Biopsy**
  Anal carcinoma. Lichen sclerosus.

- Always perform a digital rectal examination.
- Perianal candidiasis suggests diabetes. Check the blood sugar.
- Perianal warts imply an STD. Refer to a GUM clinic.
- Always take a full sexual history, including unusual sexual practices.
- Suspicious anal lesions should be biopsied to exclude anal cancer.

PYREXIA OF UNKNOWN ORIGIN

Most pyrexias result from a clearly defined illness, e.g. acute pyelonephritis or acute appendicitis, or from self-limiting viral infections, e.g. common cold. Pyrexia of unknown origin is a fever, the cause of which is undetermined after taking a history and performing a clinical examination. The fever is often prolonged.

CAUSES

BACTERIAL

- Abscess, e.g. subphrenic, pelvic
- Subacute bacterial endocarditis
- TB
- Brucellosis
- Typhoid
- Leptospirosis
- Q fever
- Cat scratch disease

VIRAL

- Influenza
- Glandular fever
- HIV
- CMV

FUNGAL

- Candidiasis
- Aspergillosis
- Pneumocystis jiroveci (formerly carinii)

PROTOZOAL

- Malaria
  - (common in Africa)
- Amoebiasis
- Toxoplasmosis

NEOPLASIA

- Hypernephroma
- Lymphoma
- Hepatoma
- Acute leukaemia

CONNECTIVE TISSUE DISEASE

- Rheumatoid arthritis
- SLE
- Polyarteritis nodosa and other vasculitis
- Temporal arteritis

GRANULOMATOUS DISEASE

- Crohn's disease
- Sarcoidosis

OTHERS

- Myocardial infarction
- Post-immunisation
- Drug induced
- Pulmonary embolism
- Familial Mediterranean fever
- Munchausen's disease (factitious)

HISTORY

A full and extensive history should be taken, noting especially travel abroad, contact with infection, contact with animals, bites, abrasions, rashes, diarrhoea. Check the drug history, including non-prescription drugs and drug abuse. Check for any recent history of surgery, particularly abdominal surgery. Is there any history of recent immunisations? Has the patient experienced night sweats, weight loss and general malaise?

EXAMINATION

A full physical examination should be carried out. This should be directed at every system of the body, checking particularly for lymphadenopathy and hepatosplenomegaly. Rectal and vaginal examination should be carried out.

INVESTIGATIONS

It may be necessary to carry out numerous and repeated investigations. It may also be necessary to withhold any drugs one at a time to see if the temperature settles.

GENERAL INVESTIGATIONS

- FBC, ESR
  Hb ↓ malignancy, anaemia of chronic disease, e.g. rheumatoid arthritis. WCC ↑ infection, leukaemia. Lymphocytes ↑ viral

infection. Platelets ↓ leukaemia. ESR ↑ malignancy, connective tissue disease, TB.

- **U&Es**
  Connective tissue disease affecting the kidneys.

- **LFTs**
  Biliary tract or liver disease, e.g. cholangitis, hepatitis.

- **Blood glucose**
  Diabetes – infections are more common in diabetics.

- **Blood culture**
  Streptococcus viridans suggests infective endocarditis. Isolation of coliforms suggests the possibility of intra-abdominal sepsis.

- **Viral antibodies**
  Hepatitis B, hepatitis C, infectious mononucleosis, HIV, CMV.

- **Sputum culture**
  Microscopy for tubercle bacilli and C&S.

- **Urine microscopy and culture**
  Microscopic haematuria in endocarditis. Haematuria in hypernephroma and blood dyscrasias. White cells – infection. Granular or red cell casts – renal inflammation, e.g. connective tissue disease. Proteinuria suggests renal disease.

- **Stool culture and microscopy**
  C&S. Ova, parasites and cysts on microscopy.

- **CXR**
  TB. Atypical pneumonia. Pneumonitis associated with HIV and *Pneumocystis jiroveci*. Secondary deposits. Hilar glands associated with sarcoidosis, TB and lymphoma.

- **ECG**
  Cardiac disease.

SPECIFIC INVESTIGATIONS

- **Rheumatoid factor**
  Rheumatoid arthritis.

- **Serological tests**
  Q fever, brucellosis, leptospirosis.

- **Autoantibodies**
  Connective tissue disease.

- **Mantoux test**
  TB.

- **Antistreptolysin O titre**
  Rheumatic fever.

- **Bone marrow aspirate**
  Leukaemia. Myeloma.

- **Lumbar puncture**
  White cells and organisms – meningitis. Blood – subarachnoid haemorrhage. Protein – Guillain–Barré syndrome.

- **US abdomen**
  Intraperitoneal abscesses.

- **Gallium scan**
  Localised infection.

- **Labelled white cell scan**
  Localised infection/abscess.

- **Liver biopsy**
  Hepatitis.

- **Renal biopsy**
  Glomerular disease. Malignancy.

- **Muscle biopsy**
  Myositis.

- **CT**
  Infection. Malignancy.

- **Exploratory laparotomy**
  This may be necessary to exclude intra-abdominal sepsis.

- Pyrexia of unknown origin presents a diagnostic challenge. Clinical signs are often non-specific and may fluctuate in severity and alter with chronicity.

- Empirical treatment is not advocated in cases of pyrexia of unknown origin with the following exceptions: cases meeting the criteria for culture-negative endocarditis; cases suggestive of cryptic disseminated TB; and cases in which temporal arteritis is suspected.

RASHES

A rash is a change in the skin which affects its colour, appearance or texture. It may be localised to one part of the body or be generalised. The cause of many rashes can be diagnosed on clinical inspection of the rash alone. The morphology of a rash is therefore important. Morphological terms include:

- Macule – a non-raised, usually well-demarcated, coloured area of skin.
- Papule – a raised, usually round, well-demarcated lesion <5 mm in diameter. It varies in colour and may become nodular, undergo transformation into a vesicle or ulcerate.
- Nodule – similar to a papule but is >5 mm in diameter.
- Blister – a lesion in the skin containing free fluid. Those <5 mm in diameter are termed vesicles; those >5 mm are termed bullae.
- Pustule – a pus-containing raised lesion <5 mm in diameter.
- Purpura – purpura describes areas of bleeding into the skin >2 mm in diameter. Petechiae are <2 mm in diameter and ecchymoses are >4 mm in diameter. They do not blanch with pressure.
- Erythema – a persistent reddening of the skin due to dilatation of superficial capillaries. It may be localised or generalised.
- Scales and plaques – represent an excess of keratinised epithelium in the skin.

CAUSES

Macules
Congenital

- Albright's syndrome
- Neurofibromatosis (multiple *cafe au lait* spots)

Drug reaction
Infection

- Virus
  - Non-specific viral exanthem
  - Measles
  - Rubella
- Fungus (pityriasis versicolor)
- Bacterial
  - Macular syphilide
  - Tuberculoid leprosy
  - Typhoid (rose spots)
  - common where typhoid is endemic

Immune mediated

- Allergic reaction
- Vitiligo

Neoplastic

- Lentigo maligna (Hutchinson's melanotic freckle)

Other

- Sun damage including freckles
- Pregnancy (chloasma)
- *Cafe au lait* spot
- Berloque dermatitis
- Mongolian spot
- Peutz–Jeghers syndrome

Papules

Congenital

- Pseudoxanthoma elasticum
- Tuberous sclerosis

Other

- Acne
- Campbell de Morgan spots
- Pityriasis lichenoides chronica
- Lichen planus
- Insect bite
- Guttate psoriasis
- Keratosis pilaris
- Darier's disease

Infection

- Scabies
- Viral illness
- Molluscum contagiosum
- Milia

Systemic illness

- Xanthomata (hyperlipidaemia)
- Acanthosis nigricans

Malignancy

- Kaposi's sarcoma

Nodules

Malignancy

- Lymphoma
- Metastatic carcinoma

Infections

- Warts
- Atypical infections
  - Leprosy
  - Syphilis
  - TB (lupus vulgaris)
  - (commoner where TB is endemic)
  - Fish-tank and swimming pool granuloma
  - Actinomycosis

Systemic disease

- Xanthoma
- Gouty tophi
- Rheumatoid nodules
- Sarcoidosis (lupus pernio)
- Vasculitis

Other

- Nodulocystic acne
- Keratoacanthoma
- Pyoderma gangrenosum

Pustules

Infection

- Bacterial
  - Staphylococcal infection
  - Impetigo, boils, folliculitis, sycosis barbae
  - Jacuzzi folliculitis (*Pseudomonas* infection)
- Viral
  - Herpes simplex
  - Herpes zoster
  - Cowpox
  - Orf
- Fungus
  - *Candida*

Other

- Acne vulgaris
- Rosacea
- Hidradenitis suppurativa
- Pustular psoriasis

- Dermatitis herpetiformis
- Behçet's syndrome

Drugs

- Reaction to medications

Blisters

Infection

- Viral
  - Herpes simplex
  - Herpes zoster (including chicken pox and shingles)
  - Hand, foot and mouth disease
- Bacterial
  - Bullous impetigo

Trauma

- Insect bites
- Burns
- Skin friction

Drugs

- Drug reactions
  - ACE inhibitors
  - Barbiturates

Systemic disease

- Dermatitis herpetiformis (coeliac disease)
- Porphyria

Other

- Eczema
- Secondary to peripheral leg oedema
- Pemphigus
- Pemphigoid
- Erythema multiforme
- Toxic epidermal necrolysis (scalded skin syndrome)
- Epidermolysis bullosa
- Allergic reaction

Purpura

Inherited

- Clotting disorders
  - Haemophilia

- Christmas disease
- von Willebrand's disease
- Collagen vascular disorders
  - Ehlers–Danlos syndrome

Trauma

- Accidental
- Non-accidental

Infection

- Infective endocarditis
- Meningococcal septicaemia
- Ebola virus

Other haematological

- Thrombocytopenia
  - Immune thrombocytopenic purpura
  - Lymphoma
  - Leukaemia
- Aplastic anaemia
- Paraproteinaemias
  - Cryoglobulinaemia
  - Hypergammaglobulinaemia
- DIC

Systemic illness

- Chronic liver disease
- Renal failure
- Vasculitis
  - Henoch–Schönlein purpura
  - SLE

Drugs

- Corticosteroids
- Warfarin
- Aspirin and NSAIDs
- Cytotoxic agents (bone marrow failure)

Other

- Senile purpura
- Increased intravascular pressure, e.g. following coughing or vomiting
- Vitamin C (scurvy) and K deficiency

Erythema

Infection

- Cellulitis, e.g. streptococcal
- Viral, e.g. measles
- HIV

Traumatic

- Burns (thermal, chemical, sunburn)

Drugs

- Antibiotics
- NSAIDs

Systemic disease

- Chronic liver disease (palmar erythema)
- SLE (butterfly rash)

Other

- Gout
- Rosacea
- Erythema ab igne
- 'Deck chair legs'

SPECIFIC ERYTHEMATOUS CONDITIONS

Erythema multiforme ('target' lesions)

Severe form is known as Stevens–Johnson syndrome

Infection

- Herpes simplex virus
- Mycoplasma
- Orf

Collagen disorders

Drugs

- Barbiturates
- Sulphonamides
- Penicillin

Erythema nodosum (raised, red, painful lesions commonly on shins)

Infection

- TB
  - (commoner where TB is endemic)

- Leprosy
- *Streptococcus*
- Various viral and fungal infections

Drugs

- Sulphonamides
- Dapsone
- Contraceptive pill
- BCG vaccination

Other

- Rheumatic fever
- Sarcoidosis
- Inflammatory bowel disease

Erythema marginatum

- acute rheumatic fever

Erythema induratum

- TB

Erythema chronicum migrans

- Lyme disease

Livido reticularis (fish net stocking-type rash)

- SLE
- Antiphospholipid syndrome

Palmar erythema

- Rheumatoid arthritis
- Chronic liver disease
- Pregnancy
- Thyrotoxicosis

Scales and plaques

Infection

- Fungal (e.g. pityriasis versicolor)
- Syphilis (secondary)

Malignancy

- Bowen's disease
- Mycosis fungoides

Drugs

- Beta blockers
- Carbamazepine

Systemic disease

- Reactive arthritis (keratoderma blenorrhagica)

Other

- Psoriasis
- Eczema
- Seborrhoeic dermatitis
- Seborrhoeic keratosis
- Lichen simplex
- Lichen planus
- Solar keratosis
- Juvenile plantar dermatosis
- Ichthyosis

HISTORY

A specific history for each condition is beyond the scope of this book and the reader is referred to a textbook of dermatology.

Important factors in the history include: duration of the rash and associated symptoms; distribution at onset and any change or spread; associated itch or pain. Determine the patient's age, racial background, occupation, sexual orientation, drug history, family history, e.g. predisposition to psoriasis, eczema or skin cancer. Take a full medical history. Enquire about any contact with infectious diseases, e.g. measles, chicken pox. Are there any associated symptoms, e.g. joint symptoms? Is there a history of exposure to the sun? Is there any history of any allergies or exposures to irritants or cosmetics? Check carefully for diabetes or immunosuppression which might suggest a fungal infection.

EXAMINATION

The patient should be examined in good light using the naked eye initially and then a magnifying glass (or dermatoscope) to inspect the rash. Ascertain the distribution of the rash. Symmetrical rashes suggest an endogenous cause, e.g. viral; asymmetrical rashes suggest an exogenous cause, e.g. local skin irritants, nappy rash. Note the morphology of the rash, i.e. macular, papular, red and scaly. Check all sites that may be affected and complete the examination by examining the scalp, eyes, mouth, hands and feet, especially the nails, and anogenital area. Check for lymphadenopathy. Is there any associated fever?

GENERAL INVESTIGATIONS

- **Urinalysis**
  Diabetes, e.g. fungal infections.

- **FBC**
  WCC ↑ infections.

- **ESR/CRP**
  Raised in autoimmune and inflammatory conditions.

- **Wood light (UV light wavelength 360 nm)**
  Pigmentary disease and fungal infections.

- **Microbiology**
  Swabs for bacteria, scrapings for fungi.

- **Patch testing**
  Allergens.

- **Aspiration of vesicles**
  Culture for bacteria, e.g. staphylococci, meningococci. PCR EM or examination for viruses, e.g. herpes simplex, herpes zoster.

- **Viral antibodies**
  Herpes simplex, herpes zoster.

- **HIV serology**
  May be positive with Kaposi's sarcoma.

- **Biopsy**
  Confirms many suspected lesions and excludes malignancy.

- **Meningococcal septicaemia is rapidly fatal if not recognised. Check with a glass that the rash does not blanch with pressure.**

- **Lentigo maligna (Hutchinson's melanotic freckle) is associated with a high risk of malignant change. Referral for a biopsy is essential.**

- **Rapid development of a new mole or change in an existing one is highly suggestive of malignant melanoma. Urgent dermatological referral is required.**

- **Severe or recurrent staphylococcal, candidal or herpetic viral infections may point to an immunosuppressed state. Further investigation is essential.**

- **Certain conditions such as pemphigus and toxic epidermal necrolysis may lead to severe illness. Urgent referral is required.**

- **Stevens–Johnson syndrome is life-threatening and patients should be admitted to hospital for careful monitoring.**

RECTAL BLEEDING

Rectal bleeding is a common symptom. The majority of patients with rectal bleeding have a simple condition such as haemorrhoids but the symptoms should always be taken seriously and investigated. Rectal bleeding with change in bowel habit and colicky abdominal pain should be regarded as due to colorectal cancer until proved otherwise.

CAUSES

ANUS

- Haemorrhoids
- Fissure-in-ano
- Carcinoma
- Trauma

COLON AND RECTUM

- Carcinoma
- Polyps
- Diverticular disease
- Inflammatory bowel disease
  - Ulcerative colitis
  - Crohn's disease
- Ischaemic colitis
- Rectal prolapse
- Angiodysplasia
- Irradiation colitis or proctitis
- Solitary rectal ulcer

SMALL BOWEL

- Meckel's diverticulum
- Intussusception
- Mesenteric infarction
- Aortoenteric fistula

UPPER GASTROINTESTINAL TRACT

- Massive haemorrhage, e.g. duodenal ulcer

OTHERS

- Anticoagulants
- Bleeding diatheses
- Uraemia

HISTORY

Anus
Haemorrhoids

Piles occur at any age. Bleeding from piles is noted either on the toilet paper or as splashes in the toilet after defecation. Uncomplicated piles are not painful.

Fissure-in-ano

Fissure-in-ano is most common under the age of 40 years. It is quite common in children. The patient experiences pain on defecation, which may persist for minutes or hours afterwards. Constipation is usually a precipitating cause, the constipation being made worse by the fissure as the patient avoids defecation because of pain. Blood is noticed on the toilet paper or streaked on the stool.

Carcinoma of the anal canal

Carcinoma of the anal canal usually occurs in the elderly. It presents with pain on defecation and streaking of blood on the stools and blood on the toilet paper. Initially, in the early stages, it may be mistaken for a fissure-in-ano.

Trauma

There may be a history of a penetrating injury to the anal canal. Sexual abuse or homosexual practices may be relevant.

Colorectal
Carcinoma

With colonic carcinoma the blood may be mixed with the stool. There is usually a history of accompanying change in bowel habit and colicky abdominal pain. With rectal cancer the blood is usually streaked on the stool and there may be a history of tenesmus, i.e. a sense of incomplete evacuation of the rectum.

Polyps

The history may be similar to that of carcinoma.

Diverticular disease

Bleeding associated with diverticular disease is typically acute, massive and fresh. There may be a past history of diverticular disease

Inflammatory bowel disease

With ulcerative colitis and Crohn's disease there is often sudden onset of diarrhoea with watery, brown motions containing mucus and fresh blood. There is usually colicky abdominal pain. With ulcerative proctitis the patient may complain of tenesmus.

Ischaemic colitis

This usually occurs in the elderly. There is colicky abdominal pain associated with the passage of dark-red venous blood PR.

Angiodysplasia

The patient is usually elderly. There is bleeding PR, which may be torrential but is more often repeated small bleeds.

Irradiation proctitis or colitis

There will be a history of irradiation, often for carcinoma of the cervix. The patient passes blood and mucus PR and complains of tenesmus.

Rectal prolapse

The patient will be aware of something hanging out of the back passage that comes down on defecation. Bleeding is due to trauma.

Solitary rectal ulcer

Bleeding occurs after defecation, usually in small volumes. This may be associated with mucus discharge and a feeling of a lump in the anus.

Small bowel

Meckel's diverticulum

This usually results in painless bleeding in young adults. The blood tends to be dark red and may on occasions have the characteristics of melaena.

Intussusception

This usually occurs in infants, but may rarely occur at any age. The child has colicky abdominal pain and draws the legs up, screams and passes a stool consisting of mixed blood and mucus ('redcurrant jelly' stool).

Mesenteric infarction

The patient is usually elderly, or a younger patient who has a history of heart disease (embolism). The patient develops severe central abdominal, colicky pain associated with diffuse tenderness and later collapse and shock.

Aortoenteric fistula

This usually occurs following repair of an infrarenal aortic aneurysm with a Dacron graft. The Dacron graft becomes infected, the fistula forms between the aorta and duodenum. Depending on the speed of the bleed, there may be either melaena or profuse red rectal haemorrhage with shock.

Upper gastrointestinal tract

Massive haemorrhage from the upper gastrointestinal tract, e.g. bleeding oesophageal varices, duodenal ulcer, may present with bright-red bleeding PR. This is due to extremely fast intestinal transit and the patient will always be shocked.

Others

Check for a history of anticoagulants. The patient may have a bleeding disorder. Check for bleeding from other sites or spontaneous bruising.

Uraemia

Rectal bleeding may occur in uraemia and this may be related to a platelet defect.

Rarely, rectal bleeding may occur with collagen diseases, particularly polyarteritis nodosa.

EXAMINATION

Anus
Haemorrhoids

There may be obvious prolapsed haemorrhoids; however, sigmoidoscopy and proctoscopy are usually required to make the diagnosis.

Fissure-in-ano

Separate the buttocks. A chronic fissure-in-ano with a sentinel pile may be seen in the midline posteriorly, or more rarely in the midline anteriorly. Digital rectal examination, if attempted, will be extremely painful.

Carcinoma

This may show a hard ulcer in the anal canal with everted edges; however, in the early stages, carcinoma of the anal canal may be difficult to distinguish from a chronic fissure-in-ano. Biopsy should be undertaken.

Trauma

Bruising may be apparent around the anal canal. There may be a split in the skin or mucosa. Digital rectal examination will be painful.

Colon and rectum
Carcinoma

An abdominal mass may be palpable. There may be signs of intestinal obstruction. Digital rectal examination may reveal a hard, irregular, ulcerating mass.

Polyps

A polyp may be palpable in the rectum. There may be no findings on physical examination.

Diverticular disease

The patient may be tender in the left iliac fossa. Often there are no abdominal findings.

Inflammatory bowel disease

There may be a palpable abdominal mass with Crohn's disease. There may be localised abdominal tenderness. If toxic dilatation has occurred, the abdomen will be distended and tender, and there may be signs of peritonitis if perforation has occurred.

Ischaemic colitis

Physical examination may show left-sided abdominal tenderness and the patient may be shocked.

Angiodysplasia

There may be little to find other than rectal bleeding. There are usually no abdominal signs.

Irradiation colitis or proctitis

There may be some abdominal tenderness. Digital rectal examination will reveal a granular mucosa and blood on the glove.

Rectal prolapse

There will be obvious prolapse of the rectum with ulcerated, bleeding rectal mucosa.

Solitary rectal ulcer

There are no abdominal findings. Digital rectal examination may give the impression of a polypoid swelling just inside the rectum, which may be mistaken for carcinoma. Proctoscopy will reveal redness and oedema of the mucosa and, in about 50% of patients, frank ulceration will be noted.

Small bowel

Meckel's diverticulum

There will usually be nothing to find on abdominal examination.

Intussusception

A mass may be palpable in the right iliac fossa. Eventually, as the intussusception proceeds, the right iliac fossa becomes 'empty'.

Mesenteric infarction

The patient may be in atrial fibrillation and this suggests embolism. There will be diffuse abdominal tenderness, later accompanied by collapse and shock.

Aortoenteric fistula

There will usually be the long midline scar of a recent aortic aneurysm repair. Otherwise there will be little to find on abdominal examination.

Upper gastrointestinal tract

Massive haemorrhage

There may be signs of liver failure associated with a massive bleed from varices. There may be epigastric tenderness associated with duodenal ulceration.

Others

With anticoagulants there may be bleeding from other orifices, as may occur also with bleeding diatheses. Look for signs of bruising. Uraemic bleeding is often seen in patients with established uraemia and they may already be on dialysis and have an arteriovenous fistula or a CAPD tube *in situ*. Rectal bleeding from collagen diseases is rare. Polyarteritis nodosa is probably the most common. Bleeding is due to necrotising vasculitis and there may be signs of vasculitis elsewhere, e.g. skin.

GENERAL INVESTIGATIONS

- **FBC, ESR**
  Hb ↓ may occur in almost any type of rectal bleeding. WCC ↑ inflammatory bowel disease, ischaemic colitis, aortoenteric fistula. Platelets ↓ in bleeding diatheses. ESR ↑ carcinoma, collagen disease.

- **U&Es**
  Urea and creatinine raised with uraemic bleeding. The urea may be raised due to absorption of blood from the bowel. Usually in this case the creatinine is normal.

- **LFTs**
  Liver failure associated with oesophageal varices.

- **Sigmoidoscopy/proctoscopy**
  Anorectal tumours. Haemorrhoids. Distal colitis. Solitary rectal ulcer. Biopsy.

- **AXR**
  Obstruction associated with carcinoma. Inflammatory bowel disease (toxic dilatation of the colon).

SPECIFIC INVESTIGATIONS

- **Barium enema**
  Carcinoma. Diverticular disease. Polyps. Inflammatory bowel disease. Ischaemic colitis.

- **Colonoscopy**
  Diverticular disease. Colonic tumours. Angiodysplasia. Colitis.

- **Angiography (in the acute bleeding phase)**
  Angiodysplasia. Bleeding Meckel's diverticulum.

- Labelled red cell scan
  Angiodysplasia. Meckel's diverticulum.

- Technetium scan
  Meckel's diverticulum.

- Haemorrhoids are common. There may be other
  causes for the bleeding. Always do a digital rectal
  examination and sigmoidoscopy.

- Change of bowel habit and weight loss in association
  with rectal bleeding requires urgent investigation.

- Painless rectal haemorrhage in the elderly is likely
  to be due to either diverticular disease (common) or
  angiodysplasia (less common).

- In a child presenting with rectal bleeding with no
  obvious cause, always consider non-accidental injury.

SCALP LESIONS

Lesions on the scalp are common; the most common are sebaceous cysts, which are often multiple.

CAUSES

TRAUMATIC

- Haematoma
- Cephalhaematoma

CYSTIC

- Sebaceous cysts

NEOPLASTIC

BENIGN
- Ivory osteoma

MALIGNANT
Primary
- Basal cell carcinoma
- Squamous cell carcinoma
- Malignant melanoma
- Leukaemia
- Myeloma

Secondary
- Breast
- Bronchus
- Thyroid
- Prostate
- Kidney

INFECTIVE

- Tinea capitis
- Cock's peculiar tumour

OTHER

- Psoriasis
- Seborrhoeic dermatitis

HISTORY

Traumatic

Check for a history of trauma. A boggy haematoma may overlie a skull fracture. A cephalhaematoma is seen in a newborn baby. It follows a traumatic delivery. The haematoma is below the periosteum of the skull

Sebaceous cyst

These may be multiple. The patient usually notices them when combing the hair.

Neoplastic

With an ivory osteoma the patient may notice a rock-hard swelling on the scalp. The patient is usually a young adult and is asymptomatic. Malignant ulcers may occur on the scalp. The patient will notice a lesion when combing the hair and bleeding may occur. These lesions present earlier in bald patients. Bony tenderness and swelling may be a presenting symptom of secondary deposits. There may be a history of a primary or a careful history must be taken to establish the site of a primary.

Infective

With Cock's peculiar tumour the patient may notice a sore, bleeding lesion on the scalp. Cock's peculiar tumour is due to a sebaceous cyst suppurating and granulation tissue appearing on its surface. It may be mistaken for a squamous cell carcinoma. Tinea capitis usually occurs in childhood. There is an itchy, red, scaly patch on the scalp and the hairs break easily, leaving patches of stubble.

Other

Psoriasis may affect the scalp. There is usually a history of lesions elsewhere on the body. Seborrhoeic dermatitis presents with a fine, scaly rash on the scalp. Hair growth is usually normal with both these lesions.

EXAMINATION

Traumatic

A knock on the head may cause a boggy haematoma. X-ray is required to exclude an underlying fracture. Cephalhaematoma occurs in the newborn; the haematoma spreads beneath the periosteum of the skull and is therefore limited by the skull suture lines.

Sebaceous cyst

Sebaceous cysts are spherical, tender, firm swellings in the scalp. They may be multiple. Rarely is a punctum visible with sebaceous cysts on the scalp.

Neoplastic

An ivory osteoma is a bony, hard, smooth swelling arising from the outer table of the skull. The skin is freely mobile over it. A squamous cell carcinoma presents as an ulcer with a hard, everted edge. A malignant melanoma is usually pigmented, ulcerated and bleeds. In both these conditions cervical lymphadenopathy may be present. A basal cell carcinoma is a raised ulcer with a rolled edge with a pearly appearance, often with superficial telangiectasia. Lesions in the skull may be secondaries from lung, breast, thyroid, prostate and kidney. Each of these areas should be examined for a possible primary.

SECTION A

Myeloma may present with painful lesions in the skull. There may be areas of localised tenderness.

Infective

Cock's peculiar tumour presents as an open, granulating sebaceous cyst. It appears angry and swollen and may be mistaken for a squamous cell carcinoma. In tinea capitis there are red, scaly patches on the scalp, with broken hairs giving a stubbled appearance.

Other

With psoriasis there are well-demarcated areas of scales heaped up over red plaque. The hair grows normally through the plaques. Check for psoriatic lesions elsewhere. Seborrhoeic dermatitis shows fine scales but the hairs remain intact.

GENERAL INVESTIGATIONS

The diagnosis of most of these lesions is made on clinical examination alone.

- **FBC, ESR**
  Hb ↓ malignancy. WCC ↑ leukaemia. ESR ↑ myeloma and other malignancies.

- **CXR**
  Primary tumour. Secondary malignancy, e.g. secondaries from malignant melanoma.

- **Skull X-ray**
  Fracture. Ivory osteoma. Pepper-pot skull – myeloma. Secondary deposits – osteolytic from lung, breast and thyroid. Osteosclerotic from prostate and occasionally kidney.

SPECIFIC INVESTIGATIONS

- **Serum protein electrophoresis**
  Monoclonal gammopathy with myeloma.

- **Bone scan**
  Bony secondaries.

- **Scalp scrapings**
  Fungal infection, e.g. tinea capitis.

- **Biopsy**
  Malignant lesions. Cock's peculiar tumour.

- **The scalp is a common site of tumour, especially in elderly, bald men and those with outside occupations. Biopsy is essential to confirm the diagnosis.**

SCROTAL PAIN

This may be due to lesions on the scrotal skin, within the scrotum, or may rarely be due to referred pain.

CAUSES

SKIN

● Infected sebaceous cyst
● Irritation (urine/faeces in the incontinent)
● Dermatitis
● Herpes simplex
● Behçet's disease
● Fournier's gangrene

INTERNAL SCROTAL SWELLINGS

● Strangulated hernia
● Testicular torsion
● Epididymo-orchitis
● Torsion of testicular appendage
● Haematocele
● Varicocele

REFERRED

● Groin strain
● Ilioinguinal nerve entrapment after hernia repair
● Idiopathic cord neuralgia
● Spinal nerve irritation

HISTORY

Skin

The patient may have noticed a skin lesion, which is itchy, sore or painful. In the elderly, confused and incontinent, pain and soreness may be due to the irritant effect of faeces and urine with superadded infection. Previous history of a superficial swelling may suggest an infected sebaceous cyst. There may be a history to suggest contact dermatitis. Painful vesicular lesions may suggest herpes. Behçet's syndrome may cause painful ulcerative lesions of the scrotum and the patient may also have similar lesions on the penis. Fournier's gangrene usually has acute onset in a young, healthy male with rapid progression to gangrene of the skin. There is often absence of a discernible cause.

Internal scrotal swellings

There may be a previous history of an inguinal hernia descending into the scrotum. Sudden onset of colicky abdominal pain and irreducibility may suggest the development of a strangulated inguinal hernia. Sudden onset of pain, redness and swelling in a teenager or young male suggests a diagnosis of testicular torsion. This may come on during vigorous exercise. This is a surgical emergency and needs urgent surgery. Gradual onset of pain, redness and tenderness will suggest epididymo-orchitis. Check for symptoms of urinary tract infection, e.g. dysuria or frequency, which may accompany epididymo-orchitis. Orchitis may be associated with mumps and this may be apparent, the patient complaining of bilateral painful parotid and submandibular glands together with painful cervical lymphadenopathy and constitutional illness. A history of trauma will suggest haematocele. A dull ache, often poorly localised, may be associated with a varicocele.

Referred pain

Rarely, the patient may complain of pain in the scrotum with no visible or palpable abnormality. Check for a history of previous inguinal hernia repair, which may have resulted in ilioinguinal nerve entrapment. Idiopathic cord neuralgia may occur but is rare. Occasionally 'groin strain' may cause scrotal pain. Referred pain from spinal lesions may rarely cause scrotal pain.

EXAMINATION

Skin

A red, scaly lesion will suggest dermatitis. There may be superadded infection. In the elderly and incontinent, the diagnosis of irritation from urine or faeces will usually be apparent. An infected sebaceous cyst will present as a localised, tender, red swelling on the scrotum. There may be purulent discharge. Herpes simplex will present with vesicular lesions. They may be present elsewhere, e.g. on the penis. Behçet's disease will present with painful ulcerative lesions on the scrotum as well as on the penis. There may be other signs of Behçet's disease, e.g. arthritis, keratitis, iritis, mouth ulcers. With Fournier's gangrene there is usually a tense, glossy oedema developing over the scrotum. Crepitations develop later before subcutaneous gangrene occurs. The gangrene may spread over the inguinal area and the lower abdominal wall. In the advanced case, the skin will have completely disappeared, leaving the testes hanging naked in the scrotum.

Internal scrotal swellings

There may be a tense, tender scrotal mass, which it is impossible to 'get above'. This would suggest a strangulated hernia. The presence of an enlarged tender testicle drawn up towards the groin suggests testicular torsion. An enlarged tender testis with redness and scrotal oedema suggests epididymo-orchitis. The parotid and submandibular glands should be checked to exclude mumps. Occasionally, torsion of a testicular appendage may occur and cause pain and scrotal swelling out of all proportion to the size of the lesion, which may be less than a few millimetres in diameter. A tender swelling with scrotal bruising and oedema following trauma will suggest a haematocele (a collection of blood between the layers of the tunica vaginalis). A varicocele may not be obvious until the patient has been standing up for 10–15 seconds. Classically it feels like a 'bag of worms' with the warm blood filling dilated veins, which are palpable through the scrotal skin. It is more common on the left-hand side. Rapid onset of a left-sided varicocele may be associated with carcinoma of the left kidney, the tumour growing down the left renal vein and obstructing the left testicular vein. Examine the abdomen for a left renal mass.

Referred pain

Check for the scar of an inguinal hernia repair. In ilioinguinal nerve entrapment there will be anaesthesia/paraesthesia below the scar and on the anterior aspect of the scrotal skin. In the rare case where scrotal pain may be referred from a spinal lesion, a full neurological examination should be carried out. Examine the lumbosacral spine for localised tenderness.

GENERAL INVESTIGATIONS

- **FBC, ESR**
  WCC ↑ infection. ESR ↑ infection, tumour.
- **US**
  Testicular lesion. Haematocele.
- **MSU**
  Urinary tract infection associated with epididymo-orchitis.
- **Swab**
  Ulcer, C&S.

SPECIFIC INVESTIGATIONS

- **Lumbosacral spine X-ray**
  Referred pain due to degenerative disease or metastases.
- **Laser Doppler**
  Check for testicular blood flow. Absent in testicular torsion.
- **Technetium scan**
  Testicular torsion (no outline of testis) versus epididymo-orchitis (good testicular blood flow).
- **US abdomen**
  Left renal carcinoma (varicocele).

SECTION A

- **MRI**
  Spinal lesion.

- **Surgery**
  Diagnostic between torsion and infection. There is rarely time or equipment to carry out laser Doppler or a technetium scan. If a testicular torsion is not dealt with within 6 hours of onset there is likely to be permanent damage to the testis. If there is any doubt in the diagnosis, assume that it is torsion and explore the scrotum surgically.

> • It is difficult, if not impossible, to distinguish between torsion and epididymo-orchitis. Urgent referral and surgical exploration is required.

SCROTAL SWELLINGS

Scrotal swellings are a common presenting complaint in the outpatient clinic. They are also therefore common in clinical examinations. It is important to be able to make a rapid diagnosis of testicular torsion and take appropriate action, i.e. surgery. It is also important to distinguish between those swellings that have underlying serious pathology (testicular tumour) and those that are simple and benign (epididymal cysts).

CAUSES

- Sebaceous cyst
- Indirect inguinal hernia
- Hydrocele
- Epididymal cyst (spermatocele)
- Epididymo-orchitis
- Testicular torsion
- Testicular tumour
- Varicocele
- Haematocele
- Sperm granuloma
- TB
  - common where TB is endemic
- Gumma

HISTORY

Sebaceous cyst

The patient may complain of several painful lumps on the scrotal skin. There may be a history of one or more of them becoming red, inflamed and tender with discharge.

Indirect inguinal hernia

The patient will be often aware of what the lump is. He may be able to reduce it. The hernia may present with a painful, irreducible swelling and signs of intestinal obstruction.

Hydrocele

An idiopathic hydrocele presents usually as a painless scrotal swelling which may become quite large. They usually occur over the age of 50 years. Occasionally there may be pain and discomfort if there is underlying testicular disease. A younger patient presenting with a hydrocele should raise the suspicion of an underlying malignancy.

Epididymal cyst

This presents as a painless scrotal swelling. Epididymal cysts may slowly enlarge over many years. They may be bilateral.

Epididymo-orchitis

The patient complains of pain and swelling, usually unilaterally. There are usually constitutional symptoms of malaise and fever. It may be accompanied by urinary tract infection with dysuria and frequency.

Testicular torsion

This usually occurs around puberty. It is rare over 25 years of age. There is sudden onset of pain in the scrotum and groin, which may radiate into the lower abdomen. This may be accompanied by nausea and vomiting. There may be a history of violent exercise, e.g. straining in the gymnasium, lifting or even masturbation. Always ascertain the exact time of onset of symptoms. To be sure of testicular salvage, surgery should be carried out within 6–8 hours of onset of symptoms.

Testicular tumour

Teratomas occur between 18 and 30 years, seminomas between 30 and 45 years. The common presentation is a feeling of heaviness in the scrotum accompanied by a painless swelling. Occasionally, symptoms are due to secondary deposits, e.g. abdominal pain from enlarged retroperitoneal lymph nodes. Occasionally, distant lymphadenopathy, e.g. cervical, may be a presenting symptom.

Varicocele

The patient (or partner) may notice varicose veins in the scrotum. Often the only symptom is a dragging ache in the scrotum and groin. Subfertility may be a presentation and is associated with bilateral varicoceles. A varicocele is more common on the left.

Haematocele

There will be a clear history of trauma.

Sperm granuloma

This may develop 2–4 months after vasectomy. The patient will complain of a small tender nodule at the site of vasectomy.

TB

This is now rare in the UK. A scrotal lump with associated dull, aching pain is the usual presentation. There may be a history of pulmonary or renal TB. There may be malaise, weight loss, haemoptysis or haematuria.

Gumma

This is extremely rare. There is a painless swelling of the testis. It needs to be distinguished from a testicular tumour. Other signs of syphilis may be present.

EXAMINATION

Sebaceous cyst

A small swelling or multiple small swellings occur in the scrotal skin. They are tense and spherical. Because of the thinness of the scrotal skin stretched over the swelling, the cheesy yellow material contained within them can be seen. There may be a small punctum surmounting the cyst.

Indirect inguinal hernia

Hernias that descend in the scrotum are invariably indirect. They may be reducible. It is impossible to get above the swelling. There is an expansile cough impulse and bowel sounds may be heard over the hernia.

Hydrocele

A hydrocele is usually unilateral. It may become very large. A hydrocele is fluctuant, transilluminates and is dull to percussion. If large enough there may be a fluid thrill. The testis cannot be palpated separately from the hydrocele. It is possible to get above the swelling except with infantile hydroceles, when the fluid extends up to the deep inguinal ring.

Epididymal cyst

An epididymal cyst usually occurs above and behind the testis. The testis can be palpated separately from it. An epididymal cyst frequently feels lobulated because often the fluid is in locules. They are fluctuant. Those containing clear fluid transilluminate. Those containing a milky opalescent fluid are called spermatoceles and do not transilluminate.

Epididymo-orchitis

The scrotal skin is hot, red and oedematous. The tenderness is initially confined to the epididymis but eventually spreads to involve the testis.

Testicular torsion

The scrotal skin is usually hot, red and oedematous. The testis is extremely tender and is often drawn up towards the groin.

Testicular tumour

There is a firm, irregular swelling in the scrotum. Often the patient notices the lump when it is very small but in other cases it may become very large before the patient presents. Rarely the tumour has been allowed to advance so far that it is attached to the scrotal skin. Check for palpable para-aortic nodes. Examine the cervical nodes, especially in the left supraclavicular fossa. Testicular tumours metastasise to the para-aortic nodes, to the mediastinal nodes, and occasionally into the cervical nodes. Inguinal nodes are not involved unless the tumour has invaded the scrotal skin, which is rare.

Varicocele

This can only be palpated with the patient standing up. The dilated veins then become visible and palpable. They are said to feel like 'a bag of worms' but actually feel more like lukewarm spaghetti. The left side is more commonly affected.

Haematocele

There is a tense, tender, fluctuant swelling. There may be obvious scrotal bruising. The testis cannot be felt separately as the blood surrounds it within the layers of the tunica vaginalis.

Sperm granuloma

There is a small, tender, painful nodule at the site of previous vasectomy.

Tuberculosis

The swelling is usually confined to the epididymis, where there is a hard lump. The spermatic cord and vas are thickened. Occasionally a sinus may have formed. Check the chest for signs of pulmonary TB. Check the neck for scars (lymph node drainage for cold abscess) or lymphadenopathy.

Gumma

A gumma is a painless swelling of the whole testis. Other signs of syphilis may be present.

GENERAL INVESTIGATIONS

- **FBC, ESR**
  Hb ↓ chronic disease, e.g. TB. WCC ↑ inflammation, e.g. epididymo-orchitis, torsion. ESR ↑ TB, syphilis, tumour.

- **CXR**
  TB. Secondary deposits from testicular tumour.

- **MSU**
  UTI associated with epididymo-orchitis.

- **US**
  Solid versus cystic. Hydrocele versus epididymal cyst. Always arrange an ultrasound of the underlying testis in the young patient with a lax hydrocele as there may be an underlying tumour.

SPECIFIC INVESTIGATIONS

- Tumour markers
  AFP, βHCG, LDH.

- EMSU
  TB.

- VDRL
  Gumma.

- US abdomen
  Carcinoma of left kidney invading the left renal vein, associated with left varicocele.

- Laser Doppler*
  Torsion versus orchitis.

- Technetium scan*
  Torsion versus epididymo-orchitis.

- Surgery
  Distinction between torsion and epididymo-orchitis.

- MRI
  Abdominal and chest MRI scan may confirm lymphadenopathy associated with secondary deposits from testicular tumours.

- It is difficult, if not impossible, to distinguish between torsion and epididymo-orchitis. Urgent surgical exploration is required.

- A hydrocele in a fit young male should raise the suspicion of an underlying malignancy. Arrange an US scan.

- A feeling of heaviness, discomfort, or a dragging sensation in the scrotum may be presenting symptoms of testicular cancer. Examine the testes carefully. If any doubt, arrange a US scan.

- Always examine the scrotum with the patient lying and standing. Allow at least 10 seconds for a varicocele to appear.

* There is rarely time or equipment to carry out these investigations. If there is any doubt about the diagnosis, assume that it is torsion and explore the scrotum surgically.

SHOCK

Shock is an abnormality of the circulation that results in inadequate organ perfusion and tissue oxygenation.

CAUSES

HYPOVOLAEMIC

- Haemorrhage
- Burns
- Gastrointestinal losses

CARDIOGENIC

- Myocardial infarction
- Acute valvular damage
- Arrhythmia

DISTRIBUTIVE

- Sepsis
- Anaphylaxis
- Neurogenic shock (spinal injury)

OBSTRUCTIVE

- Massive pulmonary embolism
- Tension pneumothorax
- Cardiac tamponade

HISTORY

Trauma

Trauma is a pertinent feature in the history as haemorrhage invariably accompanies penetrating trauma. The site and approximate amount of blood loss should be assessed. Blunt trauma to the chest is associated with tension pneumothorax, myocardial contusion and cardiac tamponade. Trauma to the pelvis and long bones can result in closed fractures, causing significant haemorrhage that may not always be apparent to the observer. Thermal injury can occur with patients involved in fires, water-heater explosions and gas explosions. Acute onset of paralysis following trauma may be due to spinal or peripheral nerve injury. Disruption to the descending sympathetic pathways with spinal injuries results in loss of vasomotor tone and consequently hypotension.

Dyspnoea

Although tachypnoea is a physiological accompaniment to blood loss, when dyspnoea is the predominant symptom you should consider pulmonary oedema from the causes of cardiogenic shock. In addition, dyspnoea is also a prominent feature of all the causes of obstructive shock.

Chest pain

The consequences of blunt trauma to the chest have been described above. In the absence of trauma, the presence of chest pain should lead you to consider myocardial infarction (central crushing) and pulmonary embolism (pleuritic).

Precipitating factors

Occasionally patients may be aware of allergens that provoke anaphylaxis. In the community, food products (shellfish, eggs, peanuts) and insect venom (bees, wasps) are common causes. In hospital, penicillin, anaesthetic agents and intravenous contrast media are the major provoking factors. Detailed systemic enquiry for presence of infection may elucidate the offending focus for patients in septic shock. A history of profuse vomiting, diarrhoea or intestinal obstruction (vomiting, constipation, colicky abdominal pain and distension) would indicate gastrointestinal losses as the cause for hypovolaemia.

EXAMINATION

Inspection

A thorough systematic inspection should be undertaken; burns and sites of bleeding from penetrating trauma may be obvious. Cyanosis is a feature of large pulmonary emboli and tension pneumothoraces. Patients with anaphylaxis often exhibit angio-oedema and urticaria.

Temperature

Patients in shock are generally cold and clammy. With septic shock, however, the skin is warm to the touch and the patient is usually pyrexial.

Pulse

A tachycardia is the earliest measurable indicator of shock; however, it may not be elevated in cases of neurogenic shock. The character of the pulse is usually weak. The rhythm may suggest an arrhythmia as the precipitating factor in cardiogenic shock. Pulsus paradoxus (decrease in amplitude of the pulse on inspiration) is consistent with cardiac tamponade.

JVP

A low JVP is a useful discriminator for hypovolaemic shock as it will usually be elevated with all causes of cardiogenic and obstructive shock.

Auscultation

Bronchospasm, and consequently wheezing, may be prominent in anaphylactic shock. Unilateral absent breath sounds indicate a pneumothorax, while muffled heart sounds are features of cardiac tamponade. The presence of a new murmur can be due to acute valvular insufficiency as a cause for cardiogenic shock.

GENERAL INVESTIGATIONS

- **Pulse oximetry**
  Although low saturation *per se* is not very discriminatory, severe impairment of oxygen saturation is associated with pulmonary embolus and pneumothorax. This may be confirmed with ABGs.

- **FBC**
  With blood loss, a low Hb may be noted, although this will not be evident immediately. A raised WCC occurs with infection. Unfortunately, it will also be raised in most causes of acute physiological stress.

- **U&Es**
  With significant gastrointestinal losses, low serum sodium and potassium accompanied by raised urea and creatinine are the usual abnormalities.

- **ECG**
  The ECG may reveal myocardial infarction or the presence of an arrhythmia as the precipitating aetiology. Electrical alternans (alternating large and small QRS complexes) is a specific indicator of pericardial tamponade. Widespread low-amplitude complexes are common in significant pericardial effusion.

- **CXR**
  May reveal a pneumothorax with deviation of the trachea (although the diagnosis of a tension pneumothorax should be clinical and relieved before a chest X-ray is performed). The cardiac silhouette may be globular in the presence of a pericardial effusion; however, tamponade is still possible with a normal-appearing chest film.

SPECIFIC INVESTIGATIONS

- **Blood cultures**
  Blood and site-specific cultures are essential in suspected septic shock. The underlying organism may be isolated.

- **Echocardiography**
  An echocardiogram will be able to demonstrate valvular dysfunction, the presence of tamponade and massive pulmonary embolism (when right heart failure is present).

- **CT pulmonary angiography**
  For the diagnosis of pulmonary embolism in the presence of shock. Emergency therapeutic measures (such as thrombolysis) may require a formal contrast pulmonary angiogram.

■ CT/MRI spine
   May be required to assess the extent and confirm the level of
   injury.

- When assessing patients in shock, it is important to
  appreciate that low blood pressure is a relatively
  late feature.

- In patients with massive haemorrhage, low blood
  count is also a late feature and cannot be relied
  upon to assess the initial degree of blood loss.

SPLENOMEGALY

The spleen must be enlarged to about three times its normal size before it becomes clinically palpable. The lower margin may feel notched on palpation. The spleen may become so massive in size that it is palpable in the right iliac fossa. Massive splenomegaly in the UK is likely to be due to chronic myeloid leukaemia, myelofibrosis or lymphoma. Splenomegaly may lead to hypersplenism, i.e. pancytopenia as cells become trapped and destroyed in an overactive spleen.

CAUSES

INFECTIVE

BACTERIAL
- Typhoid
- Typhus
- TB
- Syphilis
- Leptospirosis
- Septicaemia
- Abscess

VIRAL
- Glandular fever

PROTOZOAL
- Malaria
  - (common in Africa)

PARASITIC
- Hydatid cyst

INFLAMMATORY
- Rheumatoid arthritis
- Sarcoidosis
- Lupus
- Amyloid

NEOPLASTIC
- Metastases
- Primary tumours
- Leukaemia
- Lymphoma
- Polycythaemia vera
- Myelofibrosis

HAEMOLYTIC DISEASE

- Hereditary spherocytosis
- Acquired haemolytic anaemia
- Thrombocytopenic purpura

STORAGE DISEASES

- Gaucher's disease

DEFICIENCY DISEASES

- Severe iron-deficiency anaemia
- Pernicious anaemia

SPLENIC VEIN HYPERTENSION

- Cirrhosis
- Splenic vein thrombosis
- Portal vein thrombosis

NON-PARASITIC CYSTS

HISTORY

Infective

Most infective causes present with fever, malaise and anorexia. With typhus there will be a history of foreign travel. Typhus is conveyed between hosts by arthropods. The patient complains of severe constitutional symptoms with headache, vomiting, photophobia and toxaemia. With typhoid there will usually be a history of foreign travel or it will occur in the immigrant population. There will be a history of malaise, headache, fever, cough, constipation initially and then diarrhoea. Epistaxis and abdominal pain may occur. TB usually presents with weight loss, night sweats and a cough. If septicaemia is responsible there will usually be an obvious cause, and the patient may already be hospitalised. With splenic abscess there may be a history of endocarditis, lung abscess, drug abuse, or it may occur in an immunocompromised host. Syphilis is rare and there may be a history of contact. With leptospirosis there is often a history of contact with rats, particularly when swimming in rivers where there are rats by the riverside. Fever, jaundice, headache, haemoptysis and haematuria are presenting symptoms. With malaria there is usually a history of travel to an area where it is endemic. The patient usually presents within 2 months of travel abroad with malaise, myalgia, sweating, coldness, followed by rigors, high fever and drenching sweats. Hydatid disease occurs most frequently in rural sheep-farming regions, e.g. Wales. The commonest presentation is with a cyst in the lung causing dyspnoea, haemoptysis or anaphylaxis.

Inflammatory

Rheumatoid arthritis may be apparent. Sarcoidosis may present with lymphadenopathy, fever and malaise, as well as hepatosplenomegaly. Lupus may present with protean manifestations with cutaneous, musculoskeletal, renal, pulmonary and haematological problems. Amyloid may be primary or secondary. There may be cutaneous, cerebral, cardiac or endocrine manifestations. With secondary amyloidosis there may be a history of chronic infection, e.g. TB; inflammatory disease, e.g. rheumatoid arthritis; or neoplasia. It usually affects the kidney and liver as well as the spleen.

Neoplastic

There will often be generalised signs of malignancy. Often there will be general malaise with weight loss, and with lymphoma there will be a history of night sweats. There may also be a tendency to spontaneous bruising. Primary tumours of the spleen and splenic metastases are rare.

Haemolytic disease

Haemolytic disease usually presents with the symptoms of anaemia, namely tiredness and malaise. Jaundice may be present, although is often not very deep, merely giving a lemonish tinge to the skin. With excessive breakdown of red blood cells, pigment stones may form in the gall bladder and the disease may present with acute cholecystitis.

Storage diseases

Apart from variable hepatosplenomegaly, these may present with neurological problems, skeletal deformities or mental deterioration.

Deficiency diseases

There may be a history of pernicious anaemia. Splenomegaly is usually mild. With iron-deficiency anaemia there may be dietary deficiency, malabsorption or blood loss. Check for a history of blood loss.

Splenic vein hypertension

There may be an obvious history, with cirrhosis and signs of liver failure. Isolated splenic vein thrombosis is rare.

Non-parasitic cysts

These are rare but may arise from organised haematomas, infarcts or inflammation. They are usually isolated findings when the patient is being investigated for other conditions.

EXAMINATION

General

The spleen appears from below the tip of the left 10th rib and enlarges towards the umbilicus. It is firm and smooth and usually has a notch on its upper edge. It moves with respiration, is dull to percussion, and it is impossible to get above it.

Infective

With typhus there is only moderate splenomegaly. The patient will often be toxic with a generalised maculopapular rash. With typhoid there is moderate splenomegaly, the patient being pyrexial with a tender abdomen and with rose spots on the trunk. Again with TB the splenomegaly is only moderate. There may be chest signs. With septicaemia there is usually an obvious cause and again there is only moderate splenomegaly. With splenic abscess, again there is only moderate splenomegaly and the spleen may be tender and feel irregular. With glandular fever the patient will be pyrexial with lymphadenopathy, and occasionally there is a rash, especially if the patient has been given ampicillin. Splenomegaly is moderate. With syphilis there may be fever, malaise, lymphadenopathy, and a rash on the trunk, palms and soles. Rarely there may be hepatitis, meningism and uveitis. With leptospirosis ictohaemorrhagica the patient is usually ill with pyrexia, jaundice and purpuric rash. There may be signs of meningism. There also may be tender muscles (myositis). There may be signs of acute renal failure. With malaria there is often anaemia, jaundice and hepatosplenomegaly. With hydatid disease the liver is usually more affected than the spleen. There may be hepatomegaly in addition to splenomegaly.

Inflammatory

With inflammatory disease the spleen is rarely grossly enlarged. Changes of rheumatoid arthritis may be apparent elsewhere in the body. With sarcoidosis there may be lymphadenopathy as well as hepatosplenomegaly. With lupus there may be cutaneous manifestations as well as musculoskeletal, renal and pulmonary manifestations. With amyloid, in addition to hepatosplenomegaly, there may be signs of carpal tunnel syndrome, peripheral neuropathy, purpura and a large tongue.

Neoplastic

There may be massive splenomegaly associated with chronic myeloid leukaemia, myelofibrosis and lymphoma. Other signs such as lymphadenopathy and spontaneous bruising may be present.

Haemolytic disease

The patient may have a mild jaundice together with moderate splenomegaly. A purpuric rash may be apparent with thrombocytopenic purpura.

Storage diseases

These are rare. There may be signs of cardiac failure, skeletal deformity or neurological deficits.

Splenic vein hypertension

Signs of liver failure, e.g. spider naevi, liver palms, caput medusae and jaundice may be present.

Non-parasitic cysts

The only finding may be splenomegaly.

GENERAL INVESTIGATIONS

- **FBC, ESR, blood film**
  Hb ↓ anaemias. Hb ↑ polycythaemia. WCC ↑ infection, leukaemia, abscess. ESR ↑ infection, malignancy. WCC ↓, platelets ↓ hypersplenism. PCV ↑ polycythaemia. MCV ↑ pernicious anaemia. Blood film – spherocytosis, malaria.

- **U&Es**
  Urea ↑, creatinine ↑ renal failure, e.g. with leptospirosis, amyloid, septicaemia.

- **LFTs**
  Cirrhosis.

SPECIFIC INVESTIGATIONS

- **Rheumatoid factor**
  Rheumatoid arthritis.

- **Paul–Bunnell test**
  Glandular fever.

- **VDRL**
  Syphilis.

- **Serum iron and serum ferritin**
  ↓ iron-deficiency anaemia.

- **Parietal cell antibodies**
  Pernicious anaemia.

- **Serum vitamin B_{12}**
  Pernicious anaemia.

- **Blood culture**
  Septicaemia. Leptospirosis. Typhoid.

- **Stool culture**
  Typhoid.

- **Urine culture**
  Typhoid. Leptospirosis.

- **CSF culture**
  Leptospirosis.

- **Complement fixation test**
  Leptospirosis.

■ **ELISA/immunofluorescence**
Typhus.

■ **Bone marrow aspirate**
Myelofibrosis. Polycythaemia. Leukaemia. Gaucher's disease.

■ **US**
Cause of splenomegaly, e.g. cyst, tumour, diffuse enlargement.
Cirrhosis of the liver.

■ **CT**
Causes of splenomegaly, e.g. cyst, tumour, diffuse enlargement,
cirrhosis.

• The spleen may enlarge massively. Palpation for
suspected splenomegaly should begin in the right
lower quadrant.

STEATORRHOEA

Steatorrhoea refers to the passing of excessive amounts of fat in the faeces. The causes are listed below, according to pathogenesis.

CAUSES

LIPASE DEFICIENCY

- Impaired secretion – chronic pancreatitis
- Inactivation – excess gastric acid

BILE DEFICIENCY

- Underproduction – liver disease
- Obstruction – obstructive jaundice
- Increased degradation – bacterial overgrowth

MUCOSAL DISEASE

- Coeliac disease
- Ileal resection
- Crohn's disease

IMPAIRED FAT TRANSPORT

- Abetalipoproteinaemia

LYMPHATIC DEFICIENCY

- Lymphoma
- Whipple's disease

HISTORY

Patients with steatorrhoea often pass bulky, sticky and greasy stool that floats and is often difficult to flush away. Diarrhoea is the usual accompanying symptom (p. 97) for most of the causes. Jaundice with pale stools and dark urine implies obstruction to the flow of bile, which is essential for the absorption of fat and fat-soluble vitamins. The causes and diagnostic approach to jaundice are found on p. 240.

Abdominal pain

Vague epigastric abdominal pain experienced by patients with chronic pancreatitis may radiate to the back and is usually worse with food. Epigastric pain exacerbated by food may be a symptom of Zollinger–Ellison syndrome, which results in excessive gastric acid production (lowering the pH of gastric chyme) inactivating lipase. It usually presents with symptoms of peptic ulceration refractory to medical treatment. Abdominal pains associated with Crohn's disease are often felt in the right iliac fossa due to regional ileitis.

Associated symptoms

Patients with coeliac disease may also suffer with growth retardation and nutritional deficiencies causing anaemia and muscle wasting. Other symptoms may include bone fracture due to demineralisation, cerebellar ataxia and peripheral neuropathy. Joint pains, pyrexia, skin pigmentation and peripheral lymphadenopathy are among the varied symptoms of Whipple's disease resulting from infection with the bacterium *Tropheryma whipplei*. Steatorrhoea is the primary manifestation of intestinal lymphoma. It may be accompanied by abdominal pains and pyrexia and occasionally present with intestinal obstruction. Mouth ulcers, perianal abscesses, right iliac fossa pains and blood PR are some of the symptoms experienced by patients with Crohn's disease. Ataxia and night blindness from retinitis pigmentosa may result from abetalipoproteinaemia, which is caused by the absence of apolipoprotein B and therefore this results in defective chylomicron formation.

Past medical history

Previous surgical resection involving the terminal ileum will predispose an individual to malabsorption of fat due to decreased enterohepatic circulation of bile salts. Moreover, with decreased length of absorptive intestine, intestinal transit time decreases and there is a decrease in concomitant fat absorption. Conditions associated with intestinal stasis, hypomotility and decreased gastric acid secretion predispose to intestinal bacterial overgrowth and increased degradation of bile salts.

EXAMINATION

Steatorrhoea is often associated with malabsorption and therefore patients may appear emaciated. Mouth ulcers may be due to Crohn's or coeliac disease. Clubbing is associated with Crohn's, liver cirrhosis, coeliac disease and cystic fibrosis, which is associated with pancreatic exocrine insufficiency. Jaundice may be present with bile duct obstruction and liver disease. Bruising may result from impaired clotting due to vitamin K deficiency. The classical rash of dermatitis herpetiformis may be seen with coeliac disease. Erythema nodosum is a feature of Crohn's disease and may be accompanied by right iliac fossa tenderness, perianal abscesses and fistulae. Hepatomegaly may be found in liver disease, and splenomegaly with intestinal lymphoma.

GENERAL INVESTIGATIONS

- **Faecal fat estimation**
  Stool collections over a period of 3 days are performed with a diet consisting of ≥50 g fat per day. The normal value of faecal fat is <7 g per day.

- **FBC and blood film**
  WCC ↑ with active inflammation. Acanthocytes are present on the blood film with abetalipoproteinaemia.

- **ESR**
  ↑ with acute Crohn's disease.

- **LFTs**
  Bilirubin and alkaline phosphatase ↑ obstructive jaundice. Transaminases ↑ liver parenchymal disease. Albumin ↓ malabsorption syndromes.

- **Blood glucose**
  ↑ with diabetes, a complication of chronic pancreatitis.

- **Serum amylase**
  Usually normal with chronic pancreatitis, but may be elevated if associated with recurrent acute attacks of pancreatitis.

- **Antigliadin, antiendomysial and antireticulin antibodies**
  To detect coeliac disease.

- **AXR**
  Calcification with chronic pancreatitis.

- **Jejunal biopsy**
  Subtotal villous atrophy and crypt hyperplasia with coeliac disease, which are reversible on a gluten-free diet. Dilated lymphatics and PAS-positive macrophages in Whipple's disease. Absent villi with lymphocytic infiltration of the lamina propria and histological evidence of malignancy with intestinal lymphoma.

SPECIFIC INVESTIGATIONS

- *Tropheryma whipplei* serology
  Positive in Whipple's disease

- ^{14}C-labelled bile acid breath tests
  Screening test for bacterial overgrowth.

- **Serum gastrin assay**
  Zollinger–Ellison syndrome.

- **Small bowel enema**
  Strictures, skip lesions, fissures and fistulae with Crohn's disease.

- **Colonoscopy**
  Mucosal hyperaemia, friability, ulceration and contact bleeding with Crohn's disease.

- **CT abdomen**
  Abdominal lymphadenopathy with lymphoma.

- Always take a careful history as the patient may actually complain of diarrhoea. In steatorrhoea the stool is classically described as pale, fatty and offensive and difficult to flush away. Clear distinction between diarrhoea and steatorrhoea is important.

STRIDOR

Stridor is a high-pitched inspiratory sound produced by upper airway obstruction.

CAUSES

CONGENITAL

- Laryngomalacia (congenital flaccid larynx)

ACQUIRED

- Foreign body
- Infection
  - Epiglottitis
  - Retropharyngeal abscess
- Iatrogenic
  - Post-tracheostomy stenosis
  - Post-intubation stenosis
  - Post-thyroid surgery
- Goitre
- Laryngeal oedema
  - Anaphylaxis
  - Inhalational injury
- Cricoarytenoid rheumatoid arthritis

MALIGNANCY

- Intraluminal obstruction
  - Larynx
  - Trachea
  - Bronchus
- External compression
  - Malignant nodes

BILATERAL VOCAL CORD PALSY

- Brainstem stroke
- Thyroid carcinoma
- Oesophageal carcinoma

HISTORY

Onset

Instantaneous onset of stridor usually implies an inhaled foreign body. This is accompanied by violent bouts of coughing, and a clear history may be obtained from a witness. Stridor indicates partial obstruction, as complete occlusion of the upper airway is silent. Stridor that develops over a period of a few seconds to minutes may be due to laryngeal oedema from an anaphylactic reaction. This may be accompanied by urticaria and facial oedema. Enquiries should immediately determine known allergens and treatment can be initiated without delay. The most common cause of infantile stridor is laryngomalacia. During inspiration there is extreme infolding of the epiglottis and aryepiglottic folds due to inadequate cartilaginous support. Head flexion aggravates the stridor, whereas patency of the airway is improved by the prone position and head extension. The stridor gradually resolves in most infants within 2–3 months.

Precipitating factors

Iatrogenic causes of stridor may have clear precipitating factors. Tracheal stenosis may complicate a long period of intubation or tracheostomy. Upper airway obstruction occurring immediately after thyroid surgery may be due to laryngeal oedema, haematoma and bilateral recurrent nerve injury. Patients who have been rescued from fires may suffer inhalation injuries due to the high temperature of inhaled gases.

Associated symptoms

Respiratory obstruction may occur with massive enlargement of the tonsils, e.g. in glandular fever, or when complicated by a retropharyngeal abscess. Patients may notice swelling of the neck in the presence of a goitre and may be either euthyroid or complain of symptoms of abnormal thyroid function (p. 165). Symptoms of joint pains, stiffness and deformities occur with rheumatoid arthritis. Associated stridor can result from cricoarytenoid involvement. Weight loss can be an accompanying feature of malignancy. Hoarseness of the voice is an early symptom of laryngeal carcinoma; stridor occurs as a late feature. Chronic cough with haemoptysis in a chronic smoker usually heralds the onset of bronchial carcinoma. The location of the carcinoma may alter the quality of the wheeze. Partial intraluminal upper airway obstruction from bronchial carcinoma produces stridor, whereas partial lower airways obstruction produces the inspiratory monophonic wheeze. Rapid progressive painless dysphagia occurs with oesophageal carcinoma.

EXAMINATION

Inspection

With acute partial upper airway obstruction, patients will often appear very distressed. Immediate assessment for generalised urticaria, facial oedema, hypotension and widespread wheezing will allow the diagnosis of anaphylaxis to be made and appropriate treatment initiated. Soot on the face and singed nasal hair from thermal exposure may be present with inhalational injuries. A large goitre will be visible on inspection. Bilateral symmetrical deforming arthropathy involving the small joints of the hands (MCP, PIP) is suggestive of rheumatoid disease. Clubbing may be present in the fingers with bronchial carcinoma.

The cause of stridor may be visible on inspection of the throat. Further information is obtained on inspection using indirect laryngoscopy. With bilateral vocal cord palsy, the cords lie in a cadaveric position. A small glottic aperture is seen and does not widen on attempted inspiration. Supraglottic and glottic carcinomas may be readily visible.

Palpation and auscultation

The presence of cervical lymphadenopathy may be due to infection or carcinoma of the larynx, pharynx, bronchus or oesophagus. A goitre may also be palpable in the neck, skewing the trachea to one side due to compression effects. The chest is examined for monophonic wheezing, collapse of a segment, pleural effusion and rib tenderness, which are the thoracic manifestations of bronchial carcinoma.

GENERAL INVESTIGATIONS

General investigations should be tailored to the clinical findings.

- FBC
  WCC ↑ infection.
- ESR
  ↑ with infection and malignancy.
- TFTs
  ↑, ↓ or normal with goitres.
- Lateral soft-tissue neck X-ray
  Radio-opaque foreign bodies.
- CXR
  Both frontal and lateral views are required to identify radio-opaque foreign bodies. Bronchial carcinoma may present as a central mass, peripheral mass, collapse of a segment, consolidation of a lobe or as a pleural effusion. Hilar lymphadenopathy may be apparent, causing external compression of trachea or bronchus.

SPECIFIC INVESTIGATIONS

- Fibreoptic laryngoscopy
  Visualisation of the vocal cords, tumour masses, tracheal stenosis and allows biopsies to be taken.
- Bronchoscopy
  To screen for lesions in the distal trachea and proximal airways.

■ **Upper GI endoscopy**
To determine the presence of carcinoma that may be infiltrating both recurrent laryngeal nerves when associated symptoms of dysphagia are present.

■ **FNAC of a goitre**
To determine the underlying aetiology of a goitre.

■ **CT neck and thorax**
Define the extent and assist in staging of laryngeal carcinoma, thyroid carcinoma, oesophageal carcinoma and bronchial carcinoma.

- Stridor can be a symptom of impending airways obstruction and asphyxia. Urgent cricothyroidotomy may be required.

- The toxic child with stridor, severe sore throat, respiratory distress and difficulty in swallowing has acute epiglottitis until proved otherwise. Urgent admission and treatment is required.

- If the onset of stridor is very sudden, consider an inhaled foreign body.

SWEATING ABNORMALITIES

Excessive sweating is often brought to the attention of the physician when it becomes socially unacceptable, the underlying cause ranging from trivial to serious.

CAUSES

EXCESSIVE SWEATING

- Hypoglycaemia

INFECTIONS

- any systemic infection

MALIGNANCY

- Brain tumours
- Hodgkin's lymphoma

ENDOCRINE

- Diabetic autonomic neuropathy
- Menopause
- Thyrotoxicosis
- Carcinoid syndrome
- Phaeochromocytoma

PSYCHIATRIC

- Substance dependency/withdrawal
- Anxiety states

DEFICIENT SWEATING

- Heat stroke
- Miliaria
- Hypohidrotic ectodermal dysplasia
- Sympathetic tract lesions

HISTORY

Apart from heat stroke, the causes of deficient sweating are rare and usually arise from congenital disorders of the sweat glands, such as hypohidrotic ectodermal dysplasia, a condition associated with poor hair and teeth formation. Absent sweating can also be caused by miliaria, which is caused by plugging or rupture of the sweat ducts.

Excessive sweating is commonly encountered as it is a physiological accompaniment to pain, nausea, vomiting (p. 474) and shock (p. 406). The causes in the absence of these symptoms have been listed above. Excessive sweating may be episodic or constant. Episodic bouts of sweating may be due to hypogylcaemia, phaeochromocytoma, carcinoid syndrome and menopause. Patients with hypogylcaemia often complain of associated tremor, dizziness, anxiety and hunger. Paroxysmal release of catecholamines by phaeochromocytomas may produce attacks of sweating, hypertension, palpitations, headaches and anxiety. It usually comes to medical attention presenting as a result of hypertension. Carcinoid syndrome is produced by a variety of hormones secreted by enterochromaffin tumours, originating from the small bowel in the presence of hepatic metastases. Episodic sweating is associated with brick-red flushing, diarrhoea, wheezing and occasionally right-sided heart lesions.

Hot flushes and sweating may also be prominent symptoms experienced by women reaching the menopause; the aetiology has often been attributed to alterations in the concentrations of female reproductive hormones.

Patients with night sweats may complain of waking up with their clothes and bed sheets drenched in perspiration. Classically, these features are reported with TB and Hodgkin's disease. The accompanying symptoms of pulmonary TB include weight loss, cough and haemoptysis. With Hodgkin's disease, patients may complain of localised lymphadenopathy, weight loss, pruritus, fever and malaise.

Constant sweating and heat intolerance are features of thyrotoxicosis. This may result from increased metabolic rate and may be accompanied by symptoms of increased appetite with weight loss, emotional lability, diarrhoea and palpitations. Rarely excessive sweating may result from tumours encroaching on the hypothalamus.

Enquiries should be undertaken regarding substance dependency, as withdrawal states can produce severe sweating and hallucinations.

EXAMINATION

A psychological examination is required if an anxiety disorder is suspected. The following are specific features in the examination that may suggest an underlying cause.

Temperature

The presence of pyrexia (p. 374) would suggest infection as the underlying cause for sweating. However, it can also occur with Hodgkin's disease.

Inspection

Wide, staring eyes with lid lag may result from thyrotoxicosis causing sweating; in addition, the presence of exophthalmos or ophthalmoplegia specifically indicates Graves' disease as the underlying cause. Episodic brick-red flushing of the face may be experienced with carcinoid syndrome.

Palpation and auscultation

The thyroid is palpated to exclude enlargement of the gland. Regional lymph nodes are examined for enlargement, which may be due to infection or malignancy. A tachycardia is present with thyrotoxicosis and systemic infection. A rapid pulse may also be palpated during paroxysmal attacks with phaeochromocytoma, and the blood pressure will be markedly elevated. With primary pulmonary TB, pleural effusion or segmental collapse may be the only features found on examination. Detection of a new or changing heart murmur may imply endocarditis. However, either stenosis or regurgitation of the tricuspid or pulmonary valve have been reported with carcinoid syndrome. The presence of splenomegaly on abdominal examination may be due to Hodgkin's disease.

GENERAL INVESTIGATIONS

■ **BM stix**
Rapid assessment of blood sugar and may be confirmed by blood glucose estimation. Glucose may be ↑ with phaeochromocytoma.

■ **FBC and blood film**
WCC ↑ infection.

■ **ESR and CRP**
↑ with infection, malignancy and lymphoma.

■ **TSH and free T_4**
TSH ↓ and T_4 ↑ with thyrotoxicosis.

■ **CXR**
TB, bronchial carcinoid, chest infection.

SPECIFIC INVESTIGATIONS

■ **Mantoux test/ELISpot assay**
Diluted Mantoux test if no previous BCG immunisation has been performed to screen for TB. Serological testing is now available for TB.

■ **Urinary 5HIAA**
↑ with carcinoid tumours.

■ **Urinary catecholamines and metanephrines**
↑ with phaeochromocytoma.

■ **Lymph node excision biopsy**
Reed–Sternberg cells with Hodgkin's disease.

■ **MRI head**
Hypothalamic tumours.

- Drenching night sweats are serious as the underlying diagnosis may be lymphoma or chronic infection such as TB. Urgent investigation is required.

SYNCOPE

Syncope is the transient loss of consciousness due to impaired cerebral blood flow.

CAUSES

CARDIOVASCULAR

VASOVAGAL SYNCOPE
- Situational syncope
- Micturition syncope
- Cough syncope

ORTHOSTATIC HYPOTENSION
- Prolonged bedrest
- Drug-induced
- Hypovolaemic
- Autonomic failure

ARRHYTHMIA
- Supraventricular tachycardia
- Ventricular tachycardia
- Sick sinus syndrome
- Stokes–Adams attack

- Myocardial infarction
- Pulmonary embolism
- Cardiac outflow obstruction
- Carotid sinus syndrome

NEUROLOGICAL

- Seizure
- Hysterical syncope

METABOLIC

- Hypoxia
- Hypoglycaemia

HISTORY

Vasovagal syncope (the common faint) is the most common cause of syncope. It is associated with peripheral vasodilatation and a vagally mediated slowing of the heart rate. It may be precipitated by situations such as fear, emotion, prolonged standing or pain. The patient may complain of nausea, weakness and blurred vision, and appear pale with bradycardia on examination. Palpitations

(p. 351) preceding collapse may suggest an arrhythmia. Situational syncope are faints classified according to the precipitating factors and are often due to an excessive vagal response to the offending stimuli.

Orthostatic hypotension is a drop in blood pressure on standing. This causes a transient decrease in cerebral perfusion and therefore loss of consciousness. Prolonged bedrest can result in the deconditioning of the baroreceptors in the body, resulting in a postural drop of blood pressure. A drug history may exclude offending medication such as antihypertensives and opiates. Hypovolaemia is also a cause of postural hypotension (see Shock, p. 406); it is associated with a pallor, tachycardia and a low urine output. Disease states such as diabetes mellitus and Guillain–Barré syndrome can result in autonomic failure and inability of the body to maintain an appropriate blood pressure.

Cardiac outflow obstruction, which occurs with aortic stenosis and hypertrophic obstructive cardiomyopathy, will result in syncope on effort as the cardiac output cannot be increased on demand.

In carotid sinus syndrome, the receptors of the carotid sinus are more sensitive than normal, thus minor stimulation, such as turning the head or pressure from a tight collar, may elicit the carotid sinus reflex and precipitate syncope.

Seizures are paroxysmal discharges in the cortex which are sufficient to produce clinically detectable events, e.g. convulsions, loss of consciousness or behavioural symptoms. Although it is not strictly syncope, atonic seizures may present in a similar fashion, with a sudden loss of muscle tone and collapse. Patients may be incontinent during a seizure and drowsy or confused during the post-ictal phase.

Hysterical syncope tends to be very dramatic with normal examination findings during the attack.

Hypoglycaemia causes faintness and even results in loss of consciousness. It tends to be more common with insulin-treated diabetics but may also occur in normal individuals after an alcohol binge. Symptoms usually occur when the glucose is below 2.5 mmol/L.

EXAMINATION

Appearance

Vasovagal syncope often results in pallor of the complexion and clamminess. Convulsions may occur.

Blood pressure

Should be taken supine and standing, only then will a postural drop be noted.

Pulse

During the attack of syncope, taking the pulse is a good way to detect an arrhythmia. Bradycardia is the usual finding in vasovagal syncope. Stokes–Adams attacks result from complete heart block causing a transient period of asystole, with full recovery. The sick sinus syndrome is associated with alternating episodes of bradycardia and tachycardia. Shock, supraventricular and ventricular tachycardias may result in very rapid heart rates.

Pressure on the carotid sinus, located at the bifurcation of the carotid arteries, will cause syncope in patients with carotid sinus syndrome.

Auscultation

The soft second heart sound and an ejection systolic murmur radiating to the carotids characterises aortic valvular stenosis. An ejection systolic murmur can also be auscultated in hypertrophic obstructive cardiomyopathy, where the outflow of blood from the left ventricle is obstructed owing to hypertrophy of the cardiac muscle.

GENERAL INVESTIGATIONS

- **BM stix**
  Testing the blood for glucose with BM stix is a simple and very rapid way of obtaining a blood glucose level. More accurate readings can be confirmed with a serum sample.

- **FBC**
  Will indicate anaemia when haemorrhage is the underlying cause of hypovolaemia. Septic shock with peripheral vasodilatation may be associated with an elevated white cell count.

- **U&Es and serum glucose**
  Electrolyte abnormalities will predispose to seizures.

- **Blood glucose**
  Hypoglycaemia.

- **ECG**
  When obtained during an attack may reveal an arrhythmia. Pulseless ventricular tachycardia should be treated as ventricular fibrillation and cardiac resuscitation should commence. Q waves and ST elevations may be seen with myocardial infarction.

SPECIFIC INVESTIGATIONS

- **EEG**
  Although epilepsy is essentially a clinical diagnosis, seizures associated with specific electrical changes in the cortex can

be used to confirm the diagnosis. A negative EEG does not, however, exclude epilepsy.

- **24-hour ECG**
  May be able to document arrhythmias associated with episodes of syncope.

- **Echocardiography**
  Allows assessment of the aortic valve and diagnosis of hypertrophic obstructive cardiomyopathy.

- **V/Q scan or CT pulmonary angiography**
  Allows diagnosis of the majority of acute pulmonary emboli.

- **Tilt table testing**
  This is usually reserved for patients with recurrent syncope of indeterminate cause. In patients with vasovagal syncope, a 60° tilt will produce hypotension, bradycardia and syncope within 30 minutes.

- **Syncope should never be ignored due to the potential serious consequences of this symptom. Any suggestion of a cardiac cause requires urgent investigation and treatment.**

THIRST

True thirst as a symptom is usually associated with two other symptoms, i.e. drinking excessive amounts of water (polydipsia) and excessive urination (polyuria).

CAUSES

INADEQUATE FLUID INTAKE

- General debility
- Neurological disease
- Anorexia

EXCESSIVE FLUID LOSS

- Vomiting
- Fever
- Diarrhoea
- Blood loss sufficient to decrease blood volume
- Excessive sweating
- Burns

ENDOCRINE AND METABOLIC

- Diabetes mellitus
- Diabetes insipidus (cranial and nephrogenic)
- Chronic renal failure

DRUGS

- Diuretics (especially overdose)
- Ecstasy

CAUSES OF DRY MOUTH

- Sjögren's syndrome
- Drugs, e.g. anticholinergics, monoamine oxidase inhibitors
- Post-head and neck radiotherapy

PSYCHIATRIC

- Psychogenic polydipsia

DIET

- Salty foods
- Spicy foods

HISTORY

It is important to distinguish between thirst and a dry mouth.
Enquire about the onset of thirst, whether it is acute or chronic.

Take a full dietary history, including salt intake and ingestion of spicy foods. A history of tiredness and lethargy with weight loss will suggest diabetes mellitus. Check for signs of infection. Check for a history of vomiting or diarrhoea. A full drug history should be taken as some drugs, e.g. anticholinergics, can result in dryness of the mouth and therefore patients may ingest excessive quantities of water, giving rise to polyuria. A history of any salivary gland swelling in association with dry eyes, dry mouth and arthritis should be sought, which would suggest Sjögren's syndrome. A history of any chronic blood loss should be sought. Malignancy and hyperparathyroidism are a common cause of chronic hypercalcaemia which can lead to polyuria by an intrinsic osmotic effect or by precipitation of nephrogenic diabetes insipidus. Cranial diabetes insipidus can result from severe, blunt head injuries, craniopharyngioma, pineal gland tumours or as a transient post-operative complication following neurosurgery. Full psychological assessment may be required if psychogenic polydipsia is suspected.

EXAMINATION

Check the temperature. Look for signs of dehydration, e.g. dry coated tongue, loss of skin turgor. Look for evidence of recent weight loss. Look for signs of Sjögren's syndrome, i.e. symmetrical enlargement of the salivary glands both parotid and submandibular. Check for dry eyes and arthritis.

GENERAL INVESTIGATIONS

- **Urinalysis**
  Diabetes. Sugar and ketones in the urine.

- **FBC**
  PCV ↑ dehydration. Hb ↓ blood loss. WCC ↑ infection.

- **U&Es**
  Renal failure.

- **Serum calcium**
  ↑ Ca – causes osmotic diuresis.

- **Blood sugar**
  ↑ diabetes.

SPECIFIC INVESTIGATIONS

- **PTH**
  ↑ hyperparathyroidism

- **Water deprivation tests (see Polyuria)**
  Cranial diabetes insipidus.

- **DDAVP test**
  Urine osmolality ↑ cranial diabetes insipidus. No urine osmolality ↑ nephrogenic diabetes insipidus.
- **CT/MRI**
  Cranial diabetes insipidus, e.g. tumour/CVA.
- **US**
  Renal failure.
- **Renal biopsy**
  Renal failure.

- It is important to distinguish between true thirst and a dry mouth.

- Thirst in an acute illness may be due to dehydration. It may also herald acute onset of diabetes. Always carry out a urinalysis to exclude diabetes mellitus.

THROAT CONDITIONS

A sore throat is an extremely common symptom, especially in children and young adults. Prolonged sore throat in an elderly patient is a cause for concern as it may indicate the presence of neoplasia.

CAUSES

INFECTIVE

- Tonsillitis
  - Bacterial, e.g. *streptococcus*, gonococcus
  - Viral, e.g. glandular fever
- Pharyngitis
  - Viral
  - Fungal
- Quinsy

INFLAMMATORY

- Thyroiditis

NEOPLASTIC

- Carcinoma
  - Tonsil
  - Posterior third of the tongue
  - Larynx
    - (common in Hong Kong, Singapore)
- Lymphoma
- Haematological disorders

NEUROLOGICAL

- Glossopharyngeal neuralgia

REFERRED PAIN

- Angina
- Oesophageal spasm

OTHER

- Reflux oesophagitis
- AIDS

HISTORY

Infective

Sore throat, dysphagia, referred pain to ear, headache, malaise. A history of oral sex may suggest oropharyngeal gonorrhoea. Quinsy is a peritonsillar abscess. There is usually a history of acute tonsillitis but the patient becomes more ill with a high temperature, dysphagia and referred pain to the ear. In glandular fever the patient can present with a severe membranous tonsillitis but usually has malaise and lymphadenopathy elsewhere.

Inflammatory

Subacute thyroiditis presents with a swelling of the thyroid, with neck pain, fever, weakness and malaise. It is a rare condition.

Neoplastic

Carcinoma of a tonsil presents with painful ulceration with induration. There is often referred pain to the ear and the patient may spit blood. Occasionally, the presenting symptom is a lump in the neck representing metastatic cervical lymphadenopathy. Carcinoma of the posterior third of the tongue may present with a feeling of soreness in the throat with difficulty in swallowing. The patient may spit blood and pain may be referred to the ear. Supraglottic carcinoma may present with a feeling of a lump in the throat but there is usually a change in voice and early cervical lymphadenopathy. Lymphoma of the tonsil rarely causes pain, the patient presenting with enlargement of one tonsil. Patients with a blood dyscrasia may present with a sore throat resulting from infection consequent upon neutropenia.

Neurological

Glossopharyngeal neuralgia presents as a sharp stabbing pain at the root of the tongue, radiating into the throat and ear, triggered by swallowing or touching the pharynx.

Referred pain

Angina may cause pain in the throat. It is usually associated with exercise. There may also be pain in the chest, radiating into the jaw and down the left arm. Occasionally, diffuse oesophageal spasm gives rise to chest pain radiating into the throat and jaw.

Other

Sore throat may occur in AIDS. It may be due to a variety of infective organisms, e.g. viral or fungal. Reflux oesophagitis may cause a burning pain in the throat or a sensation of a lump in the throat.

EXAMINATION

Infective

With tonsillitis there is usually pyrexia, foetor and pus exuding from the tonsillar crypts. The pharyngeal mucosa is often inflamed. Cervical lymphadenopathy. Check for lymphadenopathy elsewhere, and splenomegaly, which may be associated with glandular fever. Quinsy is associated with trismus and the tonsil is pushed downwards and medially by the quinsy. The uvula is usually oedematous.

Inflammatory

Thyroiditis presents with a tender, diffuse swelling in the thyroid gland, which moves on swallowing. It is rare.

Neoplastic

Carcinoma of the tonsil presents as a hard, ulcerated swelling on the tonsil. Cervical lymphadenopathy may be present. In carcinoma of the posterior third of the tongue and supraglottic larynx there is usually an indurated ulcer. Laryngoscopy is required as part of the examination. Check for cervical nodes and other sites for metastases, e.g. lung, liver. Lymphoma usually presents as painless enlargement of the tonsil. Blood dyscrasias may present with lymphadenopathy and hepatosplenomegaly. Agranulocytosis results in ulceration and membrane formation on the tonsils and oral mucosa.

Neurological

The diagnosis of glossopharyngeal neuralgia is usually made from the history. Touching the palate may trigger the symptoms.

Referred pain

Angina and oesophageal spasms are usually diagnosed from the history.

Others

Pharyngitis and tonsillitis may occur as part of AIDS, due to either viral or fungal infections. Other signs of AIDS, e.g. malaise, fever, weight loss, chest infections, Kaposi's sarcoma. Diagnosis of reflux oesophagitis is usually made on a history. There is little to find on examination.

GENERAL INVESTIGATIONS

■ FBC, ESR
  Hb ↓ malignancy. WCC ↑ infection. Blood dyscrasia.
  Lymphocytosis in glandular fever. ESR ↑ malignancy. Infection.
  Thyroiditis.

- ■ **Swab**
  Culture and sensitivity – *streptococcus* and gonococcus.
- ■ **Viral antibodies**
  Glandular fever.
- ■ **ECG**
  Cardiac ischaemia.
- ■ **CXR**
  Metastases.

SPECIFIC INVESTIGATIONS

- ■ **Indirect laryngoscopy**
  Infection. Malignancy.
- ■ **OGD**
  Oesophagitis. Hiatus hernia.
- ■ **HIV testing**
  AIDS.
- ■ **Biopsy**
  Benign versus malignant.
- ■ **CT**
  Tumour. Spread of tumour.

- • Throat swabs are useful only in the management of recurrent or persistent cases.

- • Occasionally a sore throat may be the first symptom of a more serious disorder, e.g. diabetes, agranulocytosis or malignancy.

- • Prolonged and persistent sore throat in an elderly patient is a cause for concern as it may be an indication of malignancy.

TIREDNESS

Persistent tiredness or physical fatigue with no obvious cause is a common complaint. It is normal to feel tired at times, e.g. after working long hours, unaccustomed exertion or sleepless nights. It is important to differentiate between tiredness due to excessive normal activities and tiredness due to disease.

CAUSES

POST-VIRAL FATIGUE SYNDROMES

ACUTE
- Infectious mononucleosis
- Viral hepatitis

CHRONIC
- Chronic post-viral fatigue syndrome (ME)

ENDOCRINE

- Hypothyroidism
- Diabetes mellitus
- Hyperthyroidism
- Addison's disease

MAJOR ORGAN FAILURE

- Cardiac failure
- Renal failure
- Liver failure

NEOPLASTIC

- Any malignancy

CHRONIC INFECTION

- TB
- HIV
- Brucellosis

CHRONIC INFLAMMATORY DISEASE

- Rheumatoid arthritis
- Polymyalgia rheumatica
- Crohn's disease
- SLE

CHRONIC NEUROLOGICAL DISORDERS

- Multiple sclerosis
- Myasthenia gravis

DRUGS

- Beta blockers
- Diuretics

DRUG ABUSE

- Alcohol
- Benzodiazepines

OTHERS

- Stress e.g. overwork, family commitments etc
- Depressive illness
- Anaemia
- Carbon monoxide poisoning

HISTORY

The history is most important in the diagnosis. It is necessary to define exactly what is meant by tiredness or fatigue. Fatigue is sometimes known as 'tired all the time syndrome'. Take a full history to decide whether tiredness is of a physical, psychological or social nature. Note the duration of the problem. Is it getting worse? Was there any precipitating factor? Ask about previous levels of energy and how this compares with the present. Has the patient noticed any other changes, e.g. in appetite, increased urine output or thirst or sleep disturbances? Has there been any recent change in medication, e.g. beta blockers causing lethargy? Chronic fatigue syndrome is more common in teenagers and young adults, especially students. It is uncommon after early middle age. Depression is more common in women aged 30 and over. In middle-aged and elderly people the symptoms of chronic fatigue are more likely to represent underlying organic disease.

A history of previous illnesses such as infectious mononucleosis or influenza should be sought. Ask about bereavement. Weight loss may suggest malignancy or depression with episodes of fever suggesting chronic infection, e.g. TB. Cold intolerance suggests myxoedema. Heat intolerance suggests thyrotoxicosis. In chronic fatigue syndrome the illness may fluctuate from week to week and may occasionally be relieved by rest. In malignancy the symptoms are progressive and deterioration occurs. The same is true for endocrine disorders. Tiredness associated with depression may fluctuate considerably with changing circumstances. Ask about the patient's lifestyle. Is there an excessive consumption of alcohol? Alcohol itself may cause tiredness but if alcohol is being used as a coping mechanism for stress-related illness, it is likely to aggravate rather than alleviate the problem. Ask about recreational drugs. Ask about work. Has the patient's work circumstances changed and are they working very long hours together with home commitments. Take a full neurological history to exclude conditions such as multiple sclerosis and myasthenia gravis. Carbon monoxide poisoning is rare but does occur occasionally and it is appropriate to take a history about any change of health of other members of the household as carbon monoxide poisoning would be likely to affect them also.

EXAMINATION

Meticulous examination is essential. Look at the patient. Is the patient someone who looks systemically unwell or has lost weight? Is there any evidence of anxiety, tiredness or sleep deprivation? Pyrexia may indicate the presence of systemic illness, e.g. TB, HIV. In chronic fatigue syndrome and in depression, there will be no abnormal physical signs. A slight tachycardia may occur with anxiety and stress. Check for clinical signs of anaemia. Check for signs of hyperthyroidism or hypothyroidism. Anaemia and thyrotoxicosis will produce a bounding, hyperdynamic pulse. In malignancy there may be enlarged lymph nodes or the liver may be palpable. A detailed neurological examination is required to exclude neurological disease as a cause of symptoms. Postural hypotension may occur in Addison's disease.

GENERAL INVESTIGATIONS

- **Urinalysis**
  Diabetes. Renal disease.

- **FBC**
  Hb ↓ anaemia. WCC ↑ infection.

- **ESR**
  ↑ infection, inflammatory disease, malignancy.

- **U&Es**
  CRF. Addison's disease.

- **LFTs**
  Alcohol abuse, hepatitis, malignancy.

- **CXR**
  TB. Malignancy. Cardiac failure.

SPECIFIC INVESTIGATIONS

- **TFTs**
  Hypothyroidism. Hyperthyroidism.

■ **Monospot**
Infectious mononucleosis.

■ **Autoantibody screen**
Connective tissue disease.

- Only 20–30% of cases will have a discernable physical cause. Up to 50% of cases have a mainly psychological cause with tiredness as a main feature of depression.

- Tiredness as a presenting symptom in the absence of other symptoms, e.g. weight loss or weight gain, is unlikely to have a physical cause.

- Tiredness and weight loss should be taken seriously and thoroughly investigated – malignancy and hyperthyroidism are possible diagnoses.

TOE LESIONS

Lesions of the toes are extremely common. They are caused by a
variety of conditions ranging from simple ingrowing toenails to
severe pain caused by ischaemia. Deformities of the toes are also
exceptionally common, particularly in the elderly.

CAUSES

TOENAILS

- Ingrowing toenail
- Subungual haematoma
- Subungual melanoma
- Subungual exostosis
- Onychogryphosis

DEFORMITIES

- Hallux valgus
- Hallux rigidus
- Hammer toe
- Claw toes

ULCERS

ISCHAEMIC

Large vessel disease
- Arteriosclerosis
- Embolism

Small vessel disease
- Diabetes
- Raynaud's
- Buerger's
- Embolism
- Vasculitis, e.g. scleroderma, SLE, rheumatoid

NEUROPATHIC

Peripheral nerve lesions
- Diabetes
- Nerve injuries
- Leprosy
  - Common where leprosy endemic

Spinal cord lesions
- Spina bifida
- Spinal injuries

- Syringomyelia

NEOPLASTIC
- Skin tumours

DISCOLORATION
- Chilblains
- Ischaemia

HISTORY

Nails

Ingrowing toenail usually presents with pain at the sides of the nail and often with infection and local inflammation. With infection the toe is painful and throbs, especially in bed at night. With subungual haematoma there is a history of injury to the nail. Bleeding occurs beneath the nail, which is extremely painful, and occasionally the patient may faint with the pain. Subungual melanoma presents with pigmentation under the nail. With subungual exostosis there is lifting of the nail with deformity. Onychogryphosis is a 'ram's horn' deformity of the nail. The nail thickens and curves over the end. It is common in the elderly but may occur in young people after injury to the nailbed.

Deformities

A patient with hallux valgus normally presents with a 'bunion'. The first metatarsal deviates medially. It is more common in females. The patient may complain that the great toe overrides the second toe. Unsuitable, tight footwear may be a precipitating cause. Hallux rigidus is osteoarthritis of the first MTP joint. It occurs in young adults. The patient complains of pain on walking, especially when 'pushing off', and stiffness in the joint. Hammer toe usually affects the second toe. There is a fixed flexion deformity of the PIP joint and compensatory hyperextension of adjacent joints. The patient merely complains of a deformed toe, and may also complain of painful callosities that have developed where the deformed toe presses against the footwear. With clawed toes both IP joints are flexed. The tips of the toes may develop painful callosities.

Ulcers

Ulcers are usually ischaemic (painful) or neuropathic (painless). Check for a history of intermittent claudication, smoking, Raynaud's disease, cardiac disease, diabetes. With neuropathic ulcers there may be a history of diabetes, nerve injuries, spinal cord lesions. Ulcers usually occur on the pressure points over the tips of the toes. Neoplastic ulcers on the toes are extremely rare. Melanoma may occur on the toes but is usually subungual.

Discoloration

Painful discoloration, either red or shiny, white, blue or black (gangrene), suggests ischaemia. Chilblains occur in childhood and early adult life, usually in females. They are more likely in those with outdoor occupations. Painful swelling occurs on the toes, which may become itchy. They are often multiple and may develop into shallow ulcers.

EXAMINATION

Nails

With ingrowing toenails there is often a serous discharge or purulent discharge from the nailfold. The toe becomes red and swollen. Granulation tissue may be apparent at the nailfold. Subungual haematoma is usually obvious. Occasionally, however, the patient forgets the injury and presents with a brownish discoloration under the nail and this has to be distinguished from a melanoma. Haematoma is usually reddish-brown with sharp edges, the melanoma being brownish-grey with an indistinct edge. A melanoma grows out with the nail. A haematoma does not. With suspected melanoma, examine the regional lymph nodes and liver for secondaries. Subungual exostosis results in deformity of the nail, which is pushed up and deformed. The swelling between the toe and the end of the nail eventually becomes obvious. Onychogryphosis is obvious with a thick discoloured nail, which curves over at the end (ram's horn deformity).

Deformities

With hallux valgus the first metatarsal bone deviates medially, the great toe laterally. There may be a thickened bursa over the medial aspect of the joint (bunion). The great toe may override the second toe. In hallux rigidus there is a stiff, painful, enlarged, first MTP joint. With hammer toe the second toe is usually affected. There is a fixed flexed deformity of the PIP joint and compensatory hyperextension of the adjacent joint. Check for the presence of corns and callosities. In claw toes both IP joints are flexed (see Foot deformities, p. 149).

Ulcers

Punched out, painful ulcers over pressure points suggest ischaemic ulcers. Check for discoloration of the toe, capillary return and absence of foot pulses. Neuropathic ulcers are painless; the circulation is usually good, but sensation is absent or blunted locally. Carry out a full neurological examination.

Discoloration

With ischaemic toe it may be shiny red, blue, white or black with gangrene. Examine the pulses. Chilblains are usually reddish-blue, the skin being oedematous, and blistering may occur, which bursts leaving superficial ulcers.

GENERAL INVESTIGATIONS

- **FBC, ESR**
  Hb ↓ anaemia of chronic disease, e.g. rheumatoid arthritis,
  SLE. WCC ↑ infection, e.g. with diabetes. ESR ↑ vasculitis, e.g.
  rheumatoid arthritis, SLE.

- **U&Es**
  Chronic renal failure with connective tissues diseases.

- **Blood glucose**
  Ischaemia with small vessel disease in diabetes.

- **X-rays**
  Subungual exostosis. Hallux rigidus.

SPECIFIC INVESTIGATIONS

- **Antibody screen**
  Connective tissue disease.

- **Doppler studies**
  Ischaemia.

- **Arteriography**
  Arterial disease.

- **MRI**
  Spinal cord lesions with neuropathy.

- **Nerve conduction studies**
  Peripheral neuropathy.

- **Excision biopsy**
  Malignant lesions, e.g. subungual melanoma.

- Take care to distinguish between ischaemic (painful)
  and neuropathic (painless) ulcers.

- A pigmented lesion below the nail (subungual) may
  be a haematoma or melanoma. Check carefully for
  a history of trauma. A haematoma grows out with
  the nail; a melanoma does not.

- Arteriopaths who develop painful toes need urgent
  investigation. It may be due to the development
  of critical ischaemia or may be embolic.

TONGUE DISORDERS

Tongue disorders are extremely common, ranging from minor furring of the tongue to extensive inflammation and malignancy. Tongue disorders are often a manifestation of systemic disease.

CAUSES

FURRING

- Gastrointestinal disease
- Dehydration
- Mouth breathers
- Smokers
- Antibiotics

COLOUR CHANGE

- White patches, e.g. leucoplakia, thrush
- Pallor (anaemia)
- Blue (central cyanosis)
- Red
  - Pernicious anaemia
  - Vitamin B deficiency
- Pigmented
  - Addison's disease

SWELLING (MACROGLOSSIA)

- Down's syndrome
- Trauma, e.g. hot liquids, corrosive substances
- Myxoedema
- Allergy
- Cretinism
- Acromegaly

CHRONIC SUPERFICIAL GLOSSITIS

- Smoking
- Spices
- Spirits
- Sepsis
- Sharp teeth
- Syphilis

ULCERATION

- Aphthous ulcer
- Dental trauma
- Carcinoma
- Chancre
- Gumma

WASTING

- Hypoglossal nerve palsy

HISTORY

Furring

A history of gastrointestinal disease, dehydration, mouth breathing, smoking or antibiotics.

Colour change

White patches on the tongue are suggestive of leucoplakia or candidiasis, the last being associated with antibiotic therapy, chemotherapy or immunosuppression. Hairy leucoplakia is associated with EBv and is found almost exclusively in patients with HIV. A pale tongue may indicate anaemia, a blue tongue central cyanosis. The patient may present with a red, painful tongue which may occur in pernicious anaemia or other forms of vitamin B deficiency. Pigmentation may be a sign of Addison's disease.

Swelling

The patient may present with a swollen tongue, which may or may not be painful. Difficulty in articulation or swallowing may be apparent. Cretinism will be obvious (extremely rare nowadays), as will Down's syndrome. A swollen tongue may be a presentation of myxoedema. Other symptoms of myxoedema may be present, e.g. slowness, weight gain, dry skin, hoarse voice, constipation, lethargy, dislike of cold weather. Acromegaly may be obvious, the patient having noticed an increase in shoe size, change in voice and jaw changes. Infection (see below) may present with swelling, as may allergies or trauma, especially burns with hot fluids or caustic substances. Infection will result in a painful tongue, the classical predispositions to chronic superficial glossitis being the six Ss: syphilis, smoking, spices, spirits, sepsis, sharp teeth.

Chronic superficial glossitis

There is a sequence of chronic inflammatory, degenerative and hypertrophic changes in the tongue which terminate in the development of a carcinoma. There may be a history of the six Ss: syphilis, smoking, sharp tooth, spirits, spices and sepsis. The patient

SECTION A

is usually over the age of 50 and presents with a tongue that has become shiny or white, or has developed a lump on the tongue. There is usually no pain and no interference with eating.

Ulceration

Ulceration is common. Aphthous ulcers are painful and are often associated with chronic debilitating disease. Dental trauma from a sharp tooth or ill-fitting dentures may cause ulcers. Chancre and gumma associated with syphilis are rare. Carcinoma has a peak incidence at 60–70 years and presents with a painless ulcer on the tongue, often at the margins on the dorsal surface. Carcinoma of the posterior third of the tongue may present with referred pain to the ear, the pain being referred from the lingual branch of the trigeminal nerve, which supplies the tongue, to the ear via the auriculotemporal nerve.

Wasting

Wasting of the tongue is caused by paralysis of the hypoglossal nerve. Check for a history of recent trauma or surgery to the neck, which may have damaged the hypoglossal nerve. Atrophy of the tongue occurs on the same side as the lesion.

EXAMINATION

Furring

Examination will reveal uniformed furring of the tongue. Note its colour. Look for signs of gastrointestinal disease.

Colour change

This will usually be obvious. White patches on the tongue may be due to leucoplakia. The white plaques may fissure with time. This is a pre-malignant condition. Other white patches may be due to candidal infection (thrush). Unlike leucoplakia, these white plaques may be rubbed off, revealing ulcerated buccal mucosa underneath. Colour changes may be uniform (pallor and cyanosis) or patchy (the pigmentation of Addison's disease). In pernicious anaemia the tongue is red, bald and painful.

Swelling

The tongue is large and tends to protrude in Down's syndrome. Other signs of Down's syndrome will be apparent, e.g. epicanthic folds, mental retardation. Look for signs of cretinism, e.g. stunted growth, relatively large head, thick eyelids, thick broad nose, thick lips, widely spaced eyes. With myxoedema there will be dry skin, dry hair, goitre, slow relaxing reflexes, congestive cardiac failure and non-pitting oedema. With acromegaly there will be large feet, prognathism, thick spade-like hands, deep voice and possibly cardiac failure. In generalised infections the tongue will be red and swollen. Allergies may present with a swollen tongue, lips, larynx, bronchospasm and rash. There will usually be a history of exposure to an allergen. The ingestion of corrosive or hot fluids will result in inflammation not only to the tongue but also to the rest of the mouth and the pharynx.

Chronic superficial glossitis

Examination reveals a thin, grey transparent film on the tongue in the early stages. Leucoplakia occurs next and eventually overt carcinoma develops.

Ulceration

Aphthous ulcers start as tender vesicular lesions with a hyperaemic base, which ulcerate leaving a small, white, circular, deep, painful ulcer. Dental trauma will usually result in ulcers at the lateral margins of the tongue adjacent to a sharp tooth. Chancres and gummas are rare, as is tuberculous ulcer of the tongue. A carcinomatous ulcer usually occurs on the upper surface of the tongue, usually at the lateral margins. It feels hard, has an everted edge and is friable and bleeds. Local lymph nodes may be palpable, due to either secondary infection or metastases.

Wasting

Ask the patient to protrude the tongue. Wasting will be noted on the affected side and the tongue deviates to the side of the lesion. Check for scars on the neck to suggest hypoglossal nerve damage.

GENERAL INVESTIGATIONS

- **FBC, ESR, CRP**
  Hb ↓ anaemia (microcytic, macrocytic). WCC ↑ infection. ESR and CRP ↑ infection, malignancy.

- **Serum vitamin B_{12}**
  Reduced in pernicious anaemia.

- **TFTs**
  T_4 ↓, TSH ↑ in myxoedema.

- **Swab**
  Culture and sensitivity. Infection. Vincent's angina. Syphilis. Bacterial, viral and fungal infections.

SPECIFIC INVESTIGATIONS

- **VDRL**
  Syphilis.

- **Serology**
  Parietal cell antibodies in pernicious anaemia.

- **HIV test**
  Hairy leucoplakia.

- **CT/MRI**
  Pituitary tumour in acromegaly.

- **Oral glucose tolerance test with growth hormone and IGF-1 measurement**
  Acromegaly.

- **ACTH stimulation tests**
  Addison's disease.

- **Biopsy**
  Carcinoma.

- A mouth ulcer which does not settle requires further investigation for malignancy especially in smokers.
- Candidal infection may be the first manifestation of diabetes or an immunosuppressive disease, e.g. HIV infection.

TREMOR

A tremor is a rhythmic oscillation of a body part and usually refers to the movements around the small joints of the hands.

CAUSES

RESTING TREMOR

- Parkinson's disease

ACTION TREMOR

- Idiopathic
- Benign essential tremor
- Physiological
- Anxiety
- Exercise
- Chronic respiratory disease
- Thyrotoxicosis

DRUGS

- Caffeine
- Alcohol (including alcohol withdrawal)
- Drug withdrawal (benzodiazepines, opiates)
- Beta agonists
- Lithium
- Phenytoin
- Ciclosporin

INTENTION TREMOR

- Cerebellar disease

HISTORY

Tremor is divided into three groups: (1) resting tremor; (2) an action tremor, which is evident when the hand is held in a sustained position or against gravity; and (3) an intention tremor, which is present during movement. Physiological causes of tremor usually have clear precipitating factors, such as anger and exercise.

An action tremor that resolves when the limb is fully supported against gravity is characteristic of benign essential tremor; in addition it may also be relieved by alcohol and is attenuated during movement. Up to one-third of patients with benign essential tremor have a family history. In addition to tremor, patients with thyrotoxicosis may also complain of heat intolerance, palpitations, increased appetite with weight loss, anxiety and diarrhoea.

A detailed drug history will easily allow you to identify any drug that may potentially cause tremor. Enquiries should also include the amount of coffee and alcohol intake.

Associated symptoms of slowness, difficulty initiating and stopping walking, muscle rigidity and muscle fatigue (especially with writing) may be present with Parkinson's disease. With cerebellar disease, difficulties may be experienced with balance and coordination.

EXAMINATION

Tremor

Observe the patient at rest: the presence of a pill-rolling tremor is suggestive of Parkinson's disease. In addition, there may be expressionless facies, titubation and drooling of saliva. Thyrotoxic patients will be thin with wide, staring eyes, lid lag, a goitre and exophthalmos with Graves' disease.

The arms are then held outstretched; all other causes of tremor will now be visible. Fine tremors can be accentuated by placing a piece of paper on the outstretched hands. The arm should be fully supported and this will cause resolution of benign essential tremor. An intention tremor is demonstrated by the finger–nose test; a tremor is markedly increased when the finger approaches the target. In addition, there may also be past-pointing where the finger overshoots the target.

General

Following this evaluation, further examination may be required to determine the underlying cause. The gait is assessed (p. 161) and differences between the parkinsonian and ataxic gait of cerebellar disease will be obvious. Further features of cerebellar dysfunction are scanning speech, dysdiadochokinesia, nystagmus and pendular reflexes. When thyrotoxicosis is suspected, the thyroid gland is palpated, ocular movements assessed and the thyroid gland auscultated for a bruit associated with Graves' disease. Features of prolonged alcohol excess may be present (signs of chronic liver disease) and alcohol may lead to cerebellar degeneration.

GENERAL INVESTIGATIONS

- ■ TSH and free T_4
  ↓ TSH and ↑ T_4 with thyrotoxicosis.

- ■ LFTs
  Abnormalities of synthetic liver function may be present in chronic alcohol excess.

- ■ ABGs
  Hypoxia and CO_2 retention in respiratory disease.

SPECIFIC INVESTIGATIONS

■ CT/MRI head
For the evaluation of patients with impaired coordination
suggestive of cerebellar disease.

- The tremor of Parkinson's disease is often subtle and
therefore other features of this condition should be
sought.

- Always consider alcohol excess as a possible cause
of tremor.

URETHRAL DISCHARGE

Any inflammatory condition within the urethra may cause a discharge. It is important to diagnose venereal conditions so that appropriate treatment is given, not only to the patient but also to sexual contacts.

CAUSES

- Prostatitis
- Non-gonococcal urethritis
- Bacterial
  - Coliforms
  - Gonorrhoea
  - *Haemophilus ducreyi* (chancroid)
  - TB
  - Syphilis (chancre)
- Reiter's disease
- Traumatic
  - Instrumental
  - Accidental
  - Foreign body
- Chemical
- Neoplastic

HISTORY

General

For any sexually transmitted disease check for a history of sexual contact, time of last sexual intercourse, contraceptive methods, number and duration of relationships, sexual practices and unusual sexual practices.

Prostatitis

Urethral discharge is rare with acute prostatitis. With chronic prostatitis there may be a clear white urethral discharge. The patient may also complain of suprapubic pain, low back pain, perineal discomfort and pain referred to the testicles.

Non-gonococcal urethritis

The patient complains of urethral discharge, which may be thinner than with gonorrhoea. The presentation may be less acute than with gonorrhoea.

Gonorrhoea

The patient will complain of a thickish, purulent urethral discharge and dysuria. Prostatitis and epididymitis may occur, the patient complaining of deep perineal pain or scrotal swelling.

Other bacterial

Urethritis may occur with urinary tract infections. Infection with *Haemophilus ducreyi* causes chancroid or soft sore. It is a tropical infection causing painful genital ulcers and swelling of the inguinal glands. The soft sores may affect the terminal urethra, resulting in dysuria and a profuse, thin, watery discharge. TB of the urethra is very rare. It is usually secondary to TB elsewhere in the genitourinary tract. A syphilitic chancre is now rare but presents as a painful swelling involving the terminal urethra.

Reiter's disease

The patient is usually a young male with recent non-specific urethritis, or it may follow an attack of dysentery. Apart from a urethral discharge, there may be a history of conjunctivitis and joint pains.

Trauma

Urethral instrumentation or prolonged catheterisation may cause urethritis. There will be a clear history of this. Foreign bodies may be introduced by the patient. The variety of these defies description! Other foreign bodies include stones passing from the bladder or fragments of urethral catheters. The patient may be too embarrassed to confess that he has introduced a foreign body into the urethra.

Chemical

Chemical urethritis is more common in females. There may be a history of change of soap or bath oils.

Neoplastic

Urethral carcinoma is rare. The patient will complain of dysuria and bloodstained urethral discharge.

EXAMINATION

Prostatitis

There may be a tender, occasionally boggy prostate on digital rectal examination.

Non-gonococcal urethritis

Pus may again be seen at the external urethral meatus. Check for prostatitis and epididymitis.

Gonorrhoea

Often a bead of pus may be seen at the external urethral meatus. It is appropriate to check for evidence of proctitis or anal discharge (homosexuals). There may be evidence of prostatitis, there being a tender, boggy prostate on digital rectal examination. Palpation of the scrotum may reveal epididymitis.

Other bacterial

Other forms of urethritis may show a discharge at the external urethral meatus. With chancroid there may be sores on the genitals with sores around the meatus. Check for inguinal lymphadenopathy. Urethral TB is very rare. Check for evidence of TB elsewhere, e.g. lungs, kidneys, epididymis. With a syphilitic chancre the meatus is oedematous and swollen. There may be inguinal lymphadenopathy.

Reiter's disease

Examine for conjunctivitis and arthritis. There may be co-existent plantar fasciitis and Achilles tendonitis. Examine for abscesses on the soles of the feet and palms of the hands (keratoderma blenorrhagica).

Traumatic

Feel along the course of the urethra for tenderness or palpable stone or foreign body.

Neoplastic

A hard lump may be felt along the course of the urethra. Pressure on it may cause a bloodstained urethral discharge.

GENERAL INVESTIGATIONS

- ■ FBC, ESR
  WCC ↑ in infection, e.g. gonorrhoea. ESR ↑ inflammation, e.g. syphilis.
- ■ Swab
  Microscopy and culture and sensitivity of urethral discharge. This may grow gonococcus, *Chlamydia trachomatis, Trichomonas* spp, *Ureaplasma urealyticum*. Secondary infection, e.g. with *candida* or coliforms, may occur. *Haemophilus ducreyi* may be grown in chancroid. Dark-ground microscopy may reveal treponemes in syphilis.

SPECIFIC INVESTIGATIONS

- ■ EMSU
  TB.
- ■ Prostatic massage
  C&S of discharge in chronic prostatitis.
- ■ VDRL
  Syphilitic chancre.
- ■ Cystourethroscopy
  Foreign body. Urethral carcinoma.

- Always take a full sexual history, including unusual sexual practices and, if STD is suspected, refer to a GUM clinic for full assessment and contact tracing.

URINARY INCONTINENCE

Urinary incontinence is the involuntary loss of urine from the bladder. Loss of urine occurs at times and places which are inconvenient, inappropriate and socially embarrassing. Stress incontinence is loss of urine during coughing or straining. Urge incontinence is the inability to maintain urinary continence in the presence of frequent and persistent urges to void. Overflow incontinence occurs when the detrusor muscle becomes flaccid and often insensitive to stretch and the bladder distends. Weakness of the sphincter mechanism eventually leads to overflow, when urine leaks out through the urethra.

CAUSES

STRESS INCONTINENCE

PELVIC FLOOR INJURY
- Childbirth
- Prostatectomy

URGE INCONTINENCE

DETRUSOR INSTABILITY
- Cystitis
- Stones
- Prostatectomy
- Post-radiotherapy
- Tuberculo-cystitis
- Interstitial nephritis
- Tumour

OVERFLOW INCONTINENCE

LOWER MOTOR NEURONE LESIONS
- Diabetes
- Sacral centre injury
- Cauda equina injury
- Sacral nerve damage, e.g. pelvic surgery

CHRONIC OUTFLOW OBSTRUCTION
- Prostatic enlargement

NEUROLOGICAL

UPPER MOTOR NEURONE LESION
- Disc lesions

- Cerebrovascular accident
- Head injury
- Spinal cord injury above sacral centre
- Spinal tumours
- Multiple sclerosis
- Syringomyelia

ANATOMICAL

- Ectopia vesicae
- Ectopic ureter
- Vesicovaginal fistula

OTHER

- Nocturnal enuresis

HISTORY

Stress incontinence

History of multiple childbirth. Difficult delivery. Recent prostatectomy. History of loss of urine during coughing and straining.

Urge incontinence

The patient is unable to maintain urinary continence in the presence of frequent and persistent urges to void. Recent prostatectomy. Recurrent attacks of cystitis with dysuria and frequency. Past history of pelvic radiotherapy. History of TB. History of ureteric colic. Persistent suprapubic discomfort and haematuria associated with stone. Haematuria associated with tumour.

Overflow incontinence

History of spinal injury involving lumbar vertebra (sacral centre, cauda equina). History of pelvic surgery, e.g. abdominoperineal resection of rectum with damage to pelvic nerves. History of diabetes. History of prostatism with chronic retention with overflow. The patient may still be able to void reasonably normally but feels the bladder is not emptying and leakage continues.

Neurological

With upper motor neurone lesions there may be a history of spinal trauma affecting the cord above the sacral centre. History of head injury, CVA, multiple sclerosis or syringomyelia.

Anatomical

Ectopia vesicae will be obvious at birth with an abdominal wall defect and the ureter opening into exposed bladder mucosa on the lower abdominal wall. Duplex ureter may be associated with an ectopic opening of the ureter into the vagina. Vesicovaginal fistula may follow pelvic surgery or pelvic radiotherapy. It may occasionally be the presenting symptom of pelvic malignancy. Rarely ureterovaginal fistula may occur from an erosion of a ureteric calculus into a vaginal fornix. With duplex ureter, vesicovaginal fistula or ureterovaginal fistula, urine dribbles from the vagina continuously.

Other

Nocturnal enuresis occurs in up to 5% of 10-year-old children. Bed-wetting after puberty usually indicates the presence of an unstable bladder or other pathology.

EXAMINATION

Stress incontinence

Observe leakage when patient coughs. A cystocele or complete prolapse may be seen.

Urge incontinence

There may be little to find on examination.

Overflow incontinence

There may be a palpable bladder. Carry out a full neurological examination. Digital rectal examination may reveal prostatic hypertrophy.

Neurological

Reflex emptying of the bladder occurs. Carry out a full neurological examination.

Anatomical

Ectopia vesicae – ureters opening into bladder mucosa on abdominal wall. With vesicovaginal fistula, examination with a vaginal speculum may indicate the site of the fistula.

GENERAL INVESTIGATIONS

■ **FBC**
  WCC ↑ in infection.

■ **MSU**
  C&S for infection.

■ **IVU**
  Assess upper tracts, obstruction, bladder lesions, fistula.

SPECIFIC INVESTIGATIONS

- **Cystoscopy**
  Bladder stone. Neoplasia.
- **Cystography**
  Vesicovaginal fistula.
- **Urodynamics**
  Uroflowmetry – measures flow rate. Cystometry – detrusor contractions. Videocystometry – leakage of urine on straining in stress incontinence – urethral pressure profiles – sphincter function and outlet obstruction.
- **CT**
  Cord lesion. Spinal tumour.
- **MRI**
  Cord lesion. Disc lesion. Spinal tumour. Syringomyelia.

- Continuous incontinence suggests a fistula, chronic outflow problems or a neurological cause.
- Incontinence with leg weakness and saddle anaesthesia suggests a cauda equina lesion. Urgent neurosurgical referral is required.

URINARY RETENTION

Retention of urine may be acute, chronic or acute-on-chronic. Patients with acute retention present as surgical emergencies. Acute retention is the sudden inability to pass urine, with the presence of painful bladder. Chronic retention is the presence of an enlarged, painless bladder with or without difficulty in micturition.

CAUSES

LOCAL

URETHRAL LUMEN OR BLADDER NECK

- Stones
- Blood clot
- Tumours
- Urethral valves
- Meatal ulcer

URETHRAL OR BLADDER WALL

- Urethral trauma
- Urethral stricture
- Urethral tumour

OUTSIDE THE WALL

- Prostatic enlargement
- Faecal impaction
- Pregnant uterus
- Pelvic tumour

GENERAL

POST-OPERATIVE

NEUROGENIC

- Spinal cord injuries
- Spinal cord disease
  - Diabetic autonomic neuropathy
  - Multiple sclerosis
  - Spinal tumour
  - Tabes dorsalis

DRUGS

- Anticholinergic drugs
- Antidepressants
- Alcohol

HISTORY

Local

Check for a history of problems with micturition, e.g. difficulty in starting, poor stream, nocturia, frequency, dysuria. Is there any history of urinary tract infection, urethritis, ureteric colic (to suggest a stone which may have passed into the bladder and then impacted into the bladder neck or urethra) or haematuria? Is there a past history of prolonged catheterisation to suggest a urethral stricture? A history of trauma will be apparent. Has the patient fallen astride an object? Has trauma caused a pelvic fracture? Is the patient constipated, to suggest faecal impaction? A pregnant uterus will be obvious.

General

Post-operative acute retention is common, especially in elderly men. This may be due to anxiety, embarrassment, supine posture, pain, drugs, fluid overload or previous unrecognised prostatism with minimal symptoms. After urological procedures it may be due to blood clot in the bladder. Check for a history of neurological disease. Has the patient suffered spinal cord injury? Check the drug history.

EXAMINATION

Local

The patient may have a tender, palpable, painful bladder with sudden onset of retention. In acute retention the bladder rarely extends far above the pubic symphysis. In chronic retention the distended bladder is often painless and more markedly distended than in acute retention, often reaching to the umbilicus. With chronic retention there may be overflow incontinence. Feel along the course of the urethra for a stone or stricture. Perform a digital rectal examination to check for prostatic hypertrophy or pelvic tumour. Following pelvic trauma with urethral injury there will be a high 'floating' prostate on rectal examination. Check the urethral meatus for ulcer or stone. Examine the patient for signs of uraemia, which may be present with chronic retention.

General

Post-operative retention will be obvious. Occasionally it is difficult to palpate the bladder because of pain and guarding related to a surgical incision. Neurological causes of acute retention or those related to spinal trauma are often obvious. Carry out a full neurological examination.

GENERAL INVESTIGATIONS

- **FBC, ESR**
  Hb ↓ in chronic renal failure, tumours, haematuria. WCC ↑ infection. ESR ↑ malignancy and infection.

- **MSU**
  Microscopy. C&S for UTI. Cytology to confirm malignancy.

- **U&Es**
  Renal failure. Obstructive uropathy.

- **CXR**
  Pulmonary oedema (chronic renal failure). Possible tumour metastases.

- **US**
  Bladder size confirms diagnosis. Dilated upper urinary tract due to back pressure. Pregnant uterus.

SPECIFIC INVESTIGATIONS

- **Urethrography**
  Urethral valves. Stricture. Urethral trauma.

- **PSA**
  Carcinoma of the prostate.

- **Cystoscopy**
  Stone, tumour, stricture.

- **Urodynamics**
  Identification and assessment of neurological or bladder neck problems.

- Digital rectal examination is mandatory in the patient with retention.
- Faecal impaction in the elderly may be a cause of urinary retention.
- A history suggestive of disc prolapse with urinary retention suggests cord compression. An urgent neurosurgical opinion is required.
- Following catheterisation for chronic retention, do not empty the bladder rapidly. This may result in brisk haematuria from the sudden decompression. Controlled drainage is required.

VAGINAL DISCHARGE

Vaginal discharge can occur at any age but is usually a symptom of reproductive years.

CAUSES

- Candidiasis
- Bacterial vaginosis
- *Trichomonas* vaginosis
- Cervicitis, e.g. gonorrhoea, *Chlamydia*, herpes
- Excessive normal secretions
- Retained foreign body, e.g. tampon, pessary
- Intrauterine contraceptive device
- Salpingitis
- Infection of Bartholin's glands
- Neoplasm, e.g. vagina, vulva
- Pyometra
- Colovaginal fistula

HISTORY

Obtain a full history of the discharge, including timing, colour, consistency, smell and the presence or absence of itch. Intensive itch suggests thrush. An offensive smell occurs with trichomonal and bacterial vaginosis. Ask whether the patient experiences pain on intercourse. Pelvic pain, tenderness and fever suggest pelvic inflammatory disease. Take a full sexual history (young women, change of partner, multiple partners). Excessive normal secretions just feel wet. There is no discomfort.

EXAMINATION

A red, swollen, sore and itchy vulva suggests candidiasis. The character of the discharge is important. A thick yellow–brown discharge from the cervix occurs with gonorrhoea; a thinner yellow-brown cervical discharge occurs with *Chlamydia*; a thin green smelly discharge occurs with trichomoniasis; a thin grey–white fishy smelling discharge suggests bacterial vaginosis; a thick white odourless discharge occurs with candidiasis. Carry out a PV and speculum examination. This will show an inflamed cervix with trichomonal vaginosis and also with cervicitis due to gonococcus, *Chlamydia* and herpes.

GENERAL INVESTIGATIONS

- **Gram stain**
  Gram stain on cervical or urethral exudate – Gram-negative intracellular diplococci in gonorrhoea.

- **Vaginal pH testing**
  pH>4.5 in bacterial vaginosis. pH<4.5 in candidiasis.

- **Triple swabs**
  High vaginal swab – bacterial vaginosis, candidiasis, trichomonal vaginalis.
  Endocervical swab – gonorrhoea.
  Endocervical swab – *Chlamydia* DNA amplification for *Chlamydia trachomatis*.

- **Urine analysis (first catch)**
  DNA amplification for *Chlamydia*.

SPECIFIC INVESTIGATIONS

- **Hysteroscopy**
  Malignancy/menorrhagia.

- **D&C**
  Malignancy.

- **Barium enema**
  Colovaginal fistula.

- **MRI**
  Colovaginal fistula.

- Malignancy is a likely cause of vaginal discharge in post-menopausal years. Always perform a full pelvic examination.

- Always take a full sexual history and, if sexually transmitted disease is suspected, refer to the GUM clinic for full assessment and contact tracing.

- Vaginal discharge is rare before puberty. Consider foreign body or sexual abuse.

- Recurrent thrush may be a presenting symptom of diabetes mellitus.

VISUAL PROBLEMS

As the sense of sight is critical, patients who present with visual disturbance are often very distressed. Below is a list of common conditions that may give rise to visual problems, grouped according to symptoms.

CAUSES

VISUAL DISTURBANCES (FLASHING LIGHTS OR FLOATERS)

- Migraine
- Retinal detachment
- Vitreous haemorrhage
- Vitreous detachment

BLURRING OF VISION

- Refractive errors
- Head injuries
- Acute angle-closure glaucoma
- Blunt trauma to the eye

LOSS OF VISION

PARTIAL LOSS

- Homonymous hemianopia – stroke, tumour
- Peripheral field loss – glaucoma, papilloedema
- Central field loss – macular degeneration
- Bitemporal hemianopia – pituitary tumour
- Horizontal field loss – retinal vascular occlusion

TOTAL LOSS

Acute

- Amaurosis fugax
- Papilloedema
  - Raised intracranial pressure
  - Malignant hypertension
- Temporal arteritis
- Optic neuritis
- Central retinal vein occlusion
- Central retinal artery occlusion
- Posterior uveitis

Gradual

- Cataract
- Glaucoma

- Diabetic retinopathy
- Hypertensive retinopathy
- Age-related macular degeneration
- Retinitis pigmentosa
- Infectious
  - Trachoma (*Chlamydia trachomatis*)
    - (common in underdeveloped countries)
  - *Onchocerciasis* (nematode infection)
    - (common in underdeveloped countries)
- Vitamin A deficiency
  - (common in underdeveloped countries)

HISTORY

First establish if visual loss is monocular or binocular. Ocular or optic nerve pathology generally causes monocular visual loss, whereas lesions at the optic chiasma or more posteriorly cause binocular loss that will respect the vertical meridian. Loss of central vision may be due to macular or optic nerve pathology. Retinal lesions cause a 'positive' scotoma (the patient is aware that part of the field is obstructed), whereas damage posterior to the retina causes a 'negative' scotoma (the patient does not see that a segment of the visual field is missing).

Visual disturbances

Bilateral flashing lights and zigzag lines are often reported by patients suffering with attacks of migraine. This is accompanied by throbbing headache, nausea, vomiting and photophobia. Posterior vitreous detachment, vitreous haemorrhage and retinal detachment are all associated with floaters and flashing lights. Visual acuity and visual fields are normal at first but may be impaired with a large vitreous haemorrhage or advanced retinal detachment.

Blurring of vision

Errors of refraction (long- or short-sighted) are the most common cause of blurring of vision. This is a common problem and is usually corrected with glasses by optometrists. Head and eye injuries may also give rise to transient blurring of the vision. With acute angle-closure glaucoma, corneal oedema will give rise to the appearances of haloes around lights and is associated with a red and painful eye.

Loss of vision

Visual loss may be partial or total. The description of the area of partial visual field loss is very informative. Complaints of vertical visual field losses are due to lesions posterior to the optic chiasma and most commonly caused by strokes, although similar effects can be produced by space-occupying lesions such as cerebral tumours.

Horizontal visual field losses imply that the cause lies within the retina and is usually due to retinal vascular occlusions. Patients with glaucoma may complain of tunnel vision, and patients with macular degeneration may experience sudden central visual field loss.

Sudden total visual loss is usually due to a vascular aetiology. Amaurosis fugax is sudden transient monocular blindness due to atheroembolism of the ophthalmic artery. Patients classically complain of a 'curtain descending across the field of vision'. With giant cell arteritis affecting the ophthalmic artery, sudden onset of blindness can occur in conjunction with the symptoms of temporal headache, jaw claudication and scalp tenderness. It is often associated with polymyalgia rheumatica. Papilloedema may cause transient visual loss, lasting seconds, related to posture.

Monocular blindness due to optic neuritis may occur with multiple sclerosis; it is often associated with retro-orbital pain that worsens with eye movements and starts with a progressive dimming of vision over a few days.

Diabetic retinopathy is the most common cause of blindness in western society. In addition, diabetics are also more prone to develop cataracts and glaucoma. In the elderly, gradual onset of visual loss may be due to cataracts, glaucoma or age-related macular degeneration. Owing to the gradual onset of symptoms, these groups of patients may present very late. A cataract may be visible on examination of the eye.

EXAMINATION

Visual acuity unaided and corrected with a pinhole should be assessed with a Snellen chart. If visualisation of the largest letter is not possible then assess vision by counting fingers. Further tests to use are those of movement and, finally, the ability to discriminate between light and dark. With refractive errors, vision can be corrected by viewing the Snellen chart through a pinhole. Visual fields are examined by confrontational testing, and the extent of visual field loss can be assessed approximately.

Pupillary response to light (direct and consensual) allows the assessment of the visual pathway. Direct light reflex may be lost in lesions involving the unilateral optic nerve and with central retinal artery occlusion.

Colour vision will be reduced disproportionately compared with visual acuity in optic nerve diseases. This may be assessed with the use of Ishihara plates.

Fundoscopy

A wealth of information is obtained on fundoscopy. The red reflex is lost with cataracts. Examination of the retina may reveal background retinopathy with diabetes, consisting of dot and blot haemorrhages with cotton-wool spots. With hypertensive retinopathy, silver wiring, arteriovenous nipping, retinal haemorrhages and eventually papilloedema may be appreciated. Growth of new vessels on the retina indicates proliferative retinopathy. An infarcted retina appears oedematous and pale; the macula appears prominent and red (cherry-red spot). Detached retinal folds may be seen, and clots of blood are visible with vitreous haemorrhage. The margins of the optic disc become blurred with papilloedema and optic neuritis but later may appear pale. A cupped optic disc appearance occurs with chronic glaucoma.

Upon completion of the examination of the eye, a neurological examination should be performed, followed by a cardiovascular examination to exclude sources of emboli. The rhythm of the pulse is assessed for atrial fibrillation and the heart and carotids are auscultated for murmurs. The blood pressure is measured to exclude hypertension.

GENERAL INVESTIGATIONS

- **ESR and CRP**
  Giant cell arteritis.

- **Blood glucose**
  Glucose ↑ diabetes.

- **Intraocular pressure measurements**
  ↑ with glaucoma.

- **Perimetry**
  Formal charting of visual fields. Arcuate scotomas are found with glaucoma. Central scotomas may be seen with optic neuritis. Bitemporal hemianopias/homonymous hemianopias and quadrantanopias in neurological pathology.

SPECIFIC INVESTIGATIONS

- **CT/MRI head**
  Tumours, stroke, multiple sclerosis.

- **Carotid Doppler**
  Atherosclerotic plaque with amaurosis fugax.

- **Temporal artery biopsy**
  Temporal arteritis.

- **US**
  To assess retina if no visualisation of fundus behind cataract or vitreous haemorrhage.

- **Sudden onset of visual disturbance or loss is an emergency and must be investigated immediately.**
- **If temporal arteritis is suspected, immediate treatment with corticosteroids is required to avoid catastrophic irreversible blindness.**

VOICE DISORDERS

Voice disorders can be caused by a number of conditions. Change in the quality of the voice ranges from mild hoarseness to aphonia. It is extremely important to exclude laryngeal carcinoma, which is easily treated in the early stages but has a poor prognosis once metastatic spread has occurred.

CAUSES

INFECTIVE

- Laryngitis

TRAUMATIC

- Blunt trauma
- Excessive vocal use

NEOPLASTIC

- Laryngeal papilloma
- Laryngeal carcinoma

RECURRENT LARYNGEAL NERVE PALSY

- Goitre
- Bronchial carcinoma
- Post-operative – thoracic, parathyroid and thyroid surgery
- Oesophageal carcinoma
- Thoracic aortic aneurysm

AUTOIMMUNE DISEASE

- Myasthenia gravis

OTHER

- Psychogenic

HISTORY

Onset

The temporal profile of deterioration in quality of the voice is useful in discriminating between the causes. Infection and excessive vocal use may result in transient deterioration. Progressive deterioration may be due to tumours, and sustained hoarseness due to recurrent laryngeal nerve palsy.

Precipitating factors

Viral infections usually precede and cause acute laryngitis. It is most commonly due to the influenza virus. Smoking and vocal cord trauma from excessive use by singers, or simply excessive shouting, are often enough to precipitate hoarseness. A history of blunt trauma to the larynx may be evident and hoarseness from resulting laryngeal fractures may be the first indication of a precarious airway.

Past medical history

Recurrent laryngeal nerve palsy associated with a goitre is usually due to thyroid malignancy. Tumour infiltration of the recurrent nerve may also result from malignancy occurring in oesophagus and lung. Hoarseness of the voice may be the first complaint of patients with a thoracic aneurysm. Previous thyroid or thoracic surgery may have resulted in vagus or recurrent laryngeal nerve injuries.

Associated symptoms

Sore throat from pharyngitis may accompany acute laryngitis. Pain referred to the ear or dysphagia can be late presenting features of laryngeal carcinomas. Rapidly progressive dysphagia is also a symptom of oesophageal carcinoma. Nasal voice may be accompanied by ptosis, diplopia and muscle fatigue with myasthenia gravis. Bizarre associated symptoms with impaired voice intensity but normal coughing ability should lead to the consideration of a functional cause; however, this should be a diagnosis of exclusion.

EXAMINATION

Indirect laryngoscopy is performed with a mirror and headlamp. If unsuccessful, the larynx can easily be examined with a flexible fibreoptic laryngoscope under local anaesthetic. A dry erythematous larynx is seen with acute laryngitis. Vocal cord papillomas and supraglottic carcinomas may be readily visible. Recurrent laryngeal nerve injury will result in paralysis of the unilateral vocal cord. Upon observing this, a detailed examination is undertaken to determine the underlying cause. The neck should be examined for the presence of a goitre. Palpable supraclavicular lymphadenopathy may arise from oesophageal carcinoma. The chest is carefully examined for signs of collapse and effusion, which may be secondary to bronchial carcinoma.

GENERAL INVESTIGATIONS

■ FBC
   ↑ White count with laryngitis.
■ ESR
   ↑ With laryngitis, carcinoma.
■ CXR
   Bronchial carcinoma, widened mediastinum with thoracic aneurysm.

SPECIFIC INVESTIGATIONS

- **Tensilon test**
  Myasthenia gravis.
- **Endoscopy**
  Oesophageal carcinoma.
- **CT neck**
  Diagnosis and staging for laryngeal and thyroid carcinoma.
- **CT thorax**
  Lung tumours, thoracic aneurysms.
- **Arch aortography**
  Thoracic aneurysm.
- **FNAC**
  Thyroid carcinoma.

- **Abnormality of the voice in association with dysphagia, especially in a smoker, is of grave concern and urgent assessment for carcinoma is necessary.**

VOMITING

Vomiting is the forceful ejection of gastric contents through the mouth. It occurs when the vomiting centre in the medulla oblongata is stimulated. This may be due to direct stimulation of the centre (central vomiting) or via afferent fibres (reflex vomiting). Haematemesis (vomiting blood) is dealt with in a separate chapter.

CAUSES

CENTRAL VOMITING

- Drugs, e.g. narcotic analgesics, chemotherapeutic agents
- Acute infections, especially in children
- Endocrine/metabolic
  - Pregnancy
  - Uraemia
  - Diabetic ketoacidosis
  - Hypercalcaemia
  - Addison's disease

REFLEX VOMITING

GASTROINTESTINAL DISEASE

Inflammation/irritation
- Appendicitis
- Cholecystitis
- Pancreatitis
- Peptic ulceration/acute gastritis
- Peritonitis
- Biliary colic
- Ureteric colic
- Gastroenteritis
  - Viral
  - Bacteria, e.g. *Campylobacter*, *Salmonella* spp
- Drugs, e.g. aspirin, NSAIDs, alcohol, iron, antibiotics
- Emetics, e.g. sodium chloride, ipecacuanha
- Poisons, e.g. arsenic

Obstruction
- Small bowel obstruction
- Pyloric stenosis
- Large bowel obstruction

CNS CAUSES

- Raised intracranial pressure
- Labyrinthine disorders
- Head injury
- Migraine
- Motion sickness
- Ménière's disease

PSYCHOGENIC

- Offensive sights and smells
- Psychiatric disorders, e.g. hysterical, bulimia nervosa, anorexia nervosa

OTHERS

- Myocardial infarction
- Severe pain, e.g. testicular torsion, fractures
- Irradiation
- Widespread malignant disease
- Severe coughing, e.g. chronic bronchitis

HISTORY

General

Nature of the vomiting

Bright-red blood, e.g. bleeding peptic ulcer. Altered blood (coffee grounds). Bile (high small bowel obstruction), faeculent (low small or large bowel obstruction). Recently eaten food. Food several days old (pyloric stenosis), projectile vomiting (infantile pyloric stenosis).

Time of vomit

Soon after meal (gastric ulcer, gastric carcinoma). Early morning (pregnancy). Chronic chest infection (after bout of coughing).

Relief of pain by vomiting

Peptic ulcer disease.

Central vomiting

Take a careful drug history. It will be obvious if the patient is having chemotherapy. Acute infections in children will usually be obvious. Check for pregnancy. Endocrine and metabolic disorders will largely be determined by the result of blood tests.

Reflex vomiting

Gastrointestinal

There will usually be a clear history of a gastrointestinal problem, e.g. localised tenderness of peritonitis or colicky abdominal pain associated with obstruction. Take a careful drug history for irritant drugs, e.g. aspirin. Check for abuse of emetics, e.g. bulimia.

CNS

With raised intracranial pressure there will usually be headache, drowsiness and fits in addition to vomiting. With labyrinthitis there will be nausea, vomiting, vertigo and often a hearing defect. Ménière's disease presents with vertigo, tinnitus and deafness. The tinnitus is usually constant but more severe before an attack. Tinnitus may precede other symptoms by many months. Attacks of Ménière's disease may last from minutes to hours. Migraine will present with a visual aura with unilateral throbbing headache and sometimes photophobia. With motion sickness the history is usually obvious.

Psychogenic

Bulimia is eating followed by self-induced vomiting. Vomiting may also occur in anorexia nervosa but failure to eat is usually the prominent feature. Hysteria may be responsible for vomiting. Full psychiatric assessment is recommended.

Others

For other causes, the history will usually be obvious. There will usually be severe chest pain in myocardial infarction, and severe pain associated with testicular torsion or trauma. A history of a fracture will be obvious. There may be a history of severe chest infection, e.g. bronchitis or bronchiectasis, associated with coughing bouts followed by vomiting. There may be a recent history of radiotherapy for malignant disease. Widespread malignant disease may cause vomiting.

EXAMINATION

Gastrointestinal

A full gastrointestinal examination should be carried out. Look for signs of localised tenderness or signs of intestinal obstruction.

CNS

With raised intracranial pressure there will be listlessness, irritability, drowsiness, and the pulse rate will be low with a rising blood pressure. Check for papilloedema. Ultimately coma and irregular breathing will occur. With acute labyrinthitis there may be nystagmus to the opposite side from the lesion. The fistula test will be positive (pressure on the tragus causes vertigo or eye deviation by reducing movement of the perilymph). Sensorineural deafness may occur in purulent labyrinthitis. With Ménière's there will be rotatory nystagmus and unsteadiness of stance and gait during an attack, together with past-pointing.

Psychogenic

In anorexia nervosa, a wasted hirsute female will present, often with anxious parents.

Others

With myocardial infarction there may be signs of acute congestive cardiac failure. With causes of severe pain, attention will normally be drawn to the appropriate area, e.g. scrotum with testicular trauma or torsion. With irradiation there may be skin signs of recent radiotherapy. With widespread malignant disease the patient is often cachectic. A site of the primary may be obvious. With severe coughing, chest signs may be obvious.

GENERAL INVESTIGATIONS

■ FBC, ESR, CRP
   Hb ↓ gastrointestinal disease. Malignancy. Anorexia nervosa.
   WCC ↑ abdominal inflammation. ESR ↑ inflammation. Tumour.

■ U&Es
   Dehydration. Uraemia. Hyperkalaemia occurs in Addison's disease.

■ LFTs
   Biliary tract disease.

■ Serum amylase
   Pancreatitis.

■ Urinalysis
   Glucose and ketones in diabetes; blood, white cells and protein suggest UTI, blood may indicate kidney stone.

■ CXR
   Congestive cardiac failure – pulmonary oedema. Malignancy. Pneumonia. Bronchiectasis.

■ ECG
   Myocardial infarction.

■ AXR
   Obstruction.

SPECIFIC INVESTIGATIONS

■ Blood glucose
   Raised in diabetes. Low in Addison's disease.

■ Serum calcium
   Hyperparathyroidism and other causes of hypercalcaemia.

■ ABGs
   Diabetic ketoacidosis.

- **βHCG**
  Pregnancy.

- **Toxicology screen**
  Drug causes of vomiting.

- **Barium enema**
  Malignancy. Diverticular disease.

- **Small bowel enema**
  Gastrointestinal disease, e.g. Crohn's disease.

- **OGD**
  Peptic ulcer disease. Malignancy.

- **US**
  Gastrointestinal disease, e.g. gallstones.

- **CT**
  Abdominal malignancy. Cerebral haemorrhage.

- **MRI**
  Intracranial lesion associated with raised intracranial pressure.

- **Caloric tests**
  Labyrinthitis, Ménière's disease.

- **Audiometry**
  Ménière's disease, labyrinthitis.

- **Although vomiting is a frequent symptom with most cases being self-limiting, it may be a clue to serious pathology. Further investigation is required urgently if there are any associated systemic signs, e.g. neurological, abdominal.**

- **Diabetics need careful monitoring as vomiting may lead to poor sugar control.**

WEIGHT GAIN

Weight gain is extremely common and the most frequent cause is simple obesity. Excessive weight gain itself has deleterious effects on general health. With the exception of simple obesity and pregnancy other conditions account for less than 1% of patients presenting with weight gain.

CAUSES

INCREASED FAT

- Simple obesity
- Hypothyroidism
- Cushing's syndrome
- Polycystic ovarian syndrome
- Hypothalamic disease

INCREASED FLUID

- Cardiac failure
- Hepatic failure with ascites
- Renal failure – nephrotic syndrome
- Lymphatic obstruction

INCREASED MUSCLE

- Athletes, e.g. weightlifters
- Androgenic steroids
- Growth hormone

OTHER

- Pregnancy

HISTORY

General

Enquire about the possibility of pregnancy and any changes in dietary habits that may result in simple weight gain. Rapid weight gain is often secondary to increased fluid as opposed to an increase in dry weight. A drug history is taken to exclude the use of anabolic steroids and growth hormone, especially in body builders. Enquire about a family history, diet and amount of activity in relation to simple obesity.

Cushing's syndrome

Patients with Cushing's syndrome present with hair growth, acne, abdominal striae, muscle weakness, back pain, amenorrhoea, thin

SECTION A

skin, bruising and depression. A drug history should be taken to exclude exogenous corticosteroids as the cause.

Hypothyroidism

With hypothyroidism, patients may complain of lethargy, anorexia, cold intolerance, goitre, dry hair, dry skin, constipation and menorrhagia.

Polycystic ovarian syndrome

Women with this condition present with hirsutism, obesity and menstrual irregularities. It is also associated with insulin resistance.

Hypothalamic disease

Prior history of neurosurgery, craniopharyngioma or other brain tumours may have resulted in damage to the hypothalamus. As it is the regulatory centre for appetite, uncontrolled excessive eating may result.

Cardiac failure

Fluid retention from cardiac failure may be accompanied by symptoms of exertional dyspnoea, orthopnoea, paroxysmal nocturnal dyspnoea. Ascites and peripheral oedema may also result from congestive heart failure.

Renal failure

Patients with renal failure may present with lethargy, fragile pigmented skin, peripheral oedema, periorbital oedema, thirst and polyuria.

ASCITES

See p. 33.

EXAMINATION

Inspection

The distribution of body fat should be noted. Patients with Cushing's syndrome have truncal obesity with proximal muscle wasting. Hirsutism is a feature of both polycystic ovarian syndrome and Cushing's syndrome. With hypothyroidism there may be loss of the outer third of the eyebrows and a 'peaches and cream' complexion.

Inspection of the trunk may reveal thin skin with easy bruising in both Cushing's syndrome and renal failure. In addition, striae and thoracic kyphosis may be present with Cushing's from wedge fractures caused by osteoporosis.

Proximal muscle weakness is found in both Cushing's syndrome and hypothyroidism. Check for the physique of a 'body builder'.

Palpation and auscultation

Peripheral oedema may be a feature of fluid overload with renal, hepatic and cardiac failure. Non-pitting oedema is characteristically found with hypothyroidism. The JVP should be examined and will be elevated with congestive cardiac failure and fluid overload with renal or hepatic failure. The pulse is taken and bradycardia may be noted with hypothyroidism. The blood pressure is measured and hypertension may be due to incorrect cuff size or may occur as a complication of Cushing's disease. A third heart sound may be present with cardiac failure, and widespread pulmonary crepitation suggests pulmonary oedema from cardiac failure or fluid overload in renal or hepatic failure.

Further examination of the abdominal system may reveal the presence of ascites (p. 33), which may result from liver disease, malignancy or cardiac failure. A complete neurological examination is performed to screen for neurological deficits, which will warrant diagnostic imaging to look for lesions involving the hypothalamus. If there is any suspicion that a patient is taking body-building drugs, e.g. anabolic steroids, check for testicular atrophy and prostatic hypertrophy.

GENERAL INVESTIGATIONS

- **Urine dipstick**
  +++ glucose – diabetes from Cushing's syndrome or as a complication of obesity. +++ protein is present with nephrotic syndrome. Blood may be present with renal disease.
- **U&Es**
  K^+ ↓ Cushing's. Urea and creatinine ↑ renal failure.
- **LFTs**
  Deranged with liver disease
- **TFTs**
  Screen for hypothyroidism.
- **Random cortisol**
  ↑ evening levels may suggest Cushing's syndrome; a normal result does not exclude it. Although commonly performed, has little diagnostic value.

SPECIFIC INVESTIGATIONS

- **24-hour urinary free cortisol**
  ↑ with Cushing's.
- **24-hour urine collection for protein**
  >3.5 g with nephrotic syndrome.
- **Low-dose dexamethasone test**
  Failure of cortisol suppression with Cushing's.

- **US abdomen and pelvis**
  Renal disorders, polycystic ovaries, ascites.
- **Echocardiography**
  Cardiac failure.
- **CT/MRI head**
  Hypothalamic disease.
- **Renal biopsy**
  To determine the aetiology of renal parenchymal disease.

- **Every opportunity should be taken to modify compliance in order to reduce weight to an appropriate level. Advice regarding diet and exercise is a crucial first step.**

WEIGHT LOSS

Unintentional weight loss is often a manifestation of significant underlying disease and should never be ignored.

CAUSES

SYSTEMIC DISEASE

- Malignancy
- Cardiac failure
- Chronic respiratory disease
- Renal failure
- Liver failure
- Malabsorption
- Connective tissue disease (e.g., SLE, rheumatoid arthritis)

ENDOCRINE

- Diabetes mellitus
- Hyperthyroidism
- Addison's disease

INFECTIVE

- TB
  - (very common in the developing world and on the increase in the developed world)
- HIV
  - (very common in the developing world)
- Helminth (worms) infection
  - (very common in endemic areas)

PSYCHIATRIC

- Depression
- Anorexia nervosa

OTHER

- Any terminal illness
- Substance abuse (e.g. laxatives, amphetamines, opiates)
- Poor nutrition
  - (common in developing countries)

HISTORY

General

The timeframe and amount of weight loss should be noted. A dietary history is required to determine the amount and type of food ingested. Decreased dietary intake may result from loss of appetite or loss of interest in eating due to depression. On the other hand, patients with thyrotoxicosis lose weight despite a voracious appetite.

Enquiries should be undertaken regarding perception of body image, as patients with anorexia nervosa believe that they are overweight despite being severely underweight. Risk factors for HIV should be screened for and a sexual history as well as information regarding intravenous drug use should be obtained. Systemic enquiry is required to identify features suggestive of malignancy or organ failure in each system to account for unintentional weight loss. A butterfly rash may be present in cases of SLE.

Cardiorespiratory system

Dyspnoea, orthopnoea, paroxysmal nocturnal dyspnoea, peripheral oedema are symptoms suggestive of congestive cardiac failure. With long-standing cardiac failure, cardiac cachexia results from loss of total body fat and lean body mass. Currently the most common aetiology is end-stage heart failure. Dyspnoea without accompanying orthopnoea or paroxysmal nocturnal dyspnoea suggests respiratory disease. With any chronic respiratory disorder, basal metabolic rate is increased as a result of the increased work of breathing. The presence of haemoptysis may be due to malignancy or TB. A long smoking history is a strong predisposing factor for the development of bronchial carcinoma and COPD. Night sweats and weight loss may be accompanying features of both TB and Hodgkin's disease.

Gastrointestinal system

Lethargy, diarrhoea, steatorrhoea (p. 416) and abdominal discomfort are various symptoms suggestive of malabsorption. Jaundice, dark urine, pale stools, itching, prolonged bleeding, abdominal swelling from ascites and confusion are symptoms associated with liver disease. Vague abdominal pains, change in bowel habit, tenesmus, blood or mucus mixed with the stools may be due to gastrointestinal malignancy. Patients with helminth infections, such as ascaris, may complain of perianal itching and notice worms in their faeces. Although this is rare in the UK, it may be encountered in patients returning from foreign travel.

Renal system

Lethargy, anorexia, nocturia, oliguria, polyuria, haematuria, frothy urine from proteinuria, skin fragility, pruritus, oedema and bone pains are some of the multisystemic features suggestive of renal disease.

Haematological system

Localised non-tender lymphadenopathy from Hodgkin's disease may be accompanied by pyrexia and pruritus. Persistent generalised lymphadenopathy, however, is a recognised presenting feature of HIV.

Endocrine system

Polydipsia and polyuria with weight loss may be presenting features of diabetics. Patients with thyrotoxicosis may complain of tremor, staring eyes, heat intolerance, palpitations and diarrhoea. With Addison's disease, anorexia, malaise, nausea, vomiting, diarrhoea or syncope from postural hypotension may be experienced.

Connective tissue diseases

Arthritis is a very common presentation of connective tissue disease including rheumatoid arthritis and SLE. Patients may also complain of early morning joint stiffness, lethargy and poor mobility.

EXAMINATION

The causes of weight loss are varied. The following specific features identified on examination may be useful in determining an underlying cause.

Inspection

Signs suggestive of endocrine disorder may be obvious; a goitre may be visible with thyrotoxicosis, accompanied by exophthalmos and tremor. Pigmentation of the skin creases and buccal mucosa in a cachectic patient with postural hypotension are the usual findings with Addison's disease. Jaundice, caput medusae, spider naevi and gynaecomastia may be seen with liver disease. Tachypnoea and pursed-lip breathing may be evident with COPD. Clubbing may be a feature of bronchial carcinoma, suppurative lung disease, cirrhosis and inflammatory bowel disease. The JVP is elevated with congestive cardiac failure. Swelling and deformity of the small joints of the hand may be seen with connective tissue disease. In addition, a rash will frequently be present with SLE.

Palpation and auscultation

Peripheral oedema may be present with cardiac failure, malabsorption, renal and liver disease. Auscultation of the chest may reveal widespread crepitations with pulmonary oedema from cardiac failure, or uniformly decreased breath sounds with COPD. Palpation of the abdomen may reveal hepatomegaly and ascites with liver disease; ascites may also occur with cardiac failure and gastrointestinal malignancies. Lying and standing blood pressure should be measured, as a postural drop is present with Addison's disease. Joint tenderness is present with connective tissue disease.

GENERAL INVESTIGATIONS

- **Urine dipstick**
  Glucose with diabetes. Protein and blood with renal disorders.

- **FBC**
  Hb ↓ chronic disease, malabsorption, renal and liver failure and connective tissue disease

- **ESR and CRP**
  ↑ with malignancy and connective tissue disease.

- **U&Es**
  Urea and creatinine ↑ renal failure. Na^+ ↓, K^+ ↑ and HCO_3^- ↓ in Addison's disease.

- **Blood glucose**
  More than 11.1 mmol/L on two separate occasions indicates diabetes mellitus.

- **LFTs**
  Bilirubin ↑, transaminases ↑ and albumin ↓ liver failure.

- **Clotting screen**
  PT ↑ liver failure.

- **TSH and free T$_4$**
  TSH ↓ and T$_4$ ↑ thyrotoxicosis.

- **CXR**
  Malignancy, TB.

SPECIFIC INVESTIGATIONS

- **ANA, RF**
  ANA raised in SLE and RF increased in rheumatoid arthritis

- **Faecal fat estimation**
  ↑ with fat malabsorption.

- **Faecal occult blood**
  Colorectal carcinoma

- **AXR**
  Pancreatic calcification with chronic pancreatitis.

- **Joint X-rays**
  Deformity and erosions with rheumatoid arthritis

- **Colonoscopy**
  Colorectal carcinoma, inflammatory bowel disease.

- **Gastroscopy**
  Gastric carcinoma.

- **US abdomen**
  Malignancy, small kidneys with renal failure.

- **Short synacthen test**
  Failure of plasma cortisol to increase with Addison's disease.

- **Echocardiography**
  Ventricular impairment with cardiac failure.
- **Stool cultures**
  Microscopy for helminths and their ova. Helminths may occasionally be visible with the naked eye.
- **HIV antibodies**
  For the diagnosis of HIV.

- Dramatic weight loss over a short period of time raises the possibility of malignancy. Urgent investigation is mandatory.

SECTION B

BIOCHEMICAL PRESENTATIONS

BLOOD UREA NITROGEN

BUN is a useful test of renal function. However, other factors such as liver failure, dehydration and protein breakdown may alter levels of BUN. The normal level of urea is 2.5–6.6 mmol/L. However, values may be lower in pregnancy and the newborn, and in the elderly values may be slightly increased due to lack of renal concentration.

CAUSES

INCREASED BUN

- Renal failure (acute and chronic)
- Dehydration
- Shock
- Congestive cardiac failure
- Gastrointestinal haemorrhage (digested blood increases blood urea)
- Excessive protein intake
- Excessive protein catabolism

DECREASED BUN

- Malnutrition
- Liver failure
- Overhydration, e.g. prolonged i.v. fluids
- Pregnancy (increased plasma volume)
- Impaired protein absorption
- SIADH
- Anabolic steroid use

SYMPTOMS AND SIGNS

Signs of uraemia, e.g. oliguria, anuria, fatigue, confusion, thirst, bronze colour of skin, oedema (peripheral and pulmonary), uraemic frost (rare).

Signs of dehydration, e.g. dry skin, loss of skin turgor.

Signs of congestive cardiac failure, e.g. oedema, JVP ↑. GI haemorrhage, e.g. tachycardia, hypotension, haematemesis and melaena. Decreased intake, e.g. oedema, ascites.

Signs of liver failure. SIADH, e.g. head injury, small cell lung cancer.

INVESTIGATIONS

- **UEs**
  Urea ↑. Na ↓ in SIADH (<130 mEq/L).

- **Creatinine**
  Cr ↑. Disparity between creatinine and urea (urea ↑ creatinine normal) in gastrointestinal haemorrhage.

- **FBC**
  Anaemia. PCV ↑ in dehydration. PCV ↓ in overhydration.

- **LFTs**
  Liver failure. Hypoalbuminaemia.

- **MSU**
  Red cells, casts and protein in intrinsic renal disease.

- **CXR**
  Pulmonary oedema. Cardiomegaly

- **Urine electrolytes**
  See Table on p. 347 in Oliguria.

- **Urine osmolality**
  Acute renal failure versus physiological oliguria. See Table on p. 347 in Oliguria.

- **US**
  Urinary tract obstruction.

- **MAG 3 scan**
  Renal function. Renal infarction (absent outline of kidney).

- A grossly raised BUN in association with metabolic acidosis, hyperkalaemia, fluid overload and clinical symptoms, e.g. coma, pericarditis, is an indication for urgent haemodialysis.

HYPERCALCAEMIA

Hypercalcaemia is a serum calcium above 2.62 mmol/L (normal range 2.12–2.62 mmol/L). It may be an asymptomatic laboratory finding. Symptoms usually become apparent with levels >3.50 mmol/L.

CAUSES

- Malignancy
  - Solid tumour with lytic bony metastases, e.g. Ca breast, bronchus
  - Solid tumours with humoral mediation, e.g. inappropriate PTH secretion with carcinoma of the bronchus, carcinoma of the kidney
  - Multiple myeloma
- Hyperparathyroidism (primary, secondary, tertiary)
- Sarcoidosis
- Drugs, e.g. thiazide diuretics, lithium
- Excess intake of vitamin A, vitamin D or calcium
- Prolonged immobilisation
- Milk-alkali syndrome (excess calcium intake)
- Hyperthyroidism
- Addison's disease
- Paget's disease of bone
- Familial hypocalciuric hypercalcaemia

SYMPTOMS AND SIGNS

These depend on the patient's age, duration and rate of increase of plasma calcium and the presence of concurrent medical conditions. Symptoms and signs include nausea and vomiting, fatigue, depression, confusion, psychosis; abdominal pain, constipation, acute pancreatitis, peptic ulceration, polyuria/nocturia, haematuria, renal colic, renal failure, bone pain, hypertension and arrhythmias. Classical symptoms of hypercalcaemia in association with hyperparathyroidism include 'stones, bones, abdominal groans and psychiatric overtones'.

INVESTIGATIONS

- **Fasting calcium and phosphate**
  Ca ↑ PO$_4$ ↓.
- **U&Es**
  ↑ creatinine ↑ urea. Renal failure.

- **PTH levels**
  ↑ hyperparathyroidism.
- **Protein electrophoresis and Bence Jones protein**
  Multiple myeloma.
- **ECG**
  Short QT interval. Widened T waves.
- **Serum amylase**
  ↑ in acute pancreatitis associated with hyperparathyroidism.
- **AXR**
  Stones. Nephrocalcinosis.
- **US**
  Renal stones. Carcinoma of the kidney (inappropriate PTH secretion). Parathyroid lesions.
- **Skull X-ray**
  Myeloma. Abnormal sella turcica in MEN associated pituitary tumour. Paget's disease of bone.
- **Sestamibi scan**
  Hyperparathyroidism.
- **24-hour urinary calcium excretion**
  ↑ calcium excretion in hyperparathyroidism (calcium-restricted diets).

- In a patient with depression or psychosis, always check the serum calcium. Hyperparathyroidism may be a cause.
- In a patient presenting with polyuria, if diabetes has been excluded, check the serum calcium.

HYPERGLYCAEMIA

Hyperglycaemia is defined as a plasma glucose >7.0 mmol/L. By far the most common cause is diabetes mellitus.

CAUSES

ENDOCRINE
- Diabetes mellitus (types 1 and 2)

DRUGS
- Corticosteroids
- Beta blockers
- Thiazide diuretics
- Niacin
- Pentamidine
- Protease inhibitors
- L-asparaginase
- Antipsychotic agents

SYSTEMIC DISEASE
- Cushing's syndrome

SEVERE STRESS
- Stroke
- Myocardial infarction

PSYCHOGENIC
- Bulimia nervosa

PHYSIOLOGICAL
- Infection
- Inflammation

OTHER
- Pregnancy

SYMPTOMS AND SIGNS

The most common symptoms include polydipsia, polyuria, polyphagia, fatigue, weight loss and blurred vision. Acute hyperglycaemia may present as hyperventilation, stupor or coma as part of a diabetic ketoacidotic crisis. Recurrent infections are common, especially of the skin.

The patient may have a history of diabetes or the symptoms may be the first presentation of the disease. Type 1 diabetes usually occurs in younger age groups whereas type 2 generally affects older individuals, with obesity being a common accompanying condition.

A thorough drug history is important. Steroids are used for a large number of conditions and therefore the dose and duration of treatment should be evaluated. The patient may complain of features of Cushing's syndrome such as excessive appetite, weight gain and weakness.

Enquire about recent severe illness such as heart attack or stroke. Hyperglycaemia may develop during the binge phase of bulimia when a large caloric load is ingested. Ask about episodes of binge eating, vomiting, significant shifts in weight over time and possible abuse of emetics. The history of bulimia may be obtained from relatives. Enquire about current or recent pregnancy.

Examination may reveal complications of diabetes such as vascular disease, retinopathy, neuropathy and Charcot joints may be present. Skin infection is common in diabetes, especially boils and abscesses. Obesity is frequent in type 2 diabetics. Look for the features of Cushing's syndrome including central obesity, moon face, hirsutism, cataracts, weakness, striae and hypertension. Complications of myocardial infarction may be present such as heart failure. Neurological examination will reveal upper motor neurone signs following stroke.

Examination findings in bulimia include tooth decay, oral trauma, dehydration and swollen salivary glands. The latter stages of pregnancy should be self evident.

INVESTIGATIONS

- **BM stix**
  ↑ glucose.

- **Blood glucose**
  ↑ glucose.

- **Urinalysis**
  ↑ glucose and ketones in diabetic ketoacidosis.

- **Oral glucose tolerance test**
  ↑ glucose in diabetes.

- **U&Es**
  ↑ urea and creatinine with diabetic nephropathy.

- **FBC**
  ↑ WCC in infection and inflammation.

- **βHCG**
  Pregnancy.

- **HbA1c**
  ↑ diabetes.

- **ABGs**
  Diabetic ketoacidosis.

- Diabetic ketoacidosis is an emergency which is identified by clinical features and a significantly raised blood sugar level with glucose and ketones in the urine. This may be the first presentation of diabetes or may occur in a known diabetic.

- Causes for diabetic ketoacidosis, e.g. intercurrent infection or poor glucose control, should be further explored.

HYPERKALAEMIA

Hyperkalaemia is an elevated blood level of potassium above 5.0 mmol/L. Hyperkalaemia is a medical emergency due to the risk of potentially fatal arrhythmias.

CAUSES

- Excess administration of potassium, especially rapidly
- Renal failure
- Haemolysis
- Massive blood transfusion
- Crush injuries (rhabdomyolysis)
- Tissue necrosis, e.g. burns, ischaemia
- Metabolic acidosis
- Adrenal insufficiency (Addison's disease)
- Drugs interfering with urinary excretion: ACE inhibitors and angiotensin receptor blockers, potassium-sparing diuretics (spironolactone and amiloride), NSAIDs (ibuprofen, naproxen), calcineurin inhibitors for immunosuppression (ciclosporin and tacrolimus), trimethoprim, pentamidine

SYMPTOMS AND SIGNS

Cardiac arrest. Mild breathlessness (hyperkalaemia associated with metabolic acidosis). Paraesthesiae, areflexia. Weakness. Palpitations. Abdominal pain. Hypoglycaemia. Hyperpigmentation associated with Addison's disease.

INVESTIGATIONS

- **U&Es**
  K^+ >5 mmol/L (patients with chronic renal failure will tolerate higher K^+ levels) – exclude haemolysis. Chronic renal failure.

- **FBC**
  Exclude haemolysis.

- **Blood gases**
  Metabolic acidosis.

- **Blood glucose**
  Diabetic ketoacidosis.

- **ECG**
  Tall T waves, flat P waves, prolonged PR interval, wide QRS.

■ Creatine kinase
↑ in crush injuries.

■ Plasma cortisol
↓ adrenal insufficiency (Addison's disease).

• **Hyperkalaemia is a medical emergency. The first sign of hyperkalaemia may be cardiac arrest due to an arrhythmia.**

HYPOKALAEMIA

Hypokalaemia is a reduced blood level of potassium below 3.5 mmol/L.

CAUSES

INADEQUATE INTAKE

- Potassium-free i.v. fluids
- Reduced oral intake, e.g. coma, dysphagia

EXCESSIVE LOSS

- Renal
  - Diuretics
  - Renal tubular disorders
- Gastrointestinal
  - Diarrhoea
  - Vomiting
  - Fistulas
  - Laxatives
  - Villous adenoma
- Endocrine
  - Cushing's syndrome
  - Steroid therapy
  - Hyperaldosteronism

SYMPTOMS AND SIGNS

Muscle weakness. Myalgia. Constipation. Paralytic ileus. Cardiac arrhythmia (ranging from ectopics to serious arrhythmias with sudden death at very low levels of potassium).

INVESTIGATIONS

- **U&Es**
  Serum K^+ <3.5 mmol/L.

- **Blood bases**
  Metabolic alkalosis – pH ↑ HCO_3^- ↑. Blood glucose. Diabetic ketoacidosis.

- **ECG**
  Flattened T waves. ST depression. U waves. Prolonged QT intervals.

- **Serum Mg**
  Mg ↓ (magnesium is required for adequate processing of K^+).

- **Plasma aldosterone**
  Raised in Conn's syndrome.
- **Plasma renin**
  Low in Conn's syndrome.
- **Plasma cortisol**
  Diurnal variation lost in Cushing's syndrome.
- **Plasma aldosterone**
  Raised in Conn's syndrome.
- **Urinary free cortisol**
  Elevated in Cushing's syndrome.
- **ACTH levels**
  High in pituitary-dependent cases, low or undetectable with adrenal tumour; may be very high with ectopic ACTH secretion.

- In a patient with prolonged ileus post-operatively, always remember to check serum potassium.
- In a patient presenting with unexplained lethargy, fatigue and muscle weakness, check the serum potassium. Conn's syndrome is a possible diagnosis.

HYPERNATRAEMIA

The normal serum sodium level is 135–145 mmol/L.
Hypernatraemia refers to a serum sodium level >145 mmol/L.

CAUSES

DECREASED WATER INTAKE

- Confusion
- Coma

NON-RENAL WATER LOSSES

- Gastrointestinal losses (e.g. vomiting, diarrhoea)
- Pyrexia
- Burns

RENAL WATER LOSSES

- Osmotic diuresis
  - Hyperglycaemia
- Nephrogenic diabetes insipidus
  - Drugs (e.g. lithium)
  - Bence Jones proteins
  - Post-relief of obstructive uropathy
  - Recovering acute tubular necrosis
- Congenital diabetes insipidus

SODIUM EXCESS

- Excessive intravenous sodium therapy
- Chronic congestive cardiac failure
- Cirrhosis of the liver
- Steroid therapy
- Cushing's syndrome
- Primary hyperaldosteronism (Conn's syndrome)

SYMPTOMS AND SIGNS

Thirst usually occurs when the plasma sodium rises by 3–4 mmol/L
above the upper limit of normal. Severe symptoms such as coma,
seizures, muscular tremor and rigidity arise when the level is above
158 mmol/L.

INVESTIGATIONS

- **U&Es**
  Na⁺ 150–170 mEq/L usually indicates dehydration. Na⁺ >170 mEq/L usually indicates diabetes insipidus. Na⁺ >190 mEq/L usually indicates long-term salt ingestion.

- **Urine osmolality**
  Central versus nephrogenic diabetes insipidus.

- **CT head**
  Central diabetes insipidus, e.g. cerebral tumour/trauma.

- Rapid correction of hypernatraemia can lead to cerebral oedema.

- Lack of thirst is associated with central nervous system disease.

HYPONATRAEMIA

The normal serum sodium level is 135–145 mmol/L. Hyponatraemia refers to serum sodium levels of less than 135 mmol/L, and serum sodium of less than 120 mmol/L is considered severe.

CAUSES

HYPOVOLAEMIC

- Gastrointestinal losses
  - Diarrhoea
  - Vomiting
  - Fistula
  - Small bowel obstruction
  - Paralytic ileus
- Renal sodium losses
  - Diuretics
  - Osmotic diuresis (e.g. hyperglycaemia)
  - Renal failure
- Other sodium losses
  - Burns
  - Ascites
  - Crush injuries
  - Peritonitis

EUVOLAEMIC

- Endocrine
  - Severe hypothyroidism
  - Addison's disease
- Water load
  - Intravenous infusions
  - Water drinking
  - TURP (transurethral resection of prostate) syndrome
- SIADH
  - Pulmonary disease (e.g. pneumonia, lung cancer)
  - Drugs (e.g. carbamazepine)
  - Intracranial disease (e.g. tumour, head injuries)

OEDEMATOUS

- Cardiac failure
- Nephrotic syndrome

SYMPTOMS AND SIGNS

Symptoms of hyponatraemia are related to how low the serum sodium is, and how rapidly it has developed. They can range from asymptomatic to mild nausea, vomiting, headache, malaise to diminished reflexes, seizures, stupor or coma.

INVESTIGATIONS

- **U&Es**
  $\downarrow Na^+$. $\uparrow$ urea and creatinine (renal failure). $\uparrow K^+$ (Addison's disease).

- **Paired serum and urine osmolality**
  SIADH is suggested by inappropriately concentrated urine (>100 mOsm/kg) with serum hypo-osmolality (<270 mOsm/kg).

- **Paired serum and urinary sodium**
  SIADH is suggested with inappropriately concentrated urinary sodium (>20 mmol/L).

- Falsely low sodium values can occur with high circulating levels of lipids, proteins and in severe hyperglycaemia.

- Most patients with hyponatraemia do not require treatment with intravenous sodium chloride, but, if this is required, the rate of correction of serum sodium levels must be carried out with great care to minimise the risk of central pontine demyelination.

HYPOGLYCAEMIA

Hypoglycaemia is defined as a plasma glucose <2.5 mmol/L. The actual glucose level at which symptoms develop varies markedly.

CAUSES

DRUGS

- Insulin
- Sulfonylurea
- Alcohol
- Aminoglutethimide
- Quinolones
- Pentamidine
- Quinine

ENDOCRINE

- Pituitary insufficiency
- Addison's disease

NEOPLASTIC

- Pancreatic islet cell tumours; insulinoma
- Non-pancreatic tumours; retroperitoneal fibrosarcoma, haemangiopericytoma

LIVER DISEASE

- Inherited glycogen storage disorders
- Cirrhosis
- Acute liver failure
- Alcohol

OTHER

- Post-prandial dumping syndrome (post-gastrectomy, post-vagotomy and drainage)
- Immune mediated (e.g. anti-insulin receptor antibodies in Hodgkin's disease)

SYMPTOMS AND SIGNS

The most common symptoms include sweatiness, palpitations, weakness, hunger, drowsiness, restlessness, tremor, seizures and coma. Occasionally personality changes may be a presenting symptom. By far the most common cause of hypoglycaemia is an excess of insulin or oral hypoglycaemic agents in a known diabetic.

Enquire about a history of diabetes mellitus and medication. Occasionally relatives of diabetics may be covertly ingesting hypoglycaemic agents. Insulin has been used by athletes to improve stamina. Alcohol excess without food may lead to hypoglycaemia. A full medication history is important.

There may be a history of pituitary dysfunction. Causes of pituitary failure include tumour, trauma, pituitary surgery and infection. The symptoms of Addison's disease include weakness, weight loss, dizziness and pigmentation of the buccal mucosa and palmar creases. Islet cell tumours may produce symptoms of hypoglycaemia intermittently and to varying degrees. Classically, the symptoms develop during fasting. Personality or neurocognitive changes may develop. Diagnosis of insulinoma depends on the classical diagnostic triad, i.e. Whipple's triad: (1) attacks precipitated by fasting; (2) blood sugar is low during the attack; (3) symptoms are relieved by administration of glucose. Check for a history of liver failure. Dumping syndrome may occur following gastric surgery when a high osmotic load is delivered to the jejunum. A history of lymphoma may be present in immune-mediated hypoglycaemia.

Examination may reveal classic signs of hypoglycaemia. Look for complications of diabetes. Look for evidence of chronic liver disease in alcoholics. Pituitary insufficiency may lead to a variety of examination findings depending upon the deficiency and may include hypotension, loss or gain of weight, breast atrophy, hypogonadism, weakness, central obesity or dry skin. Retroperitoneal tumours may lead to renal impairment. Look for features of chronic liver disease. Lymphadenopathy and hepatosplenomegaly may be apparent in Hodgkin's disease.

INVESTIGATIONS

- **BM stix**
  ↓ glucose.

- **Blood glucose**
  Hypoglycaemia.

- **LFTs**
  ↑ bilirubin and transaminases with liver failure.

- **Toxicology screen**
  Alcohol.

- **U&Es**
  ↑ urea and creatinine with renal failure associated with retroperitoneal disease.

- **Insulin and C-peptide levels**
  Normal or ↑ insulin (insulinoma, sulfonylurea treatment). Absent C-peptide with exogenous insulin. ↓ insulin (non-pancreatic neoplasm, insulin receptor antibodies), alcohol, pituitary or adrenal failure.

- **Pituitary hormone levels**
  Reduced in pituitary failure (e.g. GH (growth hormone), TSH, LH, FSH, prolactin).

- **Prolonged oral glucose tolerance test**
  To identify dumping syndrome.

- **i.v. insulin suppression test**
  Insulinoma.

- **Arterial stimulation with venous sampling**
  Insulinoma.

- **CT/MRI**
  Insulinoma.

- **Profound hypoglycaemia is an emergency with potentially serious sequelae. It can be easily and rapidly identified by a BM stix glucose estimation.**

HYPOCALCAEMIA

Hypocalcaemia is a serum calcium of <2.0 mmol/L with an ionised fraction <0.8 mmol/L.

CAUSES

ASSOCIATED WITH HIGH SERUM PHOSPHATE

- Renal failure
- Hypoparathyroidism
- Rhabdomyolysis
- Phosphate therapy

ASSOCIATED WITH LOW OR NORMAL SERUM PHOSPHATE

- Hypomagnesaemia
- Acute pancreatitis
- Critical illness including sepsis, burns
- Osteomalacia
- Overhydration

MASSIVE BLOOD TRANSFUSION DUE TO CITRATE-BINDING

HYPERVENTILATION WITH RESPIRATORY ALKALOSIS AND REDUCTION IN IONISED PLASMA CALCIUM

DRUGS

- Bisphosphonates
- Calcitonin

SYMPTOMS AND SIGNS

Circumoral paraesthesia, peripheral tingling and paraesthesia, cramp, tetany (carpo-pedal spasm), hypotension, hyperactive tendon reflexes, Chvostek's sign (tapping over the facial nerve causes facial spasm), Trousseau's sign (inflating blood pressure cuff to above systolic pressure causes carpal spasm), laryngospasm (life-threatening), cardiac arrhythmias and rarely dystonia and psychosis.

INVESTIGATIONS

- Serum calcium and phosphate
  Ca ↓ PO_4 may be low, normal or high.
- U&Es
  ↑ creatinine ↑ urea. Renal failure.
- ABGs
  pH ↑ (hypocalcaemia associated with respiratory alkalosis).

- **Serum amylase**
  Ca ↓ associated with acute pancreatitis.

- **Serum magnesium**
  ↓ Mg – magnesium deficiency may lead to hypocalcaemia.

- **PTH levels**
  Hypoparathyroidism.

- **Serum Vitamin D**
  vitamin D deficiency.

- **ECG**
  Prolonged QT interval. Prolonged ST interval.

- **The first symptom of hypocalcaemia is circumoral paraesthesia. If this occurs after thyroid or parathyroid surgery, it is an indication for an urgent check of the serum calcium and appropriate treatment.**

HYPOMAGNESAEMIA

The normal range of serum magnesium is 0.7–1.0 mmol/L.
Hypomagnesaemia refers to a serum level below 0.7 mmol/L.

CAUSES

EXCESSIVE LOSSES

- Diuretics
- Severe diarrhoea
- Prolonged vomiting
- Polyuria (poorly controlled diabetes)
- Prolonged and excessive nasogastric aspiration

INADEQUATE INTAKE

- Starvation
- Alcoholism
- Malabsorption syndrome
- Parenteral nutrition

SYMPTOMS AND SIGNS

Symptoms of low magnesium levels are very similar to those of low
calcium with muscle weakness, lethargy, irritability, confusion,
seizures and arrhythmias. In addition, there may be co-existing
symptoms due to hypocalcaemia or hypokalaemia. Severe symptoms
do not usually occur until serum levels drop below 0.5 mmol/L.

INVESTIGATIONS

- **Serum magnesium**
  Serum magnesium level is diagnostic and can indicate level of
  severity.

- **U&Es**
  ↓ K$^+$ (Mg$^+$ and K$^+$ tend to move in and out of cells in the same
  direction).

- **Serum Ca**
  ↓ Ca (present in up to 60% of cases).

- If symptoms related to hypocalcaemia and
  hypokalaemia are resistant to calcium and potassium
  supplements, respectively, remember to check the
  serum magnesium level.

METABOLIC ACIDOSIS

Metabolic acidosis is caused by increased production of hydrogen ions from metabolic causes or from excessive bicarbonate loss (pH ↓, HCO_3^- ↓).
Compensatory mechanisms are:

- ↓ pCO_2 by hyperventilation
- ↓ H^+ by kidneys (unless in renal failure).

CAUSES

EXCESSIVE PRODUCTION OF H^+

- Diabetic ketoacidosis
- Lactic acidosis secondary to hypoxia, e.g. shock, ischaemic gut
- Septicaemia
- Starvation
- Drugs, e.g. ethanol, salicylates

DECREASED H^+ EXCRETION

- Renal failure

EXCESSIVE LOSS OF BASE

- Diarrhoea
- Fistula – pancreatic, intestinal or biliary

EXCESSIVE INTAKE OF ACID

- Parenteral nutrition

SYMPTOMS AND SIGNS

These may be non-specific. Specific symptoms include chest pain, palpitations, headache, nausea, vomiting, abdominal pain, weight loss. Deep rapid breathing (Kussmaul respirations) classically associated with diabetic ketoacidosis. Extreme acidosis may result in lethargy, stupor, coma, seizures, arrhythmias, ventricular tachycardia.

INVESTIGATIONS

- **Arterial blood gases**
  pH usually <7.35. Bicarbonate usually <12 mmol/L.

- **FBC**
  WCC ↑ in sepsis, infarction, septicaemia.

- **U&Es**
  ↑ K^+.

- **Blood glucose**
  ↑ in diabetic ketoacidosis.

■ Serum salicylate
   Salicylate poisoning.

To distinguish between the main types of metabolic acidosis it is necessary to measure the *anion gap*.

Anion gap=$([Na^+]+[K^+])-([Cl^-]+[HCO_3^-])$

This is normally about 8–16 mmol/L. An elevated anion gap, i.e. >16 mmol/L, may indicate a particular type of acidosis.

Increased anion gap

■ Lactic acidosis.

■ Ketoacidosis.

■ Chronic renal failure.

■ Intoxication, e.g. salicylate, ethanol, ethylene glycol, metformin.

■ Massive rhabdomyolysis.

• Rapidly increasing metabolic acidosis over minutes or hours is not due to renal failure. Severe sepsis, tissue hypoperfusion or tissue necrosis should be suspected, especially when there is an associated clinical deterioration.

METABOLIC ALKALOSIS

Metabolic alkalosis is caused by an increase in HCO_3^- or decrease in H^+ ($\uparrow$ pH, $\uparrow HCO_3^-$). Compensatory mechanisms are:

- $\uparrow pCO_2$ by hypoventilation (limited by hypoxia)
- $\downarrow HCO_3^-$ by kidneys.

CAUSES

EXCESS LOSS OF H⁺

- Vomiting
- Nasogastric aspiration
- Gastric fistula
- Diuretic therapy (thiazide or loop)
- Cushing's syndrome (mineralocorticoid effect)
- Conn's syndrome (mineralocorticoid excess)

EXCESSIVE INTAKE OF BASE

- Antacids, e.g. milk-alkali syndrome
- Ingestion of HCO_3^- (usually iatrogenic)

SYMPTOMS AND SIGNS

The patient is usually asymptomatic, although if breathing spontaneously will hypoventilate.

INVESTIGATIONS

- **Blood gases**
  pH >7.54 confirms diagnosis. HCO_3^- – normally high >29 mmol/L.

- **U&Es**
  K^+, Na^+ and Cl^- usually fall below normal range.

- **Plasma cortisol**
  Diurnal variation lost in Cushing's syndrome.

- **Plasma aldosterone**
  Raised in Conn's syndrome.

- Metabolic alkalosis will cause a left shift of the oxyhaemoglobin curve, reducing oxygen availability to the tissues.

RESPIRATORY ACIDOSIS

Respiratory acidosis is caused by CO_2 retention due to inadequate pulmonary ventilation ($\downarrow$ pH, $\uparrow$ pCO_2). Compensatory mechanisms are:
- $\uparrow$ HCO_3^- by bicarbonate buffer system
- $\downarrow$ H^+ by kidneys (can take several days).

CAUSES (ANY CAUSE OF HYPOVENTILATION)

CNS DEPRESSION

- Head injury
- Drugs, e.g. opiates, anaesthetics
- Coma
- Stroke
- Encephalitis

NEUROMUSCULAR DISEASE

- Myasthenia gravis
- Guillain–Barré syndrome

SKELETAL DISEASE

- Kyphoscoliosis
- Ankylosing spondylitis
- Flail chest

ARTIFICIAL VENTILATION (UNCONTROLLED AND UNMONITORED)

IMPAIRED GASEOUS EXCHANGE

- Chronic obstructive pulmonary disease
- Alveolar disease, e.g. pneumonia, ARDS (acute respiratory distress syndrome)
- Thoracic injury, e.g. pulmonary contusions

SYMPTOMS AND SIGNS

A history of the underlying disorder may be evident such as trauma or drug ingestion. The symptoms of respiratory acidosis can range from anxiety, disorientation, confusion, lethargy to somnolence. On examination, tachycardia and a bounding arterial pulse can occur with carbon dioxide retention. In severe disease, cyanosis and hypotension can result. Papilloedema may be a feature of underlying raised intracranial pressure. Features of a flail chest or any severe chest wall deformity may be evident.

INVESTIGATIONS

■ **ABGs**
pH <7.35.
pCO_2 >5.8 kPa.
↑ HCO_3^-.

■ **CXR**
Underlying pulmonary disease.

■ **Pulmonary function tests**
COPD which usually manifests as an obstructive defect (FEV1 ↓, FVC normal). Skeletal disease (reduced chest movement).

■ **EMG and nerve conduction studies**
Myasthenia gravis and Guillain–Barré syndrome.

■ **CT/MRI head**
Central (brain stem) lesion.

- **Exercise caution when correcting chronic hypercapnia. Rapid correction of hypercapnia can alkalinise the CSF causing seizures.**

- **Associated hypoxaemia secondary to hypoventilation is the major threat to life and must be reversed rapidly.**

RESPIRATORY ALKALOSIS

Respiratory alkalosis is a common disorder in critically ill patients. It occurs when carbon dioxide is lost via excessive pulmonary ventilation ($\uparrow$ pH, $\downarrow$ P_{CO_2}). Compensatory mechanisms are:

- $\downarrow$ HCO_3^- by bicarbonate buffer system
- $\uparrow$ H^+ by kidneys (slow process – may take several days).

CAUSES (any cause of hyperventilation)

CENTRAL NERVOUS SYSTEM

- Pyrexia
- Pain
- Anxiety
- Hysteria
- Head injury
- Stroke
- Encephalitis

RESPIRATORY DISORDERS

- Pneumonia
- Pulmonary oedema
- Pulmonary embolus

PHYSIOLOGICAL

- Pregnancy
- High altitude
- Severe anaemia

DRUGS

- Salicylates

OTHER CAUSES

- Sepsis
- Mechanical ventilation
- Metabolic acidosis (overcompensation)

SYMPTOMS AND SIGNS

Symptoms may include light headedness, circumoral paraesthesia, dizziness and numbness of the hands and feet. Acute development of low carbon dioxide levels can occasionally cause cerebral vasoconstriction leading to confusion, syncope, fits.

INVESTIGATIONS

■ **ABGs**
pH >7.45.
P_{CO_2} <4.4 kPa.
↓ HCO_3^- (compensatory mechanism due to bicarbonate buffer system).

■ **Serum calcium**
↓ Ca^{2+} (due to increased calcium binding to serum albumin).

■ **Serum salicylate level**
If overdose is suspected.

■ **CT/MRI head**
Intracranial lesion as a cause of hyperventilation.

• **Prolonged artificial ventilation with inadequate monitoring should be remembered as a cause of respiratory alkalosis.**

HAEMATOLOGICAL PRESENTATIONS

ANAEMIA

Anaemia is defined as a haemoglobin concentration of less than 13.5 g/dL in men and 11.5 g/dL in women. Classification of anaemia according to red cell indices is useful because specific investigations can be tailored accordingly.

CAUSES

MICROCYTIC (MCV <80 fL)

- Iron deficiency
- Anaemia of chronic disease
- Thalassaemia (more common in certain groups)

NORMOCYTIC (MCV 80–95 fL)

- Acute blood loss
- Haemolytic anaemia
  - Hereditary spherocytosis
  - Sickle cell disease (most common in sub-Saharan Africa)
  - G6PD deficiency (varies with ethnicity)
  - Autoimmune haemolytic anaemia
  - Malaria (geographic variability)
  - Drugs (e.g. dapsone, quinine, sulphonamides)
  - Red cell trauma (burns, mechanical heart valves)
- Mixed deficiencies
- Secondary anaemia (liver and renal disease)
- Bone marrow failure
- Pregnancy

MACROCYTIC (MCV >95 fL)

- Megaloblastic anaemia
  - Pernicious anaemia
  - Vitamin B_{12} deficiency
  - Folate deficiency
- Alcoholism
- Liver disease
- Hypothyroidism
- Hyperthyroidism (Graves)
- Addison's disease
- Marrow infiltration
- Drugs e.g. azathioprine, methotrexace.

SYMPTOMS AND SIGNS

Important aspects of the history are to enquire about symptoms suggestive of the diagnosis of anaemia, and to establish any underlying cause.

Symptoms of anaemia

The symptoms of anaemia are dependent on the degree of anaemia, speed of onset, age and the presence of co-existing disease. Mild to moderate chronic anaemia may be asymptomatic in young, fit individuals. Symptoms of anaemia include tiredness, lethargy and dyspnoea. Anaemia can precipitate or worsen angina and lower limb claudication.

History of the underlying disorder

Blood loss is a common cause of iron deficiency anaemia and frank bleeding can easily be established from the history. Occult bleeding from the gastrointestinal tract is an important cause of chronic blood loss. Patients may have melaena and may also experience upper abdominal pains from peptic ulceration, gastritis, gastro-oesophageal reflux or gastric carcinoma (p. 3). The causes of lower gastrointestinal bleeding are detailed on p. 308. The amount and frequency of blood loss with menstruation should be documented and the presence of haemoptysis and haematuria should be ascertained. Malabsorption can cause a deficiency of substrate or coenzyme requirements for the synthesis of haemoglobin. Gastrectomy or atrophic gastritis with pernicious anaemia may impair both iron and vitamin B_{12} absorption due to alterations in pH and effects on intrinsic factor, respectively. Impairment of vitamin B_{12} absorption may also result from extensive disease or resection involving the terminal ileum and predisposes to megaloblastic anaemia. A history of travel to areas where malaria and hookworm infections are endemic should be sought.

Dietary history

It is important to take a dietary history, as folate deficiency results from poor dietary intake. This is in contrast to iron, as dietary deficiency of iron alone rarely results in anaemia unless accompanied by increased utilisation or blood loss. Owing to intrinsic stores of vitamin B_{12}, dietary deficiencies may take up to 2 years before becoming clinically apparent. The amount of alcohol intake should also be noted because alcohol excess may result in a macrocytic anaemia.

Past medical and drug history

A number of chronic diseases can result in anaemia but it is important to exclude other concomitant causes before attributing anaemia to the effects of the primary illness. Diseases predisposing to macrocytic anaemia have been listed above. Aplasia of the marrow may occur as a complication of viral hepatitis or exposure to radiation and result in aplastic anaemia. Drugs such as chemotherapeutic agents, chloramphenicol and sulphonamides may also precipitate bone marrow failure. Respiratory tract infections with mycoplasma, infectious mononucleosis, lymphomas and connective tissue disease are associated with autoimmune haemolytic anaemia.

Family history

Haemoglobinopathies such as thalassaemia and sickle cell disease may be inherited. Alternatively, hereditary enzyme defects (G6PD) or red cell membrane defects (hereditary spherocytosis) may also result in intravascular haemolysis.

EXAMINATION

Classically, patients with anaemia have pallor of the palmar skin creases and conjunctivae; however, diagnosis based solely on these findings is unreliable. With iron deficiency, spoon-shaped nails (koilonychia) may be noted; these findings may be accompanied by angular cheilitis and glossitis. Jaundice can be a complication of haemolytic anaemia, or can result from chronic liver disease.

Subacute combined degeneration of the cord is a complication of severe vitamin B_{12} deficiency. Neurological examination reveals symmetrical loss of light touch, vibration and proprioception of the feet due to dorsal column involvement. In addition, Romberg's sign may be elicited. Less common features are peripheral neuropathy, optic atrophy and dementia.

With anaemia, examination of the cardiovascular system may reveal evidence of a hyperdynamic circulation with tachycardia, bounding pulse and a systolic flow murmur.

Splenomegaly is associated with hereditary spherocytosis, thalassaemia and sickle cell disease.

SPECIFIC INVESTIGATIONS

Microcytic anaemia

- FBC and blood film
  Low haemoglobin concentration occurs with microcytosis (MCV <80 fL) and hypochromia (MCH <27 pg). The platelet count may be raised when anaemia is associated with acute bleeding. Microcytic, hypochromic red blood cells with accompanying pencil cells may also be seen on the blood film.

- Serum iron and TIBC
  Serum iron reduced and TIBC raised with iron deficiency. With chronic disease both are reduced, and with thalassaemia both are normal.

- **Serum ferritin**
  Concentration of serum ferritin, a protein–iron complex, will be reduced with iron deficiency. It is not affected by chronic disease or thalassaemia.

- **Faecal occult blood and faecal microscopy**
  Detects blood loss from the gastrointestinal tract. Hookworm ova can be identified on microscopy.

- **Free erythrocyte protoporphyrin**
  Iron is added to protoporphyrin to form haem; therefore, in the presence of iron deficiency, protoporphyrin levels will be raised. It is a sensitive indicator of iron deficiency and is unaffected by chronic disease or thalassaemia.

- **Hb electrophoresis**
  Allows the specific diagnosis and classification of thalassaemia and sickle cell disease.

Normocytic anaemia

- **FBC and film**
  Low haemoglobin levels are accompanied by normal red cell indices (MCV 80–95 fL, MCH >27 pg), which can also occur in the presence of co-existing microcytic and macrocytic anaemia (mixed deficiency), although this will usually be picked up on the blood film. Certain haematology laboratories report RDW, which is increased in the presence of differing red corpuscle sizes. The reticulocyte count will be increased with haemolytic anaemia and following acute blood loss, and the blood film may reveal evidence of damaged red cells or sideroblasts.

- **Tests for haemolysis**
  Unconjugated bilirubin, urine urobilinogen and faecal stercobilinogen are raised with all causes of haemolysis. Serum haptoglobins are absent. Plasma haemoglobin is raised specifically with intravascular haemolysis. Reference to haematology textbooks will be required for confirmatory tests for individual haemolytic disorders.

- **Urinalysis**
  Haemosiderin and haemoglobin will be present in the urine specifically with intravascular haemolysis

- **Bone marrow aspiration**
  Aspiration of the bone marrow will reveal erythroid hyperplasia with haemolytic anaemia; with aplastic anaemia, bone marrow hypoplasia with fat replacement results.

Macrocytic anaemia

■ **FBC and film**
Low haemoglobin is accompanied by macrocytosis (MCV >95 fL).
The reticulocyte count is low and accompanying low platelet
and white cell counts may indicate megaloblastic anaemia.
Hypersegmented neutrophils may be seen on the blood film.

■ **Serum vitamin B$_{12}$ assay**
Serum levels of vitamin B$_{12}$ can be estimated and deficiency
readily ascertained. If the aetiology of vitamin B$_{12}$ deficiency is
not apparent, a Schilling test can be performed to clarify if the
problem lies within the stomach, terminal ileum, or is due to
intrinsic factor.

■ **Antiparietal cell antibodies and anti-intrinsic factor antibodies**
Pernicious anaemia results from lack of intrinsic factor
production or blocking antibodies.

■ **Serum and red cell folate**
Both of these tests are low with folate deficiency; however, in
the presence of vitamin B$_{12}$ deficiency the red cell folate may
actually be increased.

■ **Bone marrow aspiration**
Megaloblasts are seen in marrow aspirates with vitamin B$_{12}$ or
folate deficiency.

■ **Further tests**
Further tests for individual diseases responsible for macrocytosis
or secondary anaemia need to be tailored according to the
clinical presentation.

- **Examination of the peripheral blood film is an
  important guide to the type of anaemia, the
  underlying cause and the response to treatment.**

- **Remember that shortness of breath may be an early
  presenting symptom of anaemia.**

CLOTTING DISORDERS

Congenital disorders of clotting usually present with complications related to prolonged blood loss, whereas acquired disorders are usually discovered during coagulation testing.

CAUSES

CONGENITAL

- Haemophilia
- von Willebrand's disease

ACQUIRED

- Vitamin K deficiency
  - Haemorrhagic disease of the newborn
  - Obstructive jaundice
  - Fat malabsorption
- Liver disease
- Autoimmune diseases, e.g. SLE
- Drugs – heparin, warfarin, thrombolytic therapy
- DIC
- Massive transfusion

SYMPTOMS AND SIGNS

Onset and duration

The duration of symptoms and age of presentation is very useful in determining the underlying aetiology. Bleeding in the first few days of life occurs as a result of deficient vitamin K synthesis by the neonatal liver, due to immaturity. Patients with haemophilia usually present at a young age with excessive blood loss following injuries or surgical procedures, such as circumcision. Muscle haematomas and painful haemarthroses may be accompanying features.

Past medical history

Concomitant disease constitutes the majority of causes of acquired coagulation disturbances. As coagulation factors are synthesised in the liver, disease of the liver naturally predisposes to clotting abnormalities. Vitamin K is a fat-soluble vitamin essential for the production of clotting factors II, VII, IX and X. Conditions, such as obstructive jaundice, pancreatic or small bowel disease, that impair the absorption of fat will result in decreased production of the aforementioned factors.

Patients with SLE may produce antibodies such as the lupus anticoagulant, which, although prolonging clotting in *in vitro* testing, predisposes to thrombosis *in vivo*.

Severe infections, malignancy, obstetric complications and burns may give rise to DIC. This is characterised by widespread consumption of clotting factors and platelets, resulting in severe coagulation disturbances.

Drug history

Coagulation abnormalities may be iatrogenic. Therapeutic anticoagulation is achieved with heparin and warfarin. Thrombolytic agents produce severe derangement of clotting as a side-effect of therapy. Coagulation disturbances can result from dilution from massive blood transfusions (when the patient's entire circulating volume has been replaced by transfusion within 24 hours).

EXAMINATION

A general examination is performed to identify any stigmata from haemophilia. Early-onset osteoarthritis and pseudotumours may result from episodes of repeated haemorrhage. Skin necrosis and haematomas may be seen with warfarin overdosage. In acquired coagulation disorders signs of liver disease may bring attention to the underlying disorder.

GENERAL INVESTIGATIONS

■   FBC
    Low platelet count or abnormal platelet function result in prolonged bleeding time but not clotting results.

■   Clotting screen
    PT, APTT and TT are measured. Abnormalities are listed in the Table below.

Disorder	PT	APTT	TT
Haemophilia	N	↑	N
von Willebrand's disease	N	↑	N
Liver disease	↑	↑	N
Warfarin/vitamin K deficiency	↑	↑	N
Heparin	N or ↑	↑	↑
DIC	↑	↑	↑

PT, prothrombin time; APTT, activated partial thromboplastin time; TT, thrombin time; N, within normal range.

■ Bleeding time
Allows the differentiation of a primary clotting disorder (normal
bleeding time) and platelet disorders causing prolonged
bleeding.

SPECIFIC INVESTIGATIONS

■ Clotting factor assays
Clotting factor assays are required to differentiate between
haemophilia A, haemophilia B and von Willebrand's disease. Low
levels of factor VIII are found in both haemophilia A and von
Willebrand's disease. Low levels of factor IX indicate haemophilia
B. As the name implies, von Willebrand's factor is low in von
Willebrand's disease and the bleeding time is also prolonged.

■ Fibrinogen and fibrin degradation products
With DIC, the platelet count and serum fibrinogen levels are low,
whereas the fibrin degradation products such as D-dimers are
increased.

• **Prolonged bleeding can result from abnormal
platelet function despite normal platelet counts.**

LEUCOCYTOSIS

Leucocytosis is an increase in the absolute count of circulating white blood cells. The normal range is $4–11 \times 10^9$/L. It may involve any of the types of white cells but a polymorphonuclear leucocytosis, i.e. neutrophilia, is the most common.

CAUSES

NEUTROPHILIA

PHYSIOLOGICAL

- Neonates
- Exercise
- Pregnancy
- Parturition
- Lactation
- Stress

PATHOLOGICAL

SEPSIS, e.g. ACUTE APPENDICITIS, SEPTICAEMIA

ACUTE NON-INFECTIVE INFLAMMATION

- Surgery
- Burns
- Infarction, e.g. myocardial infarction, mesenteric infarction
- Crush injuries
- Rheumatoid arthritis

ACUTE HAEMORRHAGE AND HAEMOLYSIS

METABOLIC

- Uraemia
- Diabetic ketoacidosis
- Gout

CHRONIC MYELOPROLIFERATIVE DISEASE

- CML (chronic myeloid leukaemia)
- Polycythaemia rubrum vera
- Myelofibrosis

NON-HAEMATOLOGICAL MALIGNANCY

- Carcinoma
- Lymphoma

DRUGS

- Corticosteroids

MISCELLANEOUS
- Convulsions
- Electric shock
- Post-neutropenia rebound
- Post-splenectomy (temporary)

LYMPHOCYTOSIS

VIRAL INFECTIONS
- Glandular fever
- CMV
- Rubella
- Chicken pox
- Measles
- Mumps
- Influenza
- Infective hepatitis

BACTERIAL INFECTIONS
- Pertussis
- TB
- Brucellosis
- Syphilis

CHRONIC LYMPHOCYTIC LEUKAEMIA

POST-SPLENECTOMY (TEMPORARY)

MONOCYTOSIS

BACTERIAL
- TB
- Brucellosis
- Typhoid
- Infective endocarditis

PROTOZOAL
- Malaria
- Trypanosomiasis
- Leishmaniasis

MALIGNANT
- Myelodysplasia
- Leukaemia – monocytic and myelomonocytic
- Hodgkin's
- Carcinoma

EOSINOPHILIA
- Allergy, e.g. asthma
- Parasitic infections, e.g. filariasis, schistosomiasis
- Malignancy, e.g. Hodgkin's disease

BASOPHILIA
- Chronic myeloproliferative disease
- Hypersensitivity reactions
- Hypothyroidism

SYMPTOMS AND SIGNS

It is important to seek a history of symptoms of infection and to examine the patient for signs of infection or an underlying haematological malignancy. A full description of the signs and symptoms of haematological disease is beyond the scope of this book and the reader is referred to a textbook of haematology.

INVESTIGATIONS

- **FBC**
  Hb ↓ malignancy. WCC ↑. Differential count for type of white cell.

- **Blood film**
  'Toxic' granulation – infection. Immature granulocytes, blast cells – white cell dyscrasias.

- **Blood culture**
  Sepsis.

- **Bone marrow**
  Indicated for leukaemoid reaction, leucoerythroblastic blood film, leucocytosis due to blasts. Diagnosis of various types of white cell dyscrasia.

- **Mantoux test**
  TB.

- **Antibody screen**
  SLE.

- **Rheumatoid factor**
  Rheumatoid arthritis.

- **U&Es**
  ARF. CRF.

- **Blood sugar**
  Diabetic ketoacidosis.

- **CXR**
  Malignancy.

- **CT**
  Malignancy.

- **ECG**
  Myocardial infarction.

- **Monospot**
  Infectious mononucleosis.

- **VDRL**
  Syphilis.

- **Brucella agglutination test**
  Brucellosis.

- In patients with leucocytosis it is important to seek a history of symptoms of infection and to examine the patient not only for signs of infection, but also for the possibility of an underlying haematological disorder, i.e. exclude lymphadenopathy and hepatosplenomegaly.

LEUCOPENIA

Leucopenia is a reduction in circulating white blood cells. The normal range is $4-11 \times 10^9$/L. In practice the common form is neutropenia – a deficiency of neutrophil granulocytes. Neutropenia may be selective or part of a pancytopenia.

CAUSES

NEUTROPENIA

PANCYTOPENIA
- Bone marrow depression, e.g. cytotoxic agents, malignant infiltration
- Severe B_{12} or folate deficiency
- Hypersplenism

SELECTIVE NEUTROPENIA
- Physiological
  - Healthy black individuals
- Infection
  - Overwhelming sepsis, e.g. septicaemia
  - Brucellosis
  - TB
  - Typhoid
- Immune
  - SLE
  - Felty's syndrome
- Autoimmune neutropenia
- Drug induced, e.g. indomethacin, chloramphenicol, co-trimoxazole

LYMPHOPENIA
- Acute infection
- Trauma
- Surgery
- Radiotherapy
- Chemotherapy
- Steroid therapy
- SLE
- Uraemia
- Cushing's syndrome
- Hodgkin's disease
- Immunodeficiency syndromes, e.g. HIV

SYMPTOMS AND SIGNS

The history and physical examination provide a guide to the subsequent management of a patient with neutropenia. Simple observation is appropriate initially for an asymptomatic patient with an isolated mild neutropenia who has an unremarkable history and examination. Take a full drug history. Check for any recent infections or surgery. Check particularly for recent viral illnesses. Severe leucopenia may result in opportunistic infections. Patients with neutropenia may present with recurrent stomatitis, gingivitis, oral ulceration, sinusitis and perianal infection.

INVESTIGATIONS

■ **FBC**
  Hb ↓ in malignancy, bone marrow depression. WCC ↓ – type of white cell involved.

■ **U&Es**
  Uraemia. Renal involvement, e.g. SLE.

■ **Mantoux test**
  TB.

■ **Antibody screen**
  SLE.

■ **Antineutrophil antibody screen**
  Autoimmune neutropenia.

■ **Serum B_{12} and folate**
  B_{12} and folate deficiency.

■ **Rheumatoid factor**
  Felty's disease.

■ **Viral titres**
  HIV.

■ **Bone marrow**
  Bone marrow depression.

- **Neutropenia with counts of $<0.5 \times 10^9$/L may result in severe life-threatening sepsis, e.g. candidiasis, septicaemia, opportunistic infections. Patients in this group require febrile illnesses treating with broad spectrum i.v. antibiotics.**

POLYCYTHAEMIA

Polycythaemia is an increase in red cell concentration above the normal limit, usually accompanied by a corresponding increase in haematocrit and haemoglobin concentration. Polycythaemia can be 'real' due to a true increase in red cell concentration or 'apparent', due to low plasma volume (e.g. dehydration). Primary polycythaemia (polycythaemia vera) is due to a neoplasm of the myeloid series and secondary polycythaemia is due to raised erythropoietin levels and may be appropriate (chronic low oxygenation) or inappropriate (erythropoietin production from renal tumours).

CAUSES

TRUE POLYCYTHAEMIA (INCREASED RED CELL MASS)

- Primary polycythaemia
  - Polycythaemia vera
- Secondary polycythaemia
  - Appropriate erythropoietin production (hypoxia)
  - Smoking (due to carbon monoxide exposure)
  - Chronic respiratory disease
  - Long-term exposure to high altitude
  - Cyanotic heart disease
  - High-affinity haemoglobinopathy
- Inappropriate erythropoietin production
  - Renal carcinoma or cysts
  - Renal artery stenosis
  - Renal amyloidosis
  - Hepatocellular carcinoma
  - Massive uterine fibroids
  - Cerebellar haemangioblastoma

APPARENT POLYCYTHAEMIA (REDUCED PLASMA VOLUME, NORMAL RED CELL MASS)

- Low plasma volume polycythaemia
  - Dehydration
  - Burns
  - Enteropathy
- Gaisböck's syndrome

SYMPTOMS AND SIGNS

The condition may be asymptomatic for months or years. Presenting features of polycythaemia vera are fatigue, aquagenic pruritus (skin itching after a hot bath), sweating and, occasionally, weight loss. Patients may also present with complications such as stroke, deep vein thrombosis or hyperviscosity (headache, blurred vision and confusion). On examination there is plethora and, occasionally, cyanosis. Scratch marks or spontaneous bruising may be visible on the skin. The conjunctival vessels are engorged and dilated retinal veins may be evident on funduscopy. Splenomegaly may be palpable on examination of the abdomen.

INVESTIGATIONS

- **FBC**
  Hb 17.5 g/dL in men and 15.5 g/dL in women with accompanying rise in red cell count. Haematocrit more than 55% in men and 47% in women. Thrombocytosis and neutrophil leucocytosis present in up to 50% of cases of polycythaemia vera.

- **Blood film**
  Occasional metamyelocytes and myelocytes on blood film and polycythaemia vera.

- **Serum uric acid**
  ↑ uric acid in polycythaemia vera due to increased cell turnover.

- **ABG**
  O_2 concentration in blood normal in primary polycythaemia but reduced in secondary polycythaemia due to respiratory failure or cardiac disease with right to left shunt.

- **Total red cell volume**
  Red cells in a sample of blood from the patient are tagged with ^{51}Cr, and the labelled red cells are re-injected. The dilution of the isotope in a subsequent venous blood sample is used to calculate the red cell mass. The normal range is 25–35 mL/kg in men and 22–32 mL/kg in women.
  In the presence of ongoing blood loss (there is a predisposition to bleeding and peptic ulceration), iron-deficient polycythaemia results and the haemoglobin and haematocrit may be normal or low. The condition should be suspected when there are obviously iron-deficient red cells (low MCV) without anaemia and with a very high red cell count.

- **Plasma volume**
  ^{125}I-albumin is used to estimate total plasma volume, the normal range is 35–45 mL/kg. This is usually performed in conjunction with the estimation of total red cell volume to distinguish between real and apparent polycythaemia (the latter is due to low plasma volume).

■ **Bone marrow aspiration**
In polycythaemia vera there is a hypercellular bone marrow with erythroid hyperplasia. Megakaryocytes may be prominent and increased reticulin deposition is common.

- In polycythaemia vera the higher the haematocrit the greater the risk of thrombotic episodes. Repeated phlebotomy is required to maintain the haematocrit below 45%.

THROMBOCYTOPENIA

Thrombocytopenia is a low platelet count below 150×10^9/L. The causes of a low platelet count can be grouped according to reduced production, decreased survival or sequestration in the spleen.

CAUSES

REDUCED PRODUCTION

- Aplastic anaemia
- Drugs, e.g. tolbutamide, alcohol, cytotoxic agents
- Viral infections, e.g. EBV, CMV
- Myelodysplasia
- Bone marrow infiltration, e.g. carcinoma, leukaemia, myeloma, myelofibrosis
- Megaloblastic anaemia
- Hereditary thrombocytopenia

DECREASED PLATELET SURVIVAL

IMMUNE
- ITP
- Drugs, e.g. heparin, quinine, sulphonamides, penicillins, gold
- Infections
- Post-transfusion

NON-IMMUNE
- Disseminated intravascular coagulation (DIC)
- Thrombotic thrombocytopenic purpura
- Haemolytic uraemic syndrome

HYPERSPLENISM

- Sequestration of platelets

SYMPTOMS AND SIGNS

Drug history including over-the-counter drugs, e.g. quinine. Alcohol intake. Easy or spontaneous bruising, petechial rash, epistaxis, haematuria, mucosal bleeding. Cirrhosis/hypersplenism. History of malignancy with marrow infiltration. DIC.

Petechiae and bruising on examination. Signs of infection. Lymphadenopathy. Hepatosplenomegaly.

INVESTIGATIONS

- **FBC**
  Isolated thrombocytopenia likely to be due to increased destruction. Thrombocytopenia due to marrow failure likely to be associated with anaemia, leucopenia.

- **Blood film**
  Red cell fragmentation (DIC). Platelet size (large in ITP and some hereditary conditions). WBC (atypical lymphocytes/lymphoblasts).

- **Bleeding time**
  Prolonged if platelet count <80 × 10⁹/L.

- **Coagulation screen**
  Clotting times normal in autoimmune thrombocytopenia but may be abnormal in other causes, e.g. DIC.

- **Platelet function test**
  Associated abnormal platelet function, e.g. uraemia.

- **Serology**
  Antinuclear antibodies (autoimmune disease). Monospot (glandular fever). Antiplatelet antibodies (unreliable). Paul–Bunnell test (glandular fever). CMV serology.

- **U&Es, creatinine**
  Haemolytic uraemic syndrome, thrombotic thrombocytopenic purpura.

- **LFTs**
  Hepatitis, e.g. due to EBV, CMV.

- **Bone marrow**
  Megakaryocytes increased in number and size in ITP. Absence or reduction in megakaryocytes rules out ITP. Aplastic anaemia. Leukaemia. Marrow infiltration (carcinoma, lymphoma, myeloma).

- Primary haemostasis is only impaired when platelet count falls to <80 × 10⁹/L.

- Spontaneous bruising, purpura and mucosal bleeding are rare until the platelets are <20 × 10⁹/L, unless there is also a defect in platelet function.

- Always take a careful and detailed drug history.

- In the pale patient with purpura, a serious underlying bone marrow disorder is likely.

THROMBOCYTOSIS

Thrombocytosis is a high platelet count >450 × 10^9/L. It may be secondary to another pathological process or it may be due to a myeloproliferative disorder.

CAUSES

REACTIVE (SECONDARY)

- Haemorrhage
- Haemolysis
- Trauma
- Surgery
- Post-partum
- Chronic inflammation, e.g. rheumatoid arthritis, inflammatory bowel disease
- Iron deficiency anaemia
- Hyposplenism (splenectomy, splenic atrophy)

ESSENTIAL (PRIMARY)

- Essential thrombocythaemia (myeloproliferative disorder)
- Other chronic myeloproliferative disorders, e.g. chronic myeloid leukaemia, myelofibrosis, polycythaemia rubrum vera.

SYMPTOMS AND SIGNS

History of trauma, blood loss, surgery, splenectomy, chronic inflammatory disease. Increased platelet count at routine blood test. Bruising. Episodes of spontaneous arterial or venous thrombosis, e.g. stroke, DVT, venous thromboembolism. Hepatosplenomegaly.

INVESTIGATIONS

- **FBC**
  Platelets ↑. Hb ↓ (iron deficiency anaemia). Hb ↑ (polycythaemia rubrum vera). MCV ↓ (iron deficiency anaemia). PCV ↑ (polycythaemia rubrum vera). WBC ↑ (infection, chronic myeloid leukaemia).

- **Blood film**
  Microcytic hypochromic anaemia in iron deficiency. Thrombocytosis, giant platelets, platelet clumping, megakaryocyte fragments in essential thrombocythaemia.

- **ESR**
  Chronic inflammation. Malignancy. ESR very high in myeloma.

- ■ **Serum iron and TIBC**
  Serum iron ↓ TIBC ↑ in iron deficiency.

- ■ **Serum ferritin**
  Reduced in iron deficiency. Not affected by chronic disease.

- ■ **Bone marrow**
  Essential thrombocythaemia – hypercellularity, increased megakaryocytes, large megakaryocytes. Polycythaemia rubrum vera – increased cellularity due to hyperplasia for erythropoietic cells, granulocytopoietic cells and megakaryocytes. Chronic myeloid leukaemia – marked hypercellularity due to myeloid hyperplasia. Myelofibrosis – 'dry tap' (aspiration unsuccessful).

- • In myeloproliferative disorders associated with thrombocytosis, there is not only an increased risk of thrombosis but also an increased risk of haemorrhage.

- • Platelet counts over 750×10^9/L are serious enough to warrant investigation and treatment.

INDEX

Note to index: For ease of use, subjects are indexed with the section pages within which references can be found; for example, Palpitations, 351–3 (instead of 351, 352, 353).